Management and Prevention of Thrombosis in Primary Care

Edited by

John Spandorfer MD
Clinical Assistant Professor of Medicine,
Jefferson Medical College, Philadelphia, USA

Barbara A Konkle MD
Associate Professor of Medicine,
University of Pennsylvania School of Medicine,
Director, Penn Comprehensive Hemophilia and
Thrombosis Program, Philadelphia, USA

Geno J Merli MD
Clinical Professor of Medicine,
Division of Internal Medicine,
Jefferson Medical College, Philadelphia, USA

A member of the Hodder Headline Group
LONDON
Co-published in the United States of America by
Oxford University Press Inc., New York

First published in Great Britain in 2001 by
Arnold, a member of the Hodder Headline Group,
338 Euston Road, London NWI 3BH

http://www.arnoldpublishers.com

Co-published in the United States of America by
Oxford University Press Inc.,
198 Madison Avenue, New York, NY10016
Oxford is a registered trademark of Oxford University Press

Whilst the advice and information in this book are believed to be true and
accurate at the date of going to press, neither the authors nor the publisher
can accept any legal responsibility or liability for any errors or omissions
that may be made. In particular (but without limiting the generality of the
preceding disclaimer) every effort has been made to check drug dosages;
however, it is still possible that errors have been missed. Furthermore,
dosage schedules are constantly being revised and new side-effects
recognized. For these reasons the reader is strongly urged to consult the
drug companies' printed instructions before administering any of the drugs
recommended in this book.

British Library Cataloguing in Publication Data
A catalogue record for this book is available from the British Library

Library of Congress Cataloging-in-Publication Data
A catalog record for this book is available from the Library of Congress

ISBN 0 340 76125 3 (pb)

1 2 3 4 5 6 7 8 9 10

Commissioning Editor: Joanna Koster
Project Editor: Sarah de Souza
Production Editor: Rada Radojicic
Production Controller: Bryan Eccleshall
Cover Design: Mouse Mat

Typeset in 10/12 pt Minion by Scribe Design, Gillingham, Kent, UK
Printed and bound in Great Britain by Redwood Books, Trowbridge,
Wiltshire

What do you think about this book? Or any other Arnold title?
Please send your comments to feedback.arnold@hodder.co.uk

To our spouses, Amy, Peter, and Charlotte

Contents

Contributors

Barbara Alving MD
Director, Division of Blood Diseases and Resources, National Heart, Lung, and Blood Institute, National Institutes of Health, Bethesda, Maryland, USA

Rebecca J Beyth MD, MS
Assistant Professor of Medicine, Baylor College of Medicine and The Houston Center for Quality of Care and Utilization Studies, Texas, USA

Joseph Bonn MD
Associate Professor of Radiology, Jefferson Medical College of Thomas Jefferson University, Thomas Jefferson University Hospital, Philadelphia, Pennsylvania, USA

Sanjeev D Chunilal MB, ChB, FRACP, FRCPA
Research Fellow, Department of Medicine, McMaster University, Hamilton, Ontario, Canada

Cheryl Costello PA-C
Physician Assistant, Jefferson Methodist Heart Center South, Methodist Division, Thomas Jefferson University Hospital, Philadelphia, Pennsylvania, USA

Nicholas L Depace MD
Clinical Professor of Medicine, Thomas Jefferson University, Thomas Jefferson University Hospital, Philadelphia, Pennsylvania, USA

C Gregory Elliott MD
Professor of Medicine, The University of Utah School of Medicine, Salt Lake City, Utah, USA

James T Fitzpatrick MD
Assistant Clinical Professor of Medicine, Division of Cardiology, Thomas Jefferson University, Philadelphia, Pennsylvania, USA

Brian F Gage MD, MSc
Assistant Professor of Medicine, Division of General Medical Sciences, Washington University School of Medicine, St Louis, Missouri, USA

Guillermo Garcia-Manero MD
Assistant Professor of Medicine, Department of Leukemia, University of Texas, MD Anderson Cancer Center, Houston, Texas, USA and Division of Oncology, University of Texas–Houston Medical School, Houston, Texas, USA

Jeff S Ginsberg MD, FRCP(c)
Professor of Medicine, Department of Medicine, McMaster University, Hamilton, Ontario, Canada

Dawn E Havrda PharmD, BCPS
Assistant Professor, Department of Pharmacy Practice, College of Pharmacy, University of Oklahoma Health Science Center, Oklahoma City, Oklahoma, USA

Jamie C Hey MD
Assistant Professor of Medicine, University of Maryland School of Medicine, Baltimore, Maryland, USA

Amna Ibrahim MD
Medical Officer, Division of Oncologic Drug Products, Center for Drug Evaluation and Research, Food and Drug Administration, Rockville, Maryland, USA

Matthew J Killion MD
Assistant Professor of Medicine, Jefferson Medical College, Philadelphia, Pennsylvania, USA

Barbara A Konkle MD
Associate Professor of Medicine, University of Pennsylvania School of Medicine; Director, Penn Comprehensive Hemophilia and Thrombosis Program, Philadelphia, Pennsylvania, USA

Tammy L Lin MD
Chief Resident, Primary Care Training Program, Department of Internal Medicine, Washington University School of Medicine, Barnes-Jewish Hospital, St Louis, Missouri, USA

José A López MD
Associate Professor of Internal Medicine and Molecular and Human Genetics, Baylor College of Medicine, Houston, Texas, USA

Susan Lynch RN, BSN, CACP
Jefferson Antithrombotic Therapy Service, Division of Internal Medicine, Thomas Jefferson University Hospital, Philadelphia, Pennsylvania, USA

José Martinez MD
Professor of Medicine and Pharmacology, Jefferson Medical College of Thomas Jefferson University; Associate Director, Cardera Foundation for Hematologic Research, Philadelphia, Pennsylvania, USA

Edgar J Massabni MD
Fellow in Intervention Cardiology, Thomas Jefferson University Hospital, Philadelphia, Pennsylvania, USA

Abraham Matthews MD
Consultant in Hematology and Oncology, Omaha, Nebraska, USA

Geno J Merli MD
Clinical Professor of Medicine and Director, Division of Internal Medicine, Jefferson Medical College, Philadelphia, Pennsylvania, USA

William O'Hara BS, Pharm D,
Clinical Coordinator, Department of Pharmacy, Thomas Jefferson Hospital, Philadelphia, Pennsylvania, USA

Colleen Palermo BS, MT(ASCP)
Supervisor, Special Hematology and Hemostasis Laboratory, Cardeza Foundation
for Hematologic Research, Thomas Jefferson University, Philadelphia,
Pennsylvania, USA

Neal F Skop MD
Fellow in Cardiology, Thomas Jefferson University Hospital, Philadelphia,
Pennsylvania, USA

John Spandorfer MD
Clinical Assistant Professor of Medicine, Division of Internal Medicine, Jefferson
Medical College, Philadelphia, Pennsylvania, USA

Perumal Thiagarajan MD
Associate Professor of Medicine, University of Texas Health Sciences Center,
Houston, Texas, USA

Lynda Thomson BS, pharm D, CACP
Clinical Pharmacist, Infectious Disease and Anticoagulation, Thomas Jefferson
University Hospital, Philadelphia, Pennsylvania, USA

Theodore E Warkentin MD, FRCPC, FACP
Associate Professor, Department of Pathology and Molecular Medicine, and
Department of Medicine, McMaster University, Hamilton, Ontario, Canada;
Associate Head, Transfusion Medicine, Hamilton Regional Laboratory Medicine
Program, Hamilton Health Sciences Centre, Hamilton General Hospital, Hamilton,
Ontario, Canada

Richard H White MD
Professor of Clinical Medicine, Division of General Medicine, University of
California, Sacramento, California, USA

Preface

Primary care physicians are increasingly expected to care of patients who have a wide variety of medical illnesses. The clinical management of patients who have had thrombotic events or are at risk for thrombotic events is a common challenge for such physicians. *Management and Prevention of Thrombosis in Primary Care* is a book written for primary care physicians to assist them in that challenge. The readers will find this text not only well organized and practical, but also very applicable to their everyday practice.

Chapters, written by both specialists and generalists, cover a wide array of issues in thrombosis. Care has been taken to keep the scope and depth of the chapters appropriate for primary care physicians. Initial chapters describe underlying mechanisms of clotting, either in vitro, or in hereditary or acquired clotting disorders. Subsequent chapters cover the treatment and prevention of thrombosis with heparin (both unfractionated and low molecular weight), warfarin, and various antiplatelet agents. Complications, both hemorrhagic and nonhemorrhagic, of these agents are described in separate chapters. The antithrombotic management of patients with venous thromboembolic disease, atrial fibrillation, prosthetic heart valves, cardiomyopathy, and coronary artery disease is reviewed in individual chapter. Other common problems faced by the primary care physician, such as the use of inferior vena cava filters, the management of patients chronically anticoagulated who need to have an invasive procedures, and how to arrange an anticoagulation clinic, are all reviewed as well.

1

Principles of hemostasis and thrombosis

GUILLERMO GARCIA-MANERO, JOSÉ MARTINEZ

INTRODUCTION

Blood coagulation is a host mechanism involved in protecting the integrity of the vascular system. The coagulation system is composed of cellular and noncellular components. The cellular components are comprised largely of endothelial cells and platelets, and the other major component is formed by a group of coagulation proteins that participate in the formation and dissolution of the fibrin clot. Although the three components work in concert to preserve blood fluidity or to trigger the formation of the hemostatic response to vascular injury, for didactic reasons the vascular endothelium, platelets, and coagulation proteins are discussed under separate headings.

ROLE OF VASCULAR ENDOTHELIUM IN HEMOSTASIS AND THROMBOSIS

The endothelial lining of the blood vessel wall has been classically described as a passive barrier that preserves blood fluidity by controlling the passage of blood components to the extravascular compartment. However, the vascular endothelium is known to play an active dual role in blood coagulation, preventing the formation of intravascular clots under normal conditions, and at the same time participating in the formation of the blood clot in response to vascular injury.[1] The endothelial cell synthesizes inhibitors of platelet function, such as prostacyclin and nitric oxide, which interfere with the adhesion and aggregation of the circulating platelets.[2] In addition, the endothelial cell also synthesizes and expresses on its surface heparin-like substances[3] that regulate the activity of several coagulation enzymes, as well as of thrombomodulin, a protein that acts as an anticoagulant by mediating thrombin-induced activation of protein C (see below). Through these systems, the vascular endothelium plays a major role in the modulation of the coagulation system and in the maintenance of blood fluidity.[1]

In contrast, interruption of the endothelial lining leads to exposure of components of the vessel wall (i.e., the extracellular matrix proteins) that trigger the adhesion and aggregation of platelets. Discontinuity of the endothelium also allows the contact of coagulation proteins with specific components of the cell surface that initiate the activation of the coagulation system. Furthermore, when the endothelium is stimulated by certain cytokines,[4] it can switch its properties from anticoagulant to procoagulant. For example, cytokines, like tumor necrosis factor or endotoxin, can stimulate the synthesis of tissue factor, a membrane protein that initiates the activation of blood coagulation. The vascular endothelium is also involved in the dissolution of blood clots, a process mediated by the synthesis and release of tissue plasminogen activator, which activates plasminogen to plasmin, an enzyme which catalyzes dissolution of the blood clot, thereby opening the vascular lumen to blood circulation. In summary, the endothelial cell lining of the vessel wall is involved in several distinct functions of the hemostatic system, and the endothelium expresses anticoagulant and profibrinolytic properties that intervene in the preservation of blood fluidity. However, following vascular injury the endothelium participates in the formation of the hemostatic fibrin clot that intervenes in the preservation of vascular integrity and in the repair of the blood vessel.

The vascular endothelium also expresses cell adhesion molecules that mediate association of the endothelial cell with other components of the blood, such as leukocytes, or with circulating abnormal cells, such as tumor cells. The adhesion of leukocytes to the endothelium plays a fundamental role in the inflammatory response, and the association of endothelial cells with tumor cells is involved in tumor invasion and metastasis.[5]

ROLE OF PLATELETS IN HEMOSTASIS AND THROMBOSIS

Platelets are derived from megakaryocytes and normally circulate at a level of 150 000–400 000/mm^3. The circulating platelet is inactive and, under normal conditions, does not interact with other cells during its normal survival of about 9–10 days.[6,7] In the presence of vascular damage, such as trauma with loss of endothelium or vessel wall lesions, platelets adhere to the exposed subendothelial matrix proteins and cover the denuded area. During this step, termed primary hemostasis, the platelets adhere to von Willebrand factor present in the matrix. The adhesion of platelets is followed by their activation. Platelets are activated by specific agonists, of which thrombin is probably the most important. When these agonists bind to their specific receptors, termed G protein-coupled receptors, located in the cell membrane of the platelet, they trigger a cascade of intracellular signals, which are mediated by the sequential activation of several enzymes, including phospholipase C and protein kinase C (PKC).[8] This is discussed further in Chapter 6. Both the activation of PKC and the generation of thromboxane A2 are crucial for the activation of the fibrinogen receptor – known as the IIb/IIIa complex (GPIIb/IIIa).[9] Fibrinogen, by binding to the GPIIb/IIIa complex of adjacent platelets, will link one to another and thereby cause the platelets to aggregate (Fig. 1.1).[10–13] As discussed below, platelets also play an important role in the formation of the fibrin clot that interacts with platelets and with the vessel wall. For example, activated platelets expose on their surface negatively charged phospholipids that play a critical role in the binding and assembly of specific coagulation proteins. These interactions are fundamental for the activation of the coagulation system.[14] The fibrin clot, which results from the assembly and activation of the coagulation proteins on the platelet surface, is stronger and

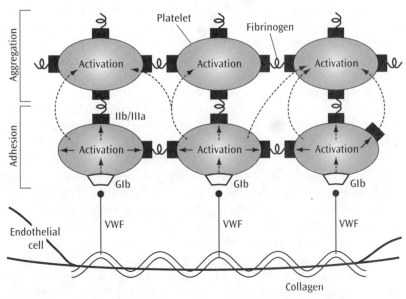

Figure 1.1 *Platelet adhesion and aggregation. In areas of endothelial damage, represented in the picture by disruption of the endothelial cell lining, von Willebrand factor (VWF), present in the subendothelial matrix, binds to glycoprotein Ib complex (GIb) located in the surface of the platelet membrane. This process is known as platelet adhesion, and provides the first layer of platelets covering the denuded area of the endothelium. The binding of VWF to GIb, and other ligands such as thrombin, to their respective receptors triggers platelet activation, with the subsequent activation of the glycoprotein IIb/IIIa receptor (IIb/IIIa) (depicted in the figure as a black rectangle on the surface of platelets). This activated receptor mediates the binding of fibrinogen and promotes platelet–platelet interaction, a process known as platelet aggregation. The expression of the IIb/IIIa receptor in the second layer of platelets is mediated by the action of agents secreted by the activated platelets (depicted in the picture by the discontinuous line).*

more stable than the primary platelet thrombus, and is usually able to stop the extravasation of blood following trauma. Other vascular responses, such as vasoconstriction, also participate in controlling bleeding following vascular injury.

The number of circulating platelets is controlled by platelet production and destruction and by the number of platelets that are stored in the tissues, mainly the spleen. The number of circulating platelets in normal individuals varies from 150 000/mm^3 to 400 0000/mm^3, and the life span of the platelet is between eight and 10 days. The number of platelets can be increased in patients with gastrointestinal bleeding, iron deficiency anemia, inflammatory processes, and following splenectomy. These elevations in platelet numbers are not considered a risk factor for thrombosis. Thrombocytosis is also seen as a manifestation of myeloproliferative disorders, including polycythemia vera, myeloid metaplasia/myelofibrosis, or essential thrombocythemia. In this setting, thrombocytosis may increase the risk for venous or arterial thrombosis, and in some instances antiplatelet therapy is indicated. However, paradoxically, some of these patients manifest a hemorrhagic tendency, and for this reason therapeutic intervention has to be individualized.[15]

Thrombocytopenia is a frequent manifestation of failure of adequate platelet production in bone marrow disorders such as aplastic anemia, leukemia, or bone marrow suppression following chemotherapy. Frequently, the cause of the thrombocytopenia is increased destruction, often by antibodies against platelets in immune thrombocytopenia[16] or by immune reactions to a variety of drugs, especially the penicillins, quinidine, sulfas, and heparin. Mucosal bleeding, whether oral, nasal, gastrointestinal, or genitourinary, is a common manifestation of thrombocytopenia. Petechiae, which are punctate hemorrhages of skin or mucosa, are a characteristic finding of severe thrombocytopenia, which usually occurs with platelet counts below 20 000/mm^3. A platelet count above 5000 to 10 000/mm^3 is considered adequate for the prevention of spontaneous bleeding, but is generally considered to be inadequate in the presence of trauma or sepsis or in patients who are receiving drugs, such as aspirin, that interfere with platelet function.[17] The critical level of platelet count for surgical procedures is not well defined. In patients with thrombocytopenia secondary to liver disease, it appears that a platelet count of 60 000/mm^3, if the prolongation of the prothrombin time (PT) is less than 2 s, is sufficient to provide adequate hemostasis for liver biopsy and paracentesis.[18–20] Thrombocytopenia can also be a manifestation of an increased storage of platelets in the spleen due to splenomegaly. In most of these cases, the platelet count is above 40 000/mm^3 and this level of thrombocytopenia does not cause bleeding disorders, except when it is combined with deficiencies of other coagulation factors.[21]

ROLE OF THE COAGULATION SYSTEM IN HEMOSTASIS AND THROMBOSIS

Overview of the coagulation cascade

The proteins that are involved in blood coagulation are present under normal conditions in inactive forms known as zymogens. The zymogens of the coagulation system are proenzymes, belonging to the group of serine proteases which are activated to enzymes by a series of sequential reactions in which one enzyme cleaves a particular proenzyme forming an active enzyme. The sequential activation of the coagulation proteins is usually referred to as the coagulation cascade because, after the initial activation, there is an amplification in the conversion of zymogens to active enzymes during each subsequent step. Table 1.1 gives details of the sites of synthesis and vitamin K dependency of the coagulation factors. The coagulation cascade hypothesis was based on the assumption that when plasma is exposed to a denuded vessel wall, factor XII (Hageman factor) is activated by contact with substances present in these tissues. The activation of factor XII by the exposed tissue is similar, according to this hypothesis, to the well-characterized activation of factor XII by artificial surfaces such as glass or kaolin, and the activation by these artificial surfaces is the basis of the activated partial thromboplastin time (aPTT) test. Activated factor XII in turn activates factor XI to factor XIa, which converts factor IX into the enzyme factor IXa. Factor IXa, in conjunction with factor VIII, acts upon factor X, converting this zymogen to factor Xa. In the final step, factor Xa, in conjunction with factor V, converts prothrombin (factor II) into thrombin (factor IIa), a specific enzyme that converts fibrinogen into fibrin.[22]

In the above scheme, the initial activation of the contact phase of blood coagulation occurs via components present in the blood, and for this reason was named 'intrinsic activation'. In the 'extrinsic pathway', the blood is exposed to factors that are not normally present there. In the extrinsic pathway, the activation occurs when a factor (which is present on the surface of different cells and hence referred to as tissue factor) binds factor VIIa, present in trace amounts in plasma. The tissue factor–VIIa complex cleaves and activates factor X to Xa, which, in the presence of factor V, cleaves and converts prothrombin to thrombin. These two distinct pathways

Table 1.1 *Sites of synthesis and vitamin K dependency of the coagulation factors*

Coagulation-involved proteins	Vitamin K dependency	Site of synthesis
Tissue factor	No	Cells in subendothelium Macrophages/tumor cells
Factor VII	Yes	Hepatocytes
Factor IX	Yes	Hepatocytes
Factor VIII	No	Liver, cell unknown
Factor XI	No	Hepatocytes
Factor X	Yes	Hepatocytes
Factor V	No	Hepatocytes/megakaryocytes
Tissue factor pathway inhibitor	No	Endothelial cells/liver
Prothrombin	Yes	Hepatocytes
Fibrinogen	No	Hepatocytes
Plasminogen	No	Hepatocytes
Tissue plasminogen activator	No	Endothelial cells
Thrombomodulin	No	Endothelial cells
Protein C	Yes	Hepatocytes
Protein S	Yes	Hepatocytes/endothelial cells
von Willebrand factor	No	Endothelial cells/megakaryocytes
Factor XIIIa subunit	No	Megakaryocytes/macrophages

of activation, the intrinsic and extrinsic pathways, explain the bleeding manifestations of patients with hemophilia A (factor VIII deficiency) and hemophilia B (factor IX deficiency), because tissue factor activation was considered complementary to the most efficient system based on activation of coagulation by the intrinsic pathway. However, this intrinsic cascade hypothesis fails to explain two major findings, namely (a) that patients with factor XII deficiency do not bleed, and (b) that patients with factor VII deficiency can have severe hemorrhagic manifestations, indicating that the extrinsic pathway is fundamental for normal hemostasis. Recent work has clarified these discrepancies by the demonstration that the tissue factor–factor VIIa complex activates factor X and also factor IX.[23] Thus, an integrated view of the coagulation system can be outlined (Fig. 1.2).[24–6]

According to this view, blood coagulation is activated via the extrinsic pathway when injury to the vascular wall allows the blood to come in contact with exposed tissue factor. Factor VIIa, which is present in trace amounts in normal plasma, binds to tissue factor, and the tissue factor–factor VIIa complex activates factor X to Xa and factor IX to IXa. Thus, the tissue factor–VIIa complex initiates the activation of both pathways. Tissue factor also binds factor VII and this binding enhances the conversion of factor VII to VIIa by small amounts of Xa or thrombin. Activation of factor

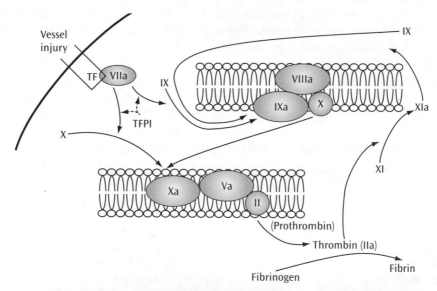

Figure 1.2 *The coagulation cascade. As described in the text, the initiation of the coagulation cascade is mediated by the binding of tissue factor (TF) to activated factor VII (VIIa). This complex activates (solid (—) arrow) the conversion of factor X to Xa and IX to IXa. This process is negatively regulated (broken (-----) arrow) by tissue factor pathway inhibitor (TFPI). The tissue factor pathway inhibitor inhibits the complex formed by tissue factor–factor VIIa, and also factor Xa (broken (----) arrow). Factor IXa activates factor X to Xa. Thus, factor Xa is generated by two distinct pathways, TF–VIIa and by factor IXa bound to factor VIIIa associated to a cell membrane (depicted in the picture as a phospholipid bilayer). Both pathways are essential for the normal activation of the coagulation cascade. In the subsequent step, factor Xa bound to Va associated with a cell membrane activates prothrombin to thrombin, which converts fibrinogen to fibrin. Thrombin also activates factor XI to XIa, which can convert factor IX into IXa.*

Xa by the tissue factor–VIIa complex is regulated by an inhibitor that circulates in association with the plasma lipoprotein fraction and is also present in endothelial cells and platelets. This inhibitor, termed tissue factor pathway inhibitor (TFPI), exerts its function by initially neutralizing factor Xa and also the tissue factor–VIIa complex. Thus, the rapid inactivation of the initial burst of formation of Xa, which is probably sufficient for basal hemostasis, must be complemented by activation of factor IX to IXa for the sustenance of a robust hemostatic response. Another mechanism for activation of factor IX is the conversion of factor XI by thrombin, and factor XIa directly activates factor IX to IXa.[25–8]

The pathways described above converge to result in the generation of factor Xa which, upon binding to factor Va, leads to the conversion of prothrombin to thrombin. Thrombin is a key enzyme in hemostasis,[29] because it possesses three fundamental functions: it converts fibrinogen into fibrin; it activates platelets; and, when it binds to thrombomodulin, it activates protein C to the anticoagulant enzyme protein Ca, which dampens the activation of the coagulation system (see below).

In the final step of blood coagulation, thrombin cleaves the fibrinopeptides of fibrinogen generating fibrin monomers that spontaneously polymerize, forming the fibrin clot. As depicted in Fig. 1.3, fibrinogen is a dimer composed of three different chains, named Aα, Bβ and γ chains, and the two halves of the molecule are linked by disulfide bonds at the center of the molecule, known as fragment E. At the other end there are two monomeric fragments known as fragment D. Thrombin cleaves the two fibrinopeptides from the central domain (E domain), producing the fibrin monomer, which spontaneously polymerizes into a fibrin clot. Thrombin cleavage of the fibrinopeptides exposes knobs in the central domain (fragment E) of the fibrin molecule which fit into a pocket exposed in fragment D of an adjacent molecule, forming a half-staggered overlap dimer. The elongation proceeds by the association of new fibrin monomers leading to the formation of double-stranded protofibrils that associate laterally to form fibrin fibers (Fig. 1.3). These interactions are based on electrical charges. The fibrin polymer is stabilized by the formation of new peptide bonds (catalyzed by factor XIIIa), between the γ chains of fragment D from two different molecules forming D–D dimers. Later, the α-chain also multimerizes via the formation of cross-linked bonds. The cross-linked clot is more stable and resistant to digestion by plasmin.[30–2]

Vitamin K-dependent coagulation factors

The vitamin K-dependent factors are procoagulants or anticoagulants that require the action of vitamin K for expression of their functional activity. Whereas factor II (prothrombin), factor VII, factor IX, and factor X belong to the procoagulant group, protein C and protein S function as anticoagulants (see Table 1.1). All the vitamin K-dependent factors contain a group of glutamic acid residues that are modified under the influence of vitamin K to γ-carboxyglutamic acids, which confer upon these factors specific functional properties. For example, without γ-carboxyglutamic acid, these factors do not bind calcium and do not properly associate with cell membrane phospholipids, an association that is necessary for the localization of these factors on the surface of platelets and other cell membranes required for their

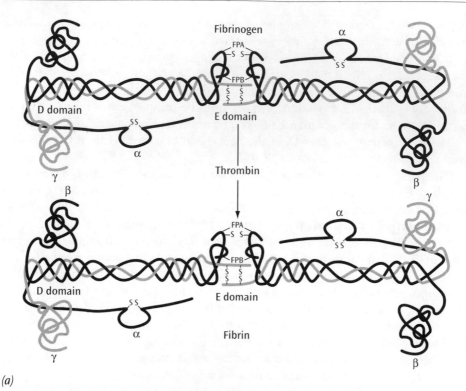

Figure 1.3 *A model of fibrinogen (a) and fibrin assembly (b). (a) Fibrinogen is a dimeric molecule and each half of the molecule is composed of three chains: Aα, Bβ, and γ. The amino terminal regions of the six chains are linked in the central domain (E domain) by disulfide bridges that form the dimer. In this region of fibrinogen, fibrinopeptides A and B (FPA and FPB) are cleaved by thrombin, which converts fibrinogen into fibrin monomers. The two nodular regions at the C terminal (D domain) contain the complementary binding sites for the central, newly exposed binding sites generated after the release of the fibrinopeptides. (Adapted with permission from Mosessen.[31])*

normal activation (Fig. 1.4).[22,33] These calcium-dependent, phospholipid-mediated interactions are also responsible for activation of coagulation in vitro. The vitamin K-dependent factors are synthesized by the hepatocyte, and reduction of their plasma level can reflect the presence of liver disease or vitamin K deficiency. The activity of the vitamin K-dependent factors is also reduced in patients taking oral anticoagulants which act by inhibiting the function of vitamin K.[18,34]

Factor VIII and factor V

These two factors have several structural and functional properties in common: they are not proenzymes; they are activated by thrombin cleavage; and their main function is to bind to cell membranes and serve as templates for the assembly of specific factors.[33,35] Factor VIIIa colocalizes factor IXa and factor X, and factor Va colocalizes factor Xa and prothrombin (Fig. 1.4).

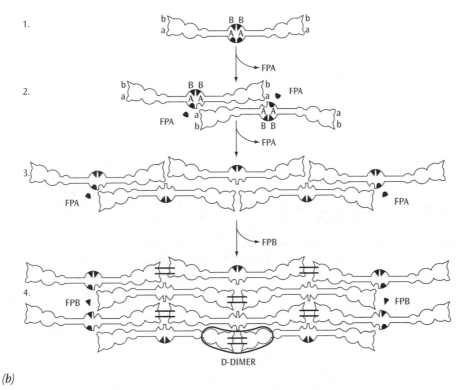

(b)

(b) A model of fibrin assembly. Semicircles represent fibrinopeptide A (FPA) and triangles fibrinopeptide B (FPB). After the cleavage of the fibrinopeptides, the binding sites are exposed, (the A site is represented by a circle and the B site by a triangle). Complementary to these sites in the E domain are those in the D domain, which are depicted as knobs (a sites are circular knobs, b sites are triangular). After cleavage of fibrinopeptide A, the A site present in the E domain of one molecule interacts with the a site of the D domain of another molecule, forming a half-staggered overlap dimer (part 2 of figure). Additional fibrin monomers associate through D:D contacts. The protofibril is formed by two rows linked by D:D interactions, and the monomers of one row are arranged in a half-staggered overlap with respect to the monomers of the other row by D:E contacts (part 3 of figure). Removal of fibrinopeptide B exposes the B sites, and the interaction with b sites promotes the lateral association of protofibrils into fibrin fibers. (Adapted with permission from Weisel.[32]) In the last stage, factor XIIIa catalyzes the formation of covalent bonds between the γ chain of two adjacent fragment D, depicted in part 4 of the figure as horizontal bars. Following the formation of D–D dimers, the α chain is also cross-linked by factor XIIIa (not shown in the figure).

Regulatory mechanisms of blood coagulation

The activation of the coagulation system is kept under tight control by several proteins that either inhibit the activation of the proenzymes or neutralize the activity of the enzymes themselves. Tissue factor pathway inhibitor, as discussed above, inhibits the first steps of blood coagulation by binding to and inactivating the Xa–VIIa–tissue factor complex.[25,26] However, the role of this inhibitor in clinical

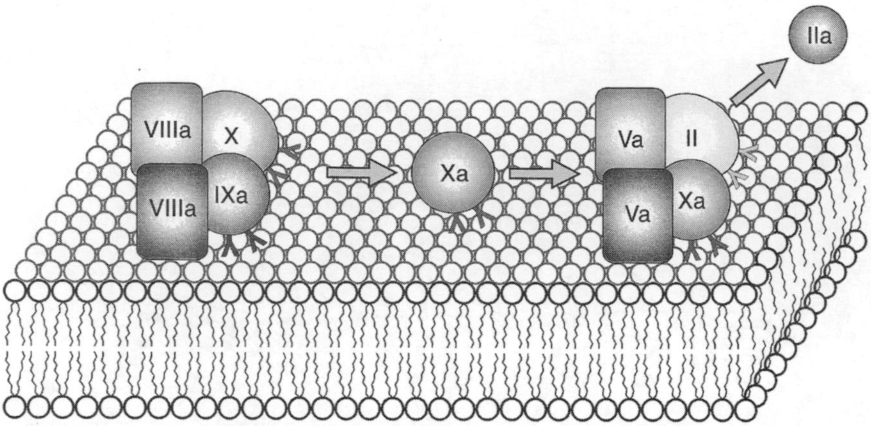

Figure 1.4 *Factors VIIIa and Va localized factors IXa, X, Xa, and II to cell membranes. Shown in this figure is the assembly of factors IXa and factor X on the complex formed by factor VIIIa, which is associated with a cell membrane, for example membranes of activated platelets, represented in the figure as a phospholipid bilayer. As seen in the figure, factors IXa and X associate with factor VIIIa and also with the phospholipid via the γ-carboxyglutamic acids (bifurcating prolongations present in factors IXa and X). Factor X is activated and in the subsequent step factors Xa and II bind to factor Va bound to cell surface phospholipids, forming a trimolecular complex. The vitamin K-dependent factors Xa and II also associate with the cell membrane phospholipids directly via their γ-carboxyglutamic acids. In this phase, factor Xa activates factor II (prothrombin) to IIa (thrombin) that in the fluid phase converts fibrinogen into fibrin. (Modified with permission from Mann et al.[33])*

disorders of blood coagulation is presently unclear. Antithrombin III is a glycoprotein that plays a major role in the inactivation of several enzymes, the most important of which are thrombin and factor Xa. The ability of antithrombin III to neutralize factors Xa and thrombin (IIa) is markedly enhanced upon its binding to heparan-like substances present on cell surfaces, or by heparin during therapeutic anticoagulation.[36] Patients with deficiency of antithrombin III (even modest reductions in the plasma level) may present with venous thrombosis, indicating that this inhibitor plays a major role in the maintenance of blood fluidity.

The second group of regulatory proteins is comprised of protein C that, in conjunction with protein S, cleaves and inactivates the two nonenzyme cofactors of blood coagulation, factor VIIIa and factor Va.[37] The cleavage of factors VIIIa and Va by activated protein C yields proteolytic products that do not support the activation of factors X and prothrombin (see above). Protein C is activated to protein Ca by thrombin which is bound to one of its endothelial cell receptors, known as thrombomodulin.[37] The functional activity of protein Ca is markedly enhanced in the presence of its cofactor, protein S (Fig. 1.5). Deficiencies of protein C or protein S are causes of a hypercoagulable state, manifested by venous thrombosis.[38,39] The importance of this mechanism in vivo has been demonstrated by the identification of patients with mutations of factor V that are resistant to the proteolytic activity of protein C, for example factor V Leiden, and these patients are at increased risk of venous thrombosis.[40,41] Other processes, such as dilution of the activated enzymes by

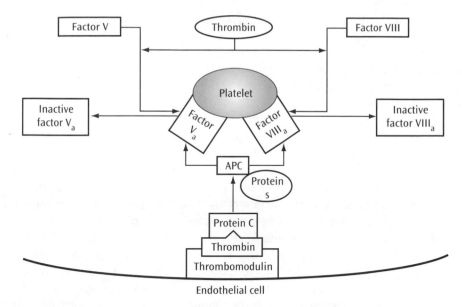

Figure 1.5 *The regulatory function in blood coagulation of proteins C and S. As described in the text, thrombin expresses both procoagulant and anticoagulant functions. In this system, the former is mediated by cleavage of factors V and VIII by thrombin, producing factors VIIIa and Va, and the latter by the activation of protein C. Activation of protein C depends upon binding of thrombin to thrombomodulin, which is present in the surface of endothelial cells. The activated protein C (APC) in conjunction with protein S inactivates factors Va and VIIIa on the surface of platelets, and the disassembly of the factor VIIIa and Va complexes dampens the activation of the coagulation cascade.*

clearance via circulating blood and their physical removal from the circulation via the reticuloendothelial system, prevent the localization of high levels of activated enzymes in isolated areas of the circulatory system, such as the deep veins of the leg. Failure of clearance of these activated factors from these areas, as can occur during prolonged immobilization with stasis of blood in these vessels, may play a role in precipitating the formation of the intravascular clot.[42]

Principles of fibrinolysis

Formation of a fibrin clot triggers a series of biochemical and cellular responses that regulate both the deposition of fibrin as well as its dissolution. These mechanisms play an important role in remodeling the vessel wall and, in the case of an intravascular fibrin clot, its dissolution by plasmin may restore luminal patency of the occluded blood vessels. One of the mechanisms for fibrinolysis involves fibrin-induced release of tissue plasminogen activator from endothelial cells.[43,44] This enzyme activates plasminogen to plasmin, which then degrades fibrin, as well as fibrinogen, into a series of well-characterized fragments known as fibrin(ogen) degradation products, which can be measured in blood as an assessment of the level of intravascular fibrinolysis.[45] When fibrin is cleaved by plasmin, the final degradation products are D–D dimer and fragment E. The D–D dimer is the result of the cross-linking of fragment D in adjacent fibrin monomers (see Fig. 1.3). In contrast, elevation of the level of fragment D monomer in plasma suggests degradation of fibrinogen (fibrinogenolysis), as opposed to fibrin. This distinction is important because it helps in the identification of fibrin formation and degradation as evidenced by high levels of D dimer.

After tissue plasminogen activator[46] is released from the vessel wall under the influence of fibrin, it binds to fibrin and activates fibrin-bound plasminogen, generating fibrin-bound plasmin, which initiates clot dissolution. The fibrinolytic process is thus localized to the area of the thrombus, with only small amounts of free plasmin in the circulation to cleave fibrinogen. For this reason, tissue plasminogen activator is considered relatively fibrin specific. In contrast, some of the therapeutic agents, notably streptokinase, activate free plasminogen (plasminogen that is not bound to fibrin) and the free plasmin that is generated degrades not only fibrin, but also fibrinogen. Plasmin also modulates the hemostatic system by cleaving factor VIII, factor V, and platelet GPIIb/IIIa, in addition to fibrinogen and fibrin.

The activity of the fibrinolytic enzymes is under the control of several inhibitors. In the case of tissue plasminogen activator, the major inhibitor is a molecule known as plasminogen activator inhibitor-1 which is synthesized and released by endothelial cells and platelets.[47] Plasmin, on the other hand, is inactivated by several inhibitors, with α2–antiplasmin playing a major role in modulating the activity of plasmin.[48]

IN CONCLUSION

The hemostatic mechanism plays a fundamental dual role. Whereas under normal conditions it serves to preserve blood fluidity, after injury to the vessel wall, the coagulation system is activated, leading to the formation of the hemostatic plug. This clot not only prevents the extravasation of blood, but also intervenes in the repair of the vessel wall. The vascular endothelium, in conjunction with specific inhibitors of blood coagulation, is involved in the preservation of blood fluidity, whereas the activated platelet and the coagulation enzymes play a crucial role in the formation of the hemostatic clot. In pathological conditions, such as in intravascular coagulation or in patients with rupture of an atheromatous plaque, the deposition of platelets and activation of the coagulation system lead to the formation of an intravascular thrombus that interferes with blood circulation, causing tissue injury, such as myocardial or cerebral infarction. Activation of the fibrinolytic pathway, either endogenously or by pharmacological means, induces the dissolution of the clot and re-establishes blood circulation. This new supply of blood can potentially induce the repair of the damaged hypoxic tissues.

ACKNOWLEDGMENTS

The authors are grateful to Mr D Likens for preparation of the figures and to Dr Stephen J Schuster for reading the manuscript.

REFERENCES

1 Wu KK. Endothelial cells in hemostasis, thrombosis, and inflammation. *Hosp Pract* 1992; **27**: 145–66.

2 Cohen RA. The role of nitric oxide and other endothelium-derived vasoactive substances in vascular disease. *Prog Cardiovasc Dis* 1995; **38**: 105–28.

3 Rosenberg RD, Rosenberg JS. Natural anticoagulant mechanisms. *J Clin Invest* 1984; **74**: 1–6.

4 Mantovani A, Sozzani S, Vecchi A, Introna M, Allavena P. Cytokine activation of endothelial cells: new molecules for an old paradigm. *Thromb Haemost* 1997; **78**: 406–14.

5 Celi A, Lorenzet R, Furie B, Furie BC. Platelet–leukocyte–endothelial cell interaction on the blood vessel wall. *Semin Hematol* 1997; **34**: 327–35.

6 Burstein SA, Harker LA. Control of platelet production. *Clin Haematol* 1983; **12**: 3–22.

7 Gewirtz AM, Hoffman R. Human megakaryocyte production: cell biology and clinical considerations. *Hematol Oncol Clin North Am* 1990; **4**: 43–64.

8 Blockmans D, Deckmyn H, Vermylen J. Platelet activation. *Blood Rev* 1995; **9**: 143–56.

9 Shattil SJ, Kashiwagi H, Pampori N. Integrin signaling: the platele paradigm. *Blood* 1998; **91**: 2645–57.

10 Bennett JS. Mechanisms of platelet adhesion and aggregation: an update. *Hosp Pract* 1992; **27**: 124–6.

11 Ruggeri ZM. New insights into the mechanisms of platelet adhesion and aggregation. *Semin Hematol* 1994; **31**: 229–39.

12 Lefkovits J, Plow EF, Topol EJ. Platelet glycoprotein IIb/IIIa receptors in cardiovascular medicine. *N Engl J Med* 1995; **332**: 1553–9.

13 Coller BS. Platelet GPIIb/IIIa antagonists: the first anti-integrin receptor therapeutics. *J Clin Invest* 1997; **100**: S57–S60.

14 Walsh PN. Platelet-mediated coagulant protein interactions in hemostasis. *Semin Hematol* 1985; **22**: 178–86.

15 Mitus AJ, Schafer AI. Thrombocytosis and thrombocythemia. *Hematol Oncol Clin North Am* 1990; **4**: 157–78.

16 George JN, Woolf SH, Raskob GE, et al. Idiopathic thrombocytopenic purpura: a practice guideline developed by explicit methods for the American Society of Hematology. *Blood* 1996; **88**: 3–40.

17 Beutler E. Platelet transfusions: the 20 000/µl trigger. *Blood* 1993; **81**: 1411–13.

18 Martinez J, Barsigian C. Coagulopathy in liver failure and vitamin K deficiency. In: Loscalzo J, Schafer AI eds *Thrombosis and hemorrhage*. Boston: Blackwell, 1994; 945–63.

19 Sharma P, McDonald GB, Banaji M. The risk of bleeding after percutaneous liver biopsy: a relation to platelet count. *J Clin Gastroenterol* 1982; **4**: 451–3.

20 Consensus conference. Platelet transfusion therapy. *JAMA* 1987; **257**: 1777–80.

21 Rutherford CJ, Frenkel EP. Thrombocytopenia. Issues in diagnosis and therapy. *Med Clin North Am* 1994; **78**: 555–75.

22 Furie B, Furie BC. Molecular and cellular biology of blood coagulation. *N Engl J Med* 1992; **326**: 800–6.

23 Osterud B, Rapaport SI. Activation of factor IX by the reaction product of tissue factor and factor VII: additional pathway for initiating blood coagulation. *Proc Natl Acad Sci USA* 1977; **74**: 5260–4.

24 Davie EW, Fujikawa K, Kisiel W. The coagulation cascade: initiation, maintenance, and regulation. *Biochemistry* 1991; **30**: 10363–70.
25 Broze GJ. The role of tissue factor pathway inhibitor in a revised coagulation cascade. *Semin Hematol* 1992; **29**: 159–69.
26 Nemerson Y. The tissue factor pathway of blood coagulation. *Semin Hematol* 1992; **29**: 170–6.
27 Broze GJ. Why do hemophiliacs bleed? *Hosp Pract* 1992; **27**: 71–86.
28 Rapaport SI, Rao LVM. Initiation and regulation of tissue factor-dependent blood coagulation. *Arterioscler Thromb* 1992; **12**: 1111–21.
29 Fenton JW, Ofosu FA, Brezniak DV, Hassouna HI. Understanding thrombin and hemostasis. *Hematol Oncol Clin North Am* 1993; **7**: 1107–19.
30 Martinez J. Congenital dysfibrinogenemia. *Curr Opin Hematol* 1997; **4**: 357–65.
31 Mosesson MW. The roles of fibrinogen and fibrin in hemostasis and thrombosis. *Semin Hematol* 1992; **29**: 177–88.
32 Weisel JW. Fibrin assembly. Lateral aggregation and the role of the pairs of fibrinopeptides. *Biophys J* 1986; **50**: 1079–93.
33 Mann KG, Nesheim ME, Church WR, Haley P, Krishnaswamy S. Surface-dependent reactions of the vitamin K-dependent enzyme complexes. *Blood* 1990; **76**: 1–16.
34 Bovill EG, Mann KG. Warfarin and the biochemistry of the vitamin K-dependent proteins. *Adv Exp Med Biol* 1987; **214**: 17–46.
35 Kane WH, Davie EW. Blood coagulation factors V and VIII: structural and functional similarities and their relationship to hemorrhagic and thrombotic disorders. *Blood* 1988; **71**: 539–55.
36 Bauer KA, Rosenberg RD. Role of antithrombin III as a regulator of in vivo coagulation. *Semin Hematol* 1991; **28**: 10–18.
37 Esmon CT. Molecular events that control the protein C anticoagulant pathway. *Thromb Haemost* 1993; **70**: 29–35.
38 Clouse L, Comp PC. The regulation of hemostasis: the protein C system. *N Engl J Med* 1986; **314**: 1298–304.
39 Dahlback B. Inherited thrombophilia: resistance to activated protein C as a pathogenic factor for venous thromboembolism. *Blood* 1995; **85**: 607–14.
40 Svensson PJ, Dahlback B. Resistance to activated protein C as a basis for venous thrombosis. *N Engl J Med* 1994; **330**: 517–22.
41 De Stefano V, Finazzi G, Mannucci PM. Inherited thrombophilia: pathogenesis, clinical syndromes, and management. *Blood* 1996; **87**: 3531–44.
42 Slack SM, Cui Y, Turitto V. The effects of flow on blood coagulation and thrombosis. *Thromb Haemost* 1993; **70**: 129–34.
43 Collen D, Lijnen HR. Basic and clinical aspects of fibrinolysis and thrombolysis. *Blood* 1991; **78**: 3114–24.
44 Runge MS, Quertermous T, Haber E. Plasminogen activators. *Circulation* 1989; **79**: 217–24.
45 Lawler CM, Bovill EG, Stump DC, Collen DJ, Mann KG, Tracy RP. Fibrin fragment D-dimer and fibrinogen Bβ peptides in plasma as markers of clot lysis during thrombolytic therapy in acute myocardial infarction. *Blood* 1990; **76**: 1341–8.
46 Loscalzo J, Braunwald E. Tissue plasminogen activator. *N Engl J Med* 1988; **319**: 925–32.
47 Krishnamurti C, Alving B. Plasminogen activator inhibitor type 1: biochemistry and evidence for modulation of fibrinolysis in vivo. *Semin Hemost Thromb* 1992; **18**: 67–80.
48 Lijnen HR, Collen D. Protease inhibitors of human plasma. Alpha-2–antiplasmin. *J Med* 1985; **16**: 225–84.

2

Laboratory evaluation of the hypercoagulable state

BARBARA A KONKLE, COLLEEN PALERMO

The clinical and special hemostasis reference laboratories serve important roles in the evaluation of patients with thrombosis. This chapter discusses the approach to laboratory testing in patients with thrombosis, including the appropriate timing for testing, important points for accurate testing, and the types of testing procedures used.

THE VALUE OF LABORATORY SCREENING TESTS

All patients with thrombosis are, by definition, hypercoagulable. As clinicians, we try to determine the reasons underlying the thrombosis. Routine admission laboratories are often useful in suggesting an underlying medical disorder, such as a malignancy or myeloproliferative disorder, particularly in older patients without a personal or family history of thrombosis. In a study evaluating patients who presented with thrombosis for an underlying malignancy, Cornuz et al. found that screening laboratory studies, including a complete blood count (CBC), chemistries, and urinalysis, combined with a basic history and physical examination detected those patients with underlying malignancy.[1] Of note, in that study of 986 patients who presented with thrombosis, 14 of the 16 who were found to have an underlying malignancy were anemic.

It is important to evaluate the patient for underlying medical conditions, particularly those that would respond to specific treatments other than anticoagulation. Acquired disorders that may be associated with abnormal screening laboratory tests and thrombosis are shown in Table 2.1.

Table 2.1 *Screening laboratory clues for acquired thrombophilic states*

Acquired condition	Possible screening laboratory findings[a]
Malignancy	Anemia, leukocytosis, hypercalcemia, hematuria
Myeloproliferative disorders polycythemia vera, essential thrombocythemia, myelofibrosis	Erythrocytosis, leukocytosis, thrombocytosis
Antiphospholipid syndrome	Elevated aPTT, thrombocytopenia
Paroxysmal nocturnal hemoglobinuria	Anemia, thrombocytopenia, neutropenia
Chronic disseminated intravascular coagulation	Increased PT and/or aPTT, thrombocytopenia, anemia
Vasculitis	Anemia, thrombocytopenia
Thrombotic thrombocytopenic purpura	Thrombocytopenia, anemia
Heparin-induced thrombocytopenia with thrombosis	Thrombocytopenia, increase aPTT if patient on heparin

[a]Screening laboratories include: complete blood count (CBC), prothrombin time (PT), activated partial thromboplastin time (aPTT), chemistry screen, and urinalysis.

APPROACH TO SPECIALIZED TESTING FOR THE HYPERCOAGULABLE STATE

Except for genetic testing, most laboratory tests used to assess patients with thrombosis are affected by the condition of the patient when the testing is performed. Acute illness and thrombosis can affect many of the tests we use to assess the underlying risk of thrombosis. Before using these tests, one must determine what is being assessed and why. For assessment of underlying risk factors to determine the length of anticoagulation, testing should be done at steady state, that is, a few months away from the episode of acute thrombosis. Testing should only be done at the time of an acute thrombosis when it would affect initial therapy. An example of this would be an assessment of apparent heparin resistance in a patient with acute thrombosis who is difficult to anticoagulate with heparin. An antithrombin III level may be checked and, if low enough, one could consider using an antithrombin III concentrate in addition to heparin. Of note, this would not make the diagnosis of an inherited disorder and testing would need to be repeated later. The study of family members can be very useful in establishing or confirming a diagnosis of an inherited disorder in an individual.

Specimen collection and handling

Accurate laboratory results, particularly in the coagulation laboratory, are highly dependent on correct specimen collection and handling. Examples of reasons for invalid results are listed in Table 2.2. For coagulation testing, it is not necessary for

Table 2.2 *Reasons for invalid results due to blood collection and handling errors*

Overfilled or underfilled blue-top tube (sodium citrate anticoagulation)
Use of wrong collection tube
Tube is not labeled or mislabeled
Specimen is clotted due to difficult venipuncture or inadequate mixing
Specimen is hemolyzed
Additive contamination due to filling tubes in wrong order
Specimen kept at incorrect temperature prior to testing
Platelet-poor plasma is not prepared in samples for which testing is delayed

the patient to fast from food or water, although it is recommended that patients do not ingest fatty substances that will result in blood specimens becoming lipemic, as that can interfere with clot-based tests assessed by light transmission.

Blood is routinely obtained by drawing through a Vacutainer device into a tube with, as appropriate for the test, an anticoagulant to prevent blood clotting. Most functional clotting tests are performed on plasma which has been anticoagulated with sodium citrate. This allows anticoagulation that can be reversed with the addition of calcium. Sodium citrate anticoagulant is in the blue-top tube in liquid form and must be mixed with the correct amount of blood for optimal anticoagulation. All tubes have a line on them to which the blood should be filled. Both overfilling and underfilling will give erroneous results. When the hematocrit is very low (< 21%) or very high (> 55%), the volume of anticoagulants must be individually prepared to compensate for the increased or decreased plasma volume. There is a certain amount of vacuum in each Vacutainer tube, which should result in appropriate filling. The collection tube should be allowed to fill until the vacuum is depleted and the contents mixed immediately by gentle inversion three or four times. Tubes should be filled with free-flowing blood. Difficult venipunctures and difficulty drawing the blood can result in partial clot activation and erroneous results.

Traditionally, it has been recommended that the blue-top tube should not be drawn first and that, if only a blue-top tube is being drawn, a discard tube (this can be a pediatric red top) should be drawn first. One study evaluated the drawing of blue-top tubes for prothrombin time (PT)/International Normalized Ratio (INR) and activated partial thromboplastin time (aPTT) determinations. In that setting, if there was a clean stick and the blood flowed freely, there was no need for a discard tube.[2] This has not been assessed for other coagulation laboratory studies. Heparinized tubes (green top) should never be filled prior to a blue-top tube using a vacutainer system, as there can be heparin contamination of the contents of the blue-top tube that can affect results. If more than one tube is being drawn, an order has been recommended to optimize results: yellow, red, blue, green, lavender, then gray.

The tourniquet should be applied just prior to specimen collection. If there appears to be difficulty in finding an appropriate site for venipuncture, the tourniquet should be released. The tourniquet should be left on no longer than two minutes, because it results in hemoconcentration, which will result in hemolysis. If there is difficulty in locating an appropriate site for venipuncture, a warm cloth may be applied to the area for a few minutes to increase blood flow. The tourniquet can then be reapplied for specimen collection.

Specimens for functional coagulation tests should be drawn from a direct venipuncture unless this is not possible due to lack of venous access. Blood drawn through lines will always have some degree of coagulation activation. Sensitive tests of clotting activation, such as the D-dimer, will demonstrate low-level positivity when drawn through a line. If drawing through a line is necessary, at least 20 cm³ of blood should be drawn before obtaining the sample for coagulation testing, and results should be interpreted with the source in mind.

Specimen temperature and transport

Appropriate handling of the specimen after collection is critical for valid laboratory assays. Coagulation factors have different stabilities at room temperature, with factors V and VIII being the least stable. In specimens from patients on stable warfarin anticoagulation, studies have documented the stability of the PT/INR when kept at room temperature for up to three days.[3,4] This is not valid, however, for aPTT determination or for other coagulation assays. The aPTT will be prolonged in samples maintained at room temperature, due to a decreasing factor VIII level. Ideally, samples should be kept on ice until the laboratory assay is performed. If the assay will not be performed within a few hours, platelet-poor plasma should be prepared and frozen until the assay is performed. If being shipped to a reference laboratory, the sample must be packaged so that it remains frozen throughout the shipping.

The International Normalized Ratio and the effect of citrate concentrations on results

The INR is a widely accepted method used to assess anticoagulation in patients on warfarin anticoagulation:

$$INR = (PT_p/PT_c)^{ISI}$$

where PT_p is the prothrombin time of the patient and PT_c is the mean prothrombin time of a normal plasma pool. The ISI is the International Sensitivity Index, which is determined for each batch of the thromboplastin reagent by comparison to an international reference on a specific instrument utilized in the testing.

The INR was adopted as a way to eliminate interlaboratory variations in test results caused by the use of thromboplastins with different sensitivities. However, there is still variability, particularly when thromboplastins are used with high ISI values and when the INR is high.[5] In addition, variability in instrumentation and the standards used when establishing the ISI can result in differing results.[6,7] Thus, it is helpful for monitoring of anticoagulation to have the testing done at the same laboratory. Unexplained variations should be discussed with the laboratory Director to find out whether procedures, instrumentation, or reagents used in the laboratory have been changed.

The concentration of citrate used to anticoagulate plasma has an effect on the INR. Tubes with 3.2% and 3.8% sodium citrate are available. The ISI of thromboplastin reagents is generally calibrated with plasma collected into 3.2% citrate. Plasma collected into 3.8% citrate has been shown to result in higher INR values.[8] There is an emerging consensus that 3.2% citrate should be used, although many laboratories still use 3.8%. Thus, this is another reason values may vary by site of testing.

LABORATORY TECHNIQUES USED FOR TESTING

The coagulation laboratory uses a number of methodologies in testing. These include clot-based, immunologic, chromogenic, and DNA-based assays. For many coagulation tests, and most notably the PT and aPTT, the endpoint of testing is the detection of clot formation. In general, automated instruments are used that signal the endpoint as a defined optical or electromechanical change.

Immunologic assays are used to quantitate the amount of a protein present in plasma. They are based on the principle of antibody recognition of an antigen. A number of different types of assays are used. Examples include latex agglutination for fibrogen degradation products, in which latex particles are coated with antibodies to fibrinogen; nephelometry, which is based on the ability of antigen–antibody complexes to scatter light; radial immunodiffusion (RID), which is based on the principle that the concentration of antigen is proportional to the rate of precipitation of antigen–antibody complex during the diffusion of an antigen in an antibody-containing gel; electroimmunodiffusion (EID), or the Laurell rocket assay, which is based on the same principles as RID but utilizes an electric current to mobilize the antigen; radioimmunoassay, in which a radioactive-tagged antibody is used to detect and quantitate antigens; and enzyme-linked immunoassays (ELISA), in which a microtiter plate is coated with a polyclonal antibody directed against an antigen and detected using a second antigen-specific antibody that is chemically coupled to an enzyme-based detection system.

Chromogenic assays are used to evaluate a specific coagulation factor in an assay that does not require all of the other components to be present in normal amounts, as is needed in clot-based assays. For these assays synthetic substrates of the enzymatic activity of the clotting factor being studied are used. The synthetic substrate is a 3–5 amino-acid peptide sequence attached to a chromophore, which, when released by cleavage, results in a measurably different optical density. For example, a chromogenic-based test for factor X activity has been proposed as a better assay to monitor warfarin therapy in patients with lupus anticoagulants, as it is not affected by the presence of a lupus anticoagulant.[9]

DNA-based tests are used to detect a change (mutation or polymorphism) in the patient's DNA. DNA is usually prepared from peripheral white blood cells collected as anticoagulated blood, although buccal mucosal smears or hair root samples, among other sources, may also be used. Most tests utilize the polymerase chain reaction (PCR) to amplify the DNA. The change is detected by using primers that differentially amplify mutant versus normal DNA, using sequence-specific primers as a probe to detect mutant versus normal DNA, or by using a restriction enzyme that cuts only normal or mutant DNA.

SPECIFIC LABORATORY TESTS

Prior to sending a patient sample to a special hemostasis reference laboratory, a number of items should be addressed. One must consider the predictive value of a positive and of a negative test. This is determined not only by sensitivity and specificity, but also by the prevalence of a particular deficiency in the population studied. Unless the specificity is close to 100%, the predictive value of a positive test is usually quite low for defects that are rare in the population. Deficiencies of type I (low protein concentration) are more common than the type II deficiencies (low functional activity, but normal protein concentration). For protein S, there are also type III deficiencies described that result in decreased free protein with normal total protein. Below are brief descriptions of frequently encountered tests. For more extensive discussions of the tests and their use in the evaluation of the patient with thrombosis, the reader is referred elsewhere.[10–14] Some conditions and therapies that affect specific laboratory assays[15–18] are shown in Table 2.3.

Table 2.3 *Medical conditions affecting laboratory assays*[15–18]

	Thrombosis/ acute illness	Liver disease	Heparin use	Warfarin use	Pregnancy/ hormonal Rx	Nephrotic syndrome
AT III	↓	↓	↓		↓/—	↓
Protein C	↑/↓/—	↓↓		↓		↑/—
Protein S	↓/—	↓		↓	↓	↑/↓/—
dRVVT		↑[a]	↑/—[a]	↑[a]		
PTT-based APC-R	↓/—[b]	↓/—[b]	↓[b]		↓/—[b]	
ACA	↓/↑/—					

[a]The dRVVT will correct with mixing if prolonged due to liver disease or warfarin, but will not consistently correct if prolongation due to heparin.
[b]The factor V-based assays, now widely used, will not be affected.
↓, decrease; ↑, increase; —, no change; Rx, treatment. AT III, antithrombin III; dRVVT, dilute Russell Viper venom time; PTT, partial thromboplastin time; APC-R, activated protein C resistance; ACA, anticardiolipin antibody.

Prothrombin time

The one-stage PT determination measures the prothrombin conversion phase of coagulation. It is used to follow the course of oral anticoagulant therapy and as a screening test for deficiencies of, or inhibitors to, the classical extrinsic pathway (fibrinogen, factors II, V, VII, and X) coagulation factors. For this test, plasma is added to a thromboplastin–calcium mixture. The time required for clot formation is measured by optical density. The PT is reported as a value in seconds, and the INR is calculated based on the ISI for the thromboplastin reagent on the instrument used.

Activated partial thromboplastin time

The aPTT screens for deficiencies of, or inhibitors to, coagulation factors in the classical intrinsic pathway, including factors VIII, IX, and X. The aPTT is also abnormal in factor XII, prekallikrein, and kininogen deficiencies. It is prolonged with abnormalities of fibrinogen and factor II and X, although it is less sensitive to abnormalities of these proteins than the PT. In this procedure, plasma is incubated with a negatively charged substance as an activator, after which calcium is added and the time required for clot formation noted.

Thrombin time and reptilase time

These tests are used in the evaluation for dysfibrinogenemia, which may be associated with thrombosis. The thrombin time is a screening test for the adequacy of fibrinogen, the presence of interfering molecules (fibrin or fibrinogen degradation products), and the presence of unfractionated heparin. It is a measure of the rate of transformation of fibrinogen to fibrin after thrombin is added and is assessed visually by clot formation.

Like thrombin, reptilase is capable of clotting fibrinogen. The reptilase time is affected less by fibrinogen/fibrin degradation products and more by abnormal fibrinogen molecules (dysfibrinogenemias) than the thrombin time. Reptilase is not inhibited by heparin; therefore, in conjunction with an elevated thrombin time, a normal reptilase time is suggestive of heparin contamination.

Protein C measurements

Testing for deficiencies of protein C begin with a test of protein C activity. If it is not abnormal, protein quantitation can be used to further classify the abnormality as a type I or type II deficiency.

FUNCTIONAL PROTEIN C

In this assay, protein C is activated in the presence of a specific activator extracted from the venom of the snake *Agkistrodon c. contortix*. The quantity of functional protein C is measured using a synthetic chromogenic substrate. The sensitivity of this assay has been estimated to be 85%, with a specificity of 95%.[19] When the test is used to rule out an inherited protein C deficiency in patients with a history of idiopathic thrombosis or thrombosis at a young age (estimated prevalence of genetic defect 3%), the predictive value of a negative test is 34% and the predictive value of a positive test is 99.6%.[12]

PROTEIN C ANTIGEN QUANTITATION

This test may be performed by a number of immunologic assays. Of these, the electroimmunodiffusion method is most sensitive as it detects all forms of protein C. Protein C studies cannot be interpreted when a patient is on warfarin and should be assessed ≥ 10 days after warfarin discontinuation. Protein C levels are very sensitive to liver dysfunction and must be interpreted in the setting of liver disease with extreme caution.

Protein S measurements

Protein S circulates in human plasma in two forms: free and complexed to C4b-binding protein. Only the free form of the molecule is biologically active. Functional protein S assays have been problematic and, at present, are not helpful in the diagnosis of protein S deficiencies. Measurement of free protein S appears to be the best test for prediction of an inherited deficiency. Low free with normal total protein S may occur with type III deficiencies or, more commonly, in a number of inflammatory states that increase C4b-binding protein and in response to hormone therapy. Protein S studies cannot be interpreted when a patient is on warfarin and should be assessed ≥ 10 days after warfarin discontinuation.

FREE PROTEIN S

Free protein S is detected by immunologic technique, usually EID, after it is separated from the bound protein S by a precipitation of the bound form using polyethylene glycol.

PROTEIN S ANTIGEN – TOTAL

This assay is performed in the same manner as for free protein S, except that free and bound protein S are not separated. In a large kindred with type I deficiency, total protein S has also been shown to increase with age into the normal range, highlighting the difficulties in using these assays to diagnose inherited deficiencies.[20] As is true for protein C assays, protein S assays are not a valid prediction of underlying thrombotic risk in patients on warfarin or with liver disease.

Antithrombin III measurements

Antithrombin III is the major thrombin inhibitor in plasma. When heparin binds to antithrombin III, it markedly enhances antithrombin III-dependent inhibitor of thrombin and other serine proteases. Assays for antithrombin III include functional assays in the presence or absence of heparin, and immunologic assays for quantitation of the protein. Antithrombin III levels may be decreased in the setting of acute thrombosis, with heparin therapy, in the nephrotic syndrome, and in patients treated with L-asparaginase.[18]

ANTITHROMBIN III ACTIVITY

Antithrombin III activity is frequently assessed using a two-step chromogenic assay. The sample is incubated with a known excess of thrombin or factor Xa in the presence of heparin. The residual enzyme activity is measured using a chromogenic substrate, and antithrombin III activity is determined from a standard curve.

IMMUNOLOGICAL ANTITHROMBIN III

A number of immunologic assays have been developed to quantitate antithrombin III. Most widely used are radial immunodiffusion, EID, and a nephelometric method.

Antiphospholipid antibody testing

Antiphospholipid antibodies comprise a heterogeneous family of autoantibodies found in patients with and without systemic lupus erythematosus that may be associated with fetal loss and thrombosis. These antibodies, which are actually directed against phospholipid-binding proteins, most notably β_2-glycoprotein 1 (β_2G1) and prothrombin, are discussed further in Chapter 4. Some of these antibodies interfere with phospholipid-dependent coagulation tests. These are termed lupus anticoagulants.

LUPUS ANTICOAGULANT TESTING

Common tests used to detect lupus anticoagulants are the dilute Russell's viper venom time (dRVVT), the kaolin clotting time (KCT), the tissue thromboplastin inhibition (TTI) test, and the dilute PT test. The methods utilized for these tests make the tests sensitive to the phospholipid component and thus sensitive to an antibody that interferes with the phospholipid. The aPTT and, less commonly, the PT may also be prolonged. Whether the aPTT is prolonged will depend, in part, on the reagent used, as some are more sensitive to lupus anticoagulants than others. If the PT is prolonged, acquired prothrombin (factor II) deficiency should be ruled out, as it can occur in this setting and be associated with bleeding.

The dRVVT utilizes the snake venom of the Russell's viper, which activates factor X directly. For both a prolonged PTT and dRVVT, a mixing study should be done, in which patient plasma and normal plasma are mixed and the test is repeated. If the prolongation is due to a factor deficiency, the mixing study will correct to normal. The dRVVT will be prolonged in patients on warfarin, but will correct with mixing. Results are less consistent with patients on heparin and the test should not be done in this setting. Specific factor inhibitors will also not correct with mixing; however, the clinical presentation should help, as these patients usually have a bleeding diathesis. Lupus anticoagulants should also affect multiple coagulation factor determinations and their levels will usually normalize with increasing dilutions. Lupus anticoagulant tests are confirmed by the addition of phospholipid, either through a platelet neutralization procedure or through the addition of hexagonal phase phospholipid. The latter is available commercially as the DVV Confirm®. The Subcommittee on Lupus Anticoagulants/Antiphospholipid Antibody of the International Society for Hemostasis and Thrombosis has recommended four criteria for the diagnosis of lupus anticoagulants:[21] (1) prolongation of a phospholipid-dependent clotting assay; (2) evidence of inhibitor demonstrated by mixing studies; (3) evidence of phospholipid dependence by correction, as described above; and (4) lack of specific inhibitor to any one coagulation factor.

ANTICARDIOLIPIN AND ANTI-β_2 GLYCOPROTEIN ANTIBODIES

Anticardiolipins are detected on ELISA plates coated with cardiolipin and blocked with serum, usually bovine or human. In the majority of patients, no reactivity is detected if serum is not present, in either the blocking agent or contributed by the patient's sample. β_2G1 is one of the proteins present in the serum and is apparently responsible for the large majority of positive anticardiolipin assays. Patients with certain infections often have ACA directed against cardiolipin itself. Anti-β_2G1 antibody testing may exclude patients with infection-related anticardiolipins, and preliminary data suggest anti-β_2G1 antibodies may be more closely associated with thrombosis than anticardiolipin or antiprothrombin antibodies.[22,23] Anticardiolipins may fluctuate with acute illnesses and may be transient. Positive anticardiolipin testing should be confirmed 6–8 weeks after the initial studies.[24] Anticardiolipin results may also vary depending on the commercial kit used, and standardization of assays is needed.[25]

Activated protein C resistance

Activated protein C resistance was first described in patients later found to have a mutation at an activated protein C cleavage site of factor V, now termed the factor V Leiden mutation.[26] This was first determined using an aPTT-based assay. Activated protein C normally prolongs the aPTT by inactivating factors V and VIII. The test determines the ratio of aPTT with activated protein C present to the aPTT without activated protein C. This ratio is decreased in a number of conditions, including pregnancy, obesity, and acute stroke, and is also affected by other conditions or therapies that would affect the aPTT. Some conditions associated with decreased response to activated protein C are associated with an increased risk of thrombosis.[27] The thrombotic risk in patients with a prolonged aPTT-based activated protein C resistance, but who are factor V Leiden negative, is currently under study.

More sensitive and specific tests for activated protein C resistance due to abnormalities of factor V, including the factor V Leiden mutation, have been developed. These utilize factor V-deficient plasma, which is mixed with patient plasma, thus making the assay dependent on the patient's factor V. A ratio with and without activated protein C is then performed. The assay is highly (> 98%) sensitive and specific for the factor V Leiden mutation and can differentiate the heterozygous from the homozygous state.[28] False positives have been reported in patients with lupus anticoagulants. Also, this assay would pick up other rare mutations in factor V resulting in activated protein C resistance, as have been described.

Factor V Leiden mutation

Studies to detect the factor V Leiden mutation and the prothrombin polymorphism (described below) are performed on patient DNA. The DNA is usually prepared from peripheral blood white blood cells and the PCR is used to amplify a segment of the factor V or prothrombin gene. The changes in DNA are detected by using differential restriction enzyme cuffing, differential primers for amplification of the DNA, or allele-specific hybridization techniques.

The factor V Leiden mutation is a single-point mutation in the gene for factor V (G to A at nucleotide position 1691), which results in replacement of an arginine in one of the activated protein C cleavage sites with a glutamine.

Prothrombin 3' untranslated polymorphism

A change in the DNA (G to A at nucleotide 20210) in the 3' end of the prothrombin gene that is transcribed (made into RNA), but not translated into protein (untranslated, UT) has been shown to be associated with an increased risk of thrombosis.[29] This is thought to be due to an increased plasma level of prothrombin, which appears to result from this polymorphism. It is detected utilizing techniques as described for the factor V Leiden mutation using prothrombin-specific primer and probes.

Anti-factor Xa

Heparins inhibit coagulation by accelerating antithrombin III-mediated inhibition of coagulation factors that are serine proteases (see Chapter 5). Whereas the degree of inhibition of thrombin (factor IIa) differs between unfractionated heparin (UFH) and low molecular weight heparin (LMWH), both inhibit factor Xa equally. The anti-Xa assay is used to determine the plasma level of UFH or LMWH activity by the measurement of the anti-Xa activity using a chromogenic substrate. The procedure is carried out with an excess of purified antithrombin III to ensure that any existing deficiency of this protein is compensated for. The test is useful in assessing the activity of LMWHs, when needed, because of their varying effect on thrombin, and thus, on the aPTT. For UFH, it is a useful direct measurement of heparin activity. Factor VIII and fibrinogen are acute phase reactants and may result in the aPTT being subtherapeutic despite adequate heparin therapy. This may be seen in a number of medical situations, most notably with malignancies. In patients with apparent heparin resistance, a test of direct heparin activity such as anti-Xa or protamine neutralization is useful.

The heparin sensitivity of aPTT reagents and instrumentation varies. For this reason, it has been recommended that laboratories establish a 'therapeutic range' of aPTT by directly comparing the aPTT to a direct measurement of activity such as anti-Xa or protamine neutralization in a group of heparinized patients. Utilizing the local laboratory reagent and instrumentation, the therapeutic range should be determined to be equivalent to an anti-Xa level of 0.3–0.7 μ/mL.[30]

CONCLUSION

The hemostasis laboratory is an important adjunct for the diagnosis and treatment of thrombotic disorders. Interpreting the tests correctly requires an understanding of the tests and of factors that influence their outcome. Optimal specialized testing requires a collaborative relationship between the physician and the hemostasis laboratory. This has become more difficult due to the constraints of managed care, the use of large reference laboratories, and the lack of control over specimen collection and handling that may ensue. However, accurate laboratory testing may prevent unnecessary anticoagulation due to erroneous diagnoses as well as recurrent thrombosis when risk factors are appropriately diagnosed and anticoagulation appropriately managed. Thus, for our patients' benefit, we must be diligent in obtaining good laboratory support.

REFERENCES

1 Cornuz J, Pearson SD, Creager MA, Cook EF, Goldman L. Importance of findings on the initial evaluation for cancer in patients with symptomatic idiopathic deep venous thromboembolism. *Ann Intern Med* 1996; **10**: 785–93.

2 Gottfried EL, Adachi MM. Prothrombin time and activated partial thromboplastin time can be performed on the first tube. *Am J Clin Pathol* 1997; **107**: 681–3.

3 Bridgen ML, Graydon C, McLeod B, Lesperance M. Prothrombin time determinations: the lack of need for discard tube and 24 hour stability. *Am J Clin Pathol* 1997; **108**: 422–6.

4 Baglin T, Luddington R. Reliability of delayed INR determinations: implications for decentralized anticoagulant care with off-site blood sampling. *Br J Haematol* 1997; **96**: 431–4.

5 Le DT, Weibert RT, Sevilla BK, Donnelly KJ, Rapaport SI. The international normalized ratio (INR) for monitoring warfarin therapy: reliability and relation to other monitoring methods. *Ann Intern Med* 1994; **120**: 552–8.

6 Van den Besselaar AMHP. Precision and accuracy of the international normalized ratio in oral anticoagulant control. *Haemostasis* 1996; **26**(Suppl. 4): 248–65.

7 Stevenson KJ, Craig S, Dufty JMK, Taberner DA. System ISI calibration: a universally applicable scheme is possible only when coumarin plasma calibrants are used. *Br J Haematol* 1997; **96**: 435–41.

8 Duncan EM, Casey CR, Duncan BM, Lloyd JV. Effect of concentration of trisodium citrate anticoagulant on calculation of the international normalized ratio and the international sensitivity index of thromboplastin. *Thromb Haemost* 1994; **72**: 84–8.

9 Moll S, Ortel TL. Monitoring warfarin therapy in patients with lupus anticoagulants. *Ann Int Med* 1997; **127**: 177–85.

10 Adcock DM, Fink L, Marlar RA. A laboratory approach to the evaluation of hereditary hypercoagulability. *Am J Clin Pathol* **108**: 434–49.

11 Lane DA, Mannucci PM, Bauer KA et al. Inherited thrombophilia: Part 1. *Thromb Haemost* 1996; **76**: 651–62.

12 Lane DA, Mannucci PM, Bauer KA et al. Inherited thrombophilia: Part 2. *Thromb Haemost* 1996; **76**: 824–34.

13 Bockenstedt PL. Laboratory methods in hemostasis. In: Loscalzo J, Schafer AI eds *Thrombosis and hemorrhage*. Baltimore: Williams and Wilkins, 1998: 517–80.

14 Beutler E, Lichtman MA, Coller BS, Kipps TJ (eds) *Williams Hematology*, New York: McGraw-Hill, 1995: L82–L105.

15 Reiter W, Ehrensberger H, Steinbrückner, Keller F. Parameters of haemostasis during acute venous thrombosis. *Thromb Haemost* 1995; **74**: 596–601.

16 Tosetto A, Missiaglia E, Gatto E, Rodeghiero F. The VITA Project: phenotypic resistance to activated protein C and FV Leiden mutation in the general population. *Thromb Haemost* 1997; **78**: 859–63.

17 Kjellberg U, Andersson NE, Rosen S, Tengborn L, Hellgren M. APC resistance and other haemostatic variables during pregnancy and puerperium. *Thromb Haemost* 1999; **81**: 527–31.

18 Bauer KA. Approach to thrombosis. In: Loscalzo J, Schafer AI eds *Thrombosis and hemorrhage*. Baltimore: Williams and Wilkins, 1998: 477–90.

19 Allaart CF, Poort SR, Rosendaal FR, Reitsma PH, Bertina RM, Briet E. Increased risk of venous thrombosis in carriers of hereditary protein C deficiency defect. *Lancet* 1993; **341**: 134–8.

20 Simmonds RE, Zoller B, Ireland H, et al. Genetic and phenotypic analysis of a large (122–member) protein S-deficient kindred provides an explanation for the familial coexistence of type I and type III plasma phenotypes. *Blood* 1997; **89**: 4364–70.

21 Brandt JT, Triplett DA, Alving B, Scharrer I. Criteria for the diagnosis of lupus anticoagulants: an update. On behalf of the Subcommittee on Lupus Anticoagulant/Antiphospholipid Antibody of the Scientific and Standardization Committee of the ISTH. *Thromb Haemost* 1995; **74**: 1185–90.

22 Forastiero RR, Martinuzzo ME, Cerrato GS, Kordich LC, Carreras LO. Relationship of anti beta2–glycoprotein I and antiprothrombin antibodies to thrombosis and pregnancy loss in patients with antiphospholipid antibodies. *Thromb Haemost* 1997; **78**: 1008–14.

23 Pengo V, Biasiolo A, Rampazzo P, Brocco T. dRVVT is more sensitive than KCT or TTI for detecting lupus anticoagulant activity of anti-beta2–glycoprotein I autoantibodies. *Thromb Haemost* 1999; **81**: 256–8.

24 Triplett DA. Antiphospholipid-protein antibodies: laboratory detection and clinical relevance. *Thromb Res* 1995; **78**: 1–31.

25 Reber G, Arvieux J, Comby E, et al. Multicenter evaluation of nine commercial kits for the quantitation of anticardiolipin antibodies. *Thromb Haemost* 1995; **73**: 444–52.

26 Hillarp A, Dahlbäck B, Zöller B. Activated protein C resistance: from phenotype to genotype and clinical practice. *Blood Rev* 1995; **9**: 201–12.

27 Koster T, Rosendaal FR, de Ronde H, Briët E, Vandenbroucke JP, Bertina RM. Venous thrombosis due to poor coagulant response to activated protein C: Leiden Thrombophilia Study. *Lancet* 1993; **342**: 1503–6.

28 Tripodi A, Negri B, Bertina RM, Mannucci PM. Screening for the FV:Q^{506} mutation – evaluation of thirteen plasma-based methods for their diagnostic efficacy in comparison with DNA analysis. *Thromb Haemost* 1997; **77**: 436–9.

29 Kapur RK, Mills LA, Spitzer SH, Hultin MB. A prothrombin gene mutation is significantly associated with venous thrombosis. *Arterioscler Thromb Vasc Biol* 1997; **17**: 2875–9.

30 Hirsh J, Warkentin TE, Raschke R, Granger C, Ohman EM, Dalen JE. Heparin and low molecular weight heparin: mechanism of action, pharmacokinetics, dosing considerations, monitoring efficacy, and safety. *Chest* 1998; **114**: 4895–5105.

3

Evaluation and treatment of patients with hereditary thrombophilia

AMNA IBRAHIM, BARBARA ALVING

INTRODUCTION

Inherited abnormalities of the coagulation system that can result in venous thrombosis were first recognized with the discovery of antithrombin III deficiency in 1965;[1] however, only in the last 5 years have the two most common inherited disorders, known as factor V Leiden and the prothrombin gene mutation, been described. Currently, an underlying hereditary risk factor for thrombosis can be found in as many as 30% of Caucasian patients who present with a first episode of venous thromboembolism.[2]

Inherited risk factors for venous thromboembolism can be broadly classified by the way in which they affect hemostasis. The first category to be discovered was that of functional deficiencies of inhibitors of coagulation factors, which include antithrombin III, protein S and protein C. Antithrombin III deficiency was the only

The views expressed by authors of this chapter are their own, and do not reflect those of the Food and Drug Administration, National Institutes of Health, or Department of Health and Human Services.

recognized inherited risk factor until the mid 1980s, when deficiencies of protein C and of protein S (which work together to inhibit factors Va and VIIIa) were reported in families with venous thrombosis.[3,4] A second inherited mechanism for thrombosis, described in 1994, is a mutation in factor V (factor V Leiden, Arg506Gln), which causes the factor Va to be resistant to inhibition by activated protein C.[5,6] A third inherited risk for thrombosis is the increased level of a clotting factor. In 1996, Poort et al.[7] described a mutation in the prothrombin gene (a guanine to adenine change in base 20 210) which results in increased levels of prothrombin. A fourth mechanism for thrombosis is increased levels of homocysteine. This may be due to an inherited abnormality in the enzymes regulating levels of homocysteine.[8]

This chapter describes the pathophysiology of these inherited disorders, as well as the clinical presentation, evaluation, and management of patients with inherited thrombophilia. The aspects of laboratory testing and the acquired conditions such as antiphospholipid syndrome are addressed in other chapters. Unless otherwise stated, the discussion focuses on the heterozygous patient.

PATHOPHYSIOLOGY

When the coagulation cascade is activated, the end product is the generation of thrombin, which converts fibrinogen to fibrin (see Chapter 1). Excessive clot formation occurs when thrombin generation is not properly inhibited or when thrombin is not rapidly inactivated. Thrombin is inhibited when it binds to thrombomodulin, a receptor on the endothelium (Fig. 3.1).[9] This prevents the clotting activity of

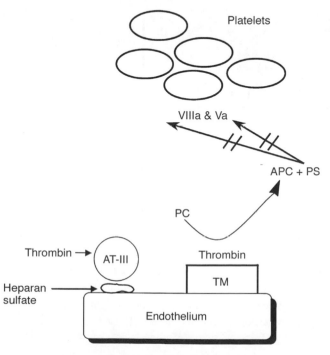

Figure 3.1 *Thrombin binds to thrombomodulin (TM) on the endothelium. Once bound, it can convert protein C (PC) to an activated form (APC) which, together with protein S (PS), can inactivate coagulation factors VIIIa and Va on a phospholipid surface such as the platelet. Antithrombin III (AT-III) also inhibits thrombin as well as factors XIIa, XIa, Xa, and IXa. The inhibitory activity of AT-III is greatly accelerated by its interaction with heparan sulfate, which coats the endothelium.*

thrombin and the thrombin can then convert protein C to an activated form, which then will act with protein S to prevent further generation of thrombin by inhibiting factors Va and VIIIa. This pathway is not effective if patients are deficient in protein C or protein S, both of which are vitamin K-dependent proteins made in the liver.[10] The pathway is also defective if a patient has factor V Leiden, also known as activated protein C resistance. Antithrombin III also has a direct and heparin-mediated inhibitory action on thrombin as well as on other coagulation factors in the cascade; thus, deficiency of antithrombin III is another important factor in hypercoagulability. As appears evident with the prothrombin gene mutation, increased levels of prothrombin can also increase the risk for thrombosis.

Homocysteine is generated from methionine. High levels are prevented in vivo by conversion of homocysteine to methionine through a pathway that utilizes the enzyme methylene tetrahydrofolate reductase along with cofactors folate and vitamin B12 (Fig. 3.2).[11] Homocysteine can also be converted to cystathionine by cystathionine β-synthase and vitamin B6. Thus, elevated levels of homocysteine can be due to several mechanisms. Acquired causes are mostly due to nutritional deficiency of cobalamin, folate, or pyridoxine, which are the essential cofactors for the metabolism of homocysteine.

Hereditary causes of hyperhomocysteinemia include cystathionine β-synthetase deficiency, which produces a more severe clinical picture but is relatively infrequent. The homozygotes occur at a frequency of less than one in 200 000 births. A more frequent but milder defect (C to T substitution at base 677) results in a heat-labile form of 5,10–methelenetetrahydrofolate reductase (MTHFR); this mutation renders the enzyme relatively inactive and probably increases the folate requirements for

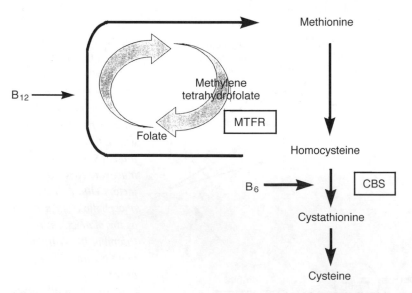

Figure 3.2 *Homocysteine is generated from methionine and is metabolized by one of two pathways. It can be converted to cystathionine by the action of cystathionine β synthase (CBS) and vitamin B$_6$, or it can be recycled to methionine by the action of methylene tetrahydrofolate reductase, which requires folate and vitamin B$_{12}$. (MTFR = methylene tetrahydrofolate reductase.)*

those who have the abnormality.[8,12] The homozygous form is present in as many as 5% of the general population.[8] The mechanisms by which elevated levels of homocysteine induce thrombosis are poorly understood, but probably involve endothelial injury.[11]

EVALUATION

How common are the inherited disorders in Caucasian patients who present with venous thrombosis?

Factor V Leiden is present in approximately 5% of the Caucasian population and is lower in African Americans (1%) as well as in Asian Americans and Native Americans.[13] The prothrombin gene mutation is present in 1–2% of Caucasians,[2,14] and probably in 1–2% of African Americans as well. In one study that included all patients (age range 17–88 years) referred to an anticoagulant clinic in the UK for treatment of a first or recurrent episode of venous thromboembolism between 1995 and 1997, factor V Leiden was present in 14% and the prothrombin gene mutation in 5%.[2] Together, deficiencies of antithrombin III, protein C, and protein S accounted for an additional 10% of the inherited abnormalities.

What are the clinical manifestations?

The most common clinical manifestations of hereditary thrombophilia, regardless of the etiology, are deep venous thrombosis, pulmonary embolism, superficial thrombophlebitis, or any combinations of these.[3,15–19] Other sites of thromboses can be pelvic veins, inferior vena cava, retinal veins, hepatic and portal veins, as well as axillary veins, and cerebral veins. Approximately 50% of thrombotic episodes occur during a high-risk period for thrombosis, such as surgery, pregnancy, trauma, or during the use of oral contraceptives. The median age of presentation can vary, depending on whether or not other risks for thrombosis are present. According to one report of patients with factor V Leiden, the mean age at the time of the first thrombotic episode was 41 years (range 17–79 years).[19]

How are homozygotes affected?

Homozygous protein C deficiency is manifested as neonatal purpura fulminans.[20] The newborns develop thrombosis of small vessels with subsequent subcutaneous ischemic necrosis. Infants have been treated successfully with purified protein C concentrates;[21] however, protein C concentrates have not yet been licenced in the USA. At least one infant with purpura fulminans who was homozygous for protein S deficiency has been described.[22] Homozygous antithrombin III deficiency is also rare, and severe thrombosis often affecting arteries can occur. Some of the antithrombin III subtypes appear to be incompatible with life.

Because of the high prevalence of factor V Leiden, homozygosity may be as frequent as 1:5000 in the general population. These homozygous individuals may be asymptomatic, even as adults;[23] however, they are at high risk for thrombosis when exposed to additional risk factors, such as the use of oral contraceptives.[24]

Laboratory testing for hypercoagulability: which tests to order and for which patients?

Evaluation for thrombophilia is most useful if it will result in productive screening of family members or influence duration or type of therapy. The presence or absence of a family history of thrombosis is not always helpful, because many patients do not have a detailed knowledge of their family medical histories. Currently, a very appropriate way to determine who should be screened may be based on the patient's age and type of thrombosis (Table 3.1).[25] The general recommendation is that patients who are younger (i.e., less than 45 years of age) at the time of the first venous thrombosis should undergo testing for all of the inherited hypercoagulable states listed in the table, including measurement of the fasting homocysteine level. (Testing for the heat-labile form of methylene tetrahydrofolate reductase is not clinically useful; rather, the homocysteine level is the important measurement.) Assessment should also be made of the lupus anticoagulant and the anticardiolipin antibody. When an initial evaluation is being performed in these younger patients with venous thrombosis, testing for all of the appropriate potential abnormalities is recommended, because patients with more than one risk factor have a greatly increased chance of developing recurrent thrombosis.[26] Furthermore, some of these risks can be altered by medications other than warfarin (i.e., folic acid).

For those who have their first venous thrombosis at age 45 years or older, testing could be done for factor V Leiden, the prothrombin gene mutation, the antiphospholipid syndrome, and homocysteine (see Table 3.1).[25] However, if these patients have a strong family history of thrombosis or describe having venous thromboembolism before the age of 45 years as well, then studies for antithrombin III, protein C, and protein S deficiency should probably be included. Once one or more abnormalities are found in the patient, additional family members can chose if they also

Table 3.1 *Summary of approach to laboratory testing in hypercoagulability*

Venous thromboembolism (age < 45 years)[a]	Arterial thrombosis
1 Factor V Leiden (DNA test)	1 Homocysteine level[b]
2 Prothrombin gene mutation (DNA test)	2 Lupus anticoagulant
3 Homocysteine level[b]	3 Anticardiolipin antibody
4 Lupus anticoagulant	4 Consider factor V Leiden and prothrombin gene mutation for young women (< 44 years) who smoke and have myocardial infarction
5 Anticardiolipin antibody	
6 Antithrombin III deficiency	
7 Protein C deficiency	
8 Protein S deficiency	

[a]For patients > than 45 years at the time of their first venous thrombosis and who have no family history of venous thrombosis, the first five tests listed would be most appropriate.
[b]Hyperhomocysteinemia can also be an acquired abnormality, as can deficiencies of antithrombin III, protein S, and protein C, all of which are synthesized by the liver.
Adapted from Alving (1998).[25]

wish to undergo evaluation.[27] Because it is possible that these abnormalities can be present in any patient with hypercoagulability, we recommend that testing is not based on ethnicity, but rather on age, as described above.[13]

All of the inherited disorders are transmitted in an autosomal dominant fashion. However, some are much more mildly expressed than are others. For example, patients with factor V Leiden frequently do not have a strong history of venous thrombosis and do not have a first venous thrombosis until they are middle aged. This may be due to the fact that this abnormality confers only a small risk for thrombosis, which is increased only in the presence of other risk factors. Ridker et al. have shown in an analysis of participants in the Physicians' Health Study that the incidence rate differences for venous thromboembolism between men with factor V Leiden and those without the mutation increased from 1.23 for those under 50 years to 6 for those aged 70 and older.[28] However, this was true only for venous thrombosis that was idiopathic, i.e., not due to underlying surgery, trauma, or cancer.

Testing for hypercoagulability is probably best initiated when the patient has completed a course of anticoagulation. If the physician wants to continue anticoagulation with warfarin indefinitely, and yet still test for protein C and protein S deficiency, the patient can be changed to outpatient heparin prophylaxis while the warfarin is eliminated, and then testing performed for these two vitamin K-dependent inhibitors. Acquired causes for thrombosis should also be considered, based on the patient's risk factors (see Chapter 4), and appropriate testing performed.[29]

Issues with hyperhomocysteinemia

Mild hyperhomocysteinemia (total plasma homocysteine levels $> 17 \mu M$) increases the risk for idiopathic venous thromboembolism (i.e., thrombosis in the absence of cancer or surgery) by 3.4-fold.[30] For individuals who have both factor V Leiden and hyperhomocysteinemia, the risk for idiopathic venous thrombosis may be increased by 20–fold.[30] The increased risk for venous thrombosis with mild hyperhomocysteinemia has also been confirmed in other studies.[31]

Mild elevations of homocysteine have also been implicated in arterial vascular disease.[11,32–4] In one study of patients with established coronary artery disease, fasting homocysteine levels were predictors of mortality.[32] The relationship between plasma homocysteine levels and cardiovascular death was linear between $5 \mu M$ and $20 \mu M$, with the slope increasing at $15 \mu M$. Thus, treatment of hyperhomocysteinemia with at least 1 mg folate daily may have a substantial impact on cardiovascular morbidity.[34]

Testing patients with arterial thrombosis

Arterial thromboses are rare in patients with deficiencies of antithrombin III, protein C, or protein S and testing for these abnormalities should not usually be included in the evaluation of patients who have only arterial thromboses. A more appropriate evaluation includes measurement of fasting homocysteine levels, testing for lupus anticoagulant and anticardiolipin antibody, and obtaining a lipid profile. Men in the Physicians' Health Study who were heterozygous for factor V Leiden were not at increased risk for stroke or myocardial infarction.[35] However, young women (below the age of 44 years) who have had a myocardial infarction and are smokers should be considered for testing for factor V Leiden and the prothrombin gene mutation, based on studies by Rosendaal et al., who found that, in this specific population, the prothrombin gene abnormality and factor V Leiden were risk factors for myocardial infarction.[36,37] This increased risk was confined to women who were current smokers at the time of the infarction and these results have not been confirmed in other studies.[38] For patients who are homozygous for factor V Leiden, an increased incidence of arterial thrombosis has not been found.[16] Rather, these patients have a higher risk for venous thromboembolism compared to those who are heterozygous, and the first episode occurs at a younger median age (31 years compared to 44 years for the heterozygotes).[16]

TREATMENT

Acute thrombosis

The treatment for acute thrombosis in patients with hereditary thrombophilia is the same as for patients in a similar situation without this condition. Heparin is initiated; ideally, this is by a weight-based protocol with the goal of achieving an activated partial thromboplastin time (aPTT) that has been calibrated such that a 'therapeutic aPTT' is one in which a corresponding plasma antifactor Xa activity is between 0.3 and 0.7 units/ml. Warfarin is initiated when the heparin levels are therapeutic; the International Normalized Ratio (INR) is maintained between 2 and 3 or at 2.5–3.5 if the patient has the antiphospholipid syndrome.

Although clinical trials with low molecular weight heparin (LMW) have generally excluded patients with inherited or acquired thrombophilia, nonetheless these patients are very likely to have received LMWH during an episode of acute venous thromboembolism before a hypercoagulable state was confirmed by laboratory testing. Additional studies are needed to determine if the efficacy of LMWH in this group of patients is different from that in patients considered not to have a hypercoagulable state.

Patients with factor V Leiden who have had one episode of venous thrombosis are at increased risk for recurrence. In men in the Physicians' Health Study who developed venous thromboembolism, the recurrence rate was increased by four-fold in those who were heterozygous for factor V Leiden compared to those who were not carriers of that mutation.[39] In an additional study in which patients with factor V Leiden and a first episode of venous thromboembolism were followed, the recurrence during an eight-year observation period was 40% in those with factor V Leiden, compared to 18% for those who had no evidence of the carrier state.[40]

For those patients who have undergone one episode of venous thromboembolism and have a documented inherited thrombophilia, indefinite anticoagulation should be considered; however, the risk of long-term anticoagulation needs to be weighed against the benefits of preventing further thrombosis.[41] Thus, the decision to continue warfarin indefinitely should be made on an individual basis. If patients with a documented hypercoagulable state have had a thrombosis at a time when they did not have additional risk factors, are at low risk for bleeding due to any other comorbid conditions, and can be monitored carefully for anticoagulation with warfarin, indefinite anticoagulation is justified. Young women with an inherited hypercoagulable state who have had thrombosis while taking oral contraceptives or in association with pregnancy may not need to take anticoagulation indefinitely. However, indefinite anticoagulation would be quite justified for patients who have had two episodes of thrombosis (regardless of any underlying documented hypercoagulability). For those individuals who do not choose to take warfarin indefinitely, anticoagulant strategies can be developed to provide protection during periods of increased thrombotic risk (pregnancy and postpartum period, surgery). Frequently, issues of lifestyle are the determining factors in a patient's willingness to undergo anticoagulation, as well as excessive concern for bleeding from warfarin (or clotting if not receiving warfarin).

Prophylactic treatments other than warfarin and heparin

We currently recommend folic acid (1 mg daily) for patients with thrombosis or cardiovascular disease who have total homocysteine levels of approximately 15 μM or higher. It is not known if such patients should have supplementation with vitamins B6 and B12 as well (no controlled trials have been performed). Food forti-fication with folic acid has just begun. A recent study reported a significant increase in mean folate concentrations (4.6 to 10.0 ng/ml) and a decrease in the prevalence of high homocysteine concentrations (> 13 μM/L) from 18.7% to 9.8% in subjects eating fortified foods and not taking vitamin supplements.[42] Areas of ongoing research include definition of the best tests for the measurement of homocysteine (i.e., should methionine loading be performed?) and whether or not additional vitamins such as B6 and B12 should be recommended.

Highly purified, virally inactivated antithrombin III concentrates are now commer-cially available from several different companies. They should be reserved for patients with antithrombin III deficiency who are to undergo surgery or labor and delivery.[43,44]

Measures to prevent and manage postphlebitic syndrome

Approximately 60% of patients who have a first episode of proximal deep venous thrombosis may develop post-thrombotic (also known as postphlebitic) syndrome during a two-year period.[45] Symptoms range from pain in the calf or thigh on stand-ing or walking to edema and ulceration. A recent prospective study in such patients has shown that wearing graduated compression hose reduces this complication by 50%. Graduated compression hose, however, do not decrease the risk for recurrent thromboses.[45] Thus, graduated compression hose as well as warfarin is an essential combination in the treatment of patients with proximal deep venous thrombosis.

Issues with respect to family planning and hormonal replacement therapy

Women with thrombophilia who wish to have birth control need to know that oral contraceptives significantly increase the risk of venous thromboembolism. For example, in women who are heterozygous for factor V Leiden, the risk is approximately 28–50/10 000 women-years of use, compared to 2–4/10 000 women-years for those who do not have recognized thrombophilia.[26] In one study, the median time of onset of thrombosis after initiation of oral contraceptives was 42 months, with a range of 3–228 months for women heterozygous for factor V Leiden.[46] For women with thrombophilia, options such as barrier methods or administration of medroxyprogesterone (DepoProvera) 150 mg intramuscularly every 3 months can be considered.

A major issue for the primary care physician is whether or not to screen women for thrombophilia before initiating oral contraceptives. Taking a careful family history for thrombosis would appear to be useful; however, it has only a 50% sensitivity, at best, for revealing factor V Leiden.[46] Thus, to detect the most common of the inherited clotting disorders (factor V Leiden), universal screening would have to be initiated and this does not appear to be cost effective, nor are the public health implications known of denying every woman who is a carrier of factor V Leiden access to oral contraceptives.[46] Screening should be recommended if a women has a personal history or strong family history of venous thrombosis.

The options for a woman who is taking warfarin and is also considering a pregnancy include initiation of heparin and discontinuation of warfarin once a pregnancy is planned. However, conception may take some time, and this method would expose the patient to prolonged heparin and the risk of heparin-induced osteoporosis. Warfarin could be continued (with vigilant monitoring for pregnancy) and replaced with heparin within 6 weeks of conception. The patient, if she elects to proceed in this fashion, should know that the risk of warfarin embryopathy is small, but still present, during this time.[47]

Women with thrombophilia, especially those with antithrombin III deficiency or who have combined abnormalities, have a risk for stillbirth that is increased by five-fold to 14-fold above those of women without these abnormalities.[48] Guidelines have been established for the prophylaxis of the pregnant woman based on thrombotic risk; it is not known if anticoagulation will reduce the risk for stillbirth.[49] Women with antithrombin III deficiency should receive replacement therapy with purified concentrates at the time of delivery.[44] Due to the high risk of thrombosis during the postpartum period, anticoagulation should be continued for at least 4–6 weeks after delivery.[50] Warfarin can be used in women who are nursing, because it is not expressed in breast milk.[51]

The estimated risk for venous thromboembolism in women receiving hormone replacement therapy (HRT) is 2–3/10 000 women-years.[52,53] Whether or not the risk is significantly increased beyond this for women with thrombophilia is not known. HRT is administered at estrogen doses that are much lower than those used in oral contraceptives. The beneficial effects of HRT may include reduction in the risk for fatal or nonfatal myocardial infarction,[54] increase in bone density,[55] and perhaps a reduction in the relative risk for Alzheimer's disease.[56] Because the potential benefits of HRT are significant, women with thrombophilia should be counseled on the limits of the knowledge concerning the risk for thrombosis, but should not categorically be denied access to HRT.[57]

CONCLUSION

The known inherited risk factors for venous thromboembolism now include factor V Leiden and the prothrombin gene mutation; DNA-based assays are commercially available for the detection of both abnormalities. Cost-effective testing for an inherited hypercoagulable state can be based on the age of the patient at the time of the initial thrombosis and on the type of thrombosis (arterial or venous). Individuals with underlying inherited thrombophilia may remain asymptomatic throughout their lives or become symptomatic only during periods of increased thrombotic risk. The rates of recurrent thrombosis have been established for some of the inherited thrombophilias (i.e., older males with factor V Leiden). These data provide valuable, albeit limited, information to guide the duration of anticoagulation in patients with hypercoagulability. The duration of anticoagulation is based on many factors and requires thoughtful discussions of the risk and benefits of long-term warfarin between the patient and the physician.

REFERENCES

1 Egberg O. Inherited anti-thrombin III deficiency causing thrombophilia. *Thromb Diath Haemorrh* 1965; **13**: 516–30.
2 Cumming AM, Keeney S, Salden A, et al. The prothrombin gene G20210A variant: prevalence in a U.K. anticoagulant clinic population. *Br J Haematol* 1997; **98**: 353–5.
3 Simmonds R, Ireland H, Lane D, et al. Clarification of the risk for venous thrombosis associated with hereditary protein S deficiency by investigation of a large kindred with a characterized gene defect. *Ann Intern Med* 1998; **128**: 8–14.
4 Allaart CF, Swibertus PR, Rosendaal FR, et al. Increased risk of venous thrombosis in carriers of hereditary protein C deficiency defect. *Lancet* 1993; **341**: 134–8.
5 Bertina RM, Koeleman RPC, Koster T, et al. Mutation in blood coagulation factor V associated with resistance to activated protein C. *Nature* 1994; **369**: 64–7.
6 Dahlback B, Hildebrand B. Inherited resistance to activated protein C is corrected by anticoagulant cofactor activity found to be a property of factor V. *Proc Natl Acad Sci USA* 1994; **91**: 1396–400.
7 Poort SR, Rosendaal FR, Reitsma PH, Bertina RM. A common genetic variation in the 3'-untranslated region of the prothrombin gene is associated with elevated plasma prothrombin levels and an increase in venous thrombosis. *Blood* 1996; **88**: 3698–703.
8 Arruda VR, von Zuben PM, Chiaparini LC, Annichino-Bizzacchi JM, Costa FF. The mutation Ala677Val in the methylene tetrahydrofolate reductase gene: a risk factor for arterial disease and venous thrombosis. *Thromb Haemost* 1997; **77**: 818–21.
9 Dittman WA, Majerus PW. Structure and function of thrombomodulin: a natural anticoagulant. *Blood* 1990; **75**: 329–36.
10 Aiach M, Borgel D, Gaussen P, Emmerich J, Alhenc-Gelas M, Gandrille S. Protein C and protein S deficiencies. *Semin Hematol* 1997; **34**: 205–17.
11 D'Angelo A, Selhub J. Homocysteine and thrombotic disease. *Blood* 1997; **90**: 1–11.
12 Froost P, Blom HJ, Milos R, et al. A candidate genetic risk factor for vascular disease: a common mutation in methylenetetrahydrofolate reductase. *Nat Genet* 1995; **10**: 111–13.
13 Ridker PM, Miletich JP, Hennekens CH, Buring JE. Ethnic distribution of factor V Leiden in 4047 men and women: implications for venous thromboembolism screening. *JAMA* 1997; **277**: 1305–7.

14 Brown K, Luddington R, Williamson D, et al. Risk of venous thromboembolism associated with a G to A transition at position 20210 in the 3'-untranslated region of the prothrombin gene. *Br J Haematol* 1997; **98**: 907–9.

15 van Boven HH, Lane DA. Antithrombin and its inherited deficiency states. *Semin Hematol* 1997; **34**: 188–204.

16 Price DT, Ridker PM. Factor V Leiden mutation and the risks for thromboembolic disease: a clinical perspective. *Ann Intern Med* 1997; **127**: 895–903.

17 Bolan CD, Krishnamurti C, Tang DB, Carrington LR, Alving BM. Association of protein S deficiency with thrombosis in a kindred with increased levels of plasminogen activator inhibitor-1. *Ann Intern Med* 1993; **119**: 779–85.

18 Demers C, Ginsberg J, Hirsh J, et al. Thrombosis in antithrombin-III-deficient persons: report of a large kindred and literature review. *Ann Intern Med* 1992; **116**: 754–61.

19 Middeldorp S, Henkens CMA, Koopman M, et al. The incidence of venous thromboembolism in family members of patients with factor V Leiden mutation and venous thrombosis. *Ann Intern Med* 1998; **128**: 15–20

20 Marlar RA, Montgomery RR, Broekmans AW, et al. Diagnosis and treatment of homozygous protein C deficiency: report of the Working Party on Homozygous Protein C Deficiency of the Subcommittee on Protein C and Protein S International Committee on Thrombosis and Haemostasis. *J Pediatr* 1989; **114**: 528–34.

21 Dreyfus M, Magny JF, Bridey F, et al. Treatment of homozygous protein C deficiency and nenonatal purpura fulminans with a purified protein C concentrate. *N Engl J Med* 1991; **325**: 1565–8.

22 Mahasandana C, Suvatte V, Marlar RA, Manco-Johnson M, Jacobson LJ, Hathaway WE. Neonatal purpura fulminans associated with homozygous protein S deficiency. *Lancet* 1990; **335**: 61–2.

23 Greengard J, Eichinger S, Griffin J, Bauer K. Brief report: variability of thrombosis among homozygous siblings with resistance to activated protein C due to an Arg→Gln mutation in the gene for factor V. *N Engl J Med* 1994; **331**: 1559–62.

24 Rintelen C, Mannhalter C, Ireland H, et al. Oral contraceptives enhance the risk of clinical manifestation of venous thrombosis at a young age in females homozygous for factor V Leiden. *Br J Haematol* 1996; **93**: 487–90.

25 Alving B. Update on management of patients with acquired or inherited hypercoagulability. *Comp Ther* 1998; **24**: 302–9.

26 Rosendaal FR. Risk factors for venous thrombosis: prevalence, risk, and interaction. *Semin Hematol* 1997; **34**: 171–87.

27 Price DT, Ridker PM. Factor V Leiden mutation and the risks for thromboembolic disease: a clinical perspective. *Ann Intern Med* 1997; **127**: 895–903.

28 Ridker PM, Glynn RJ, Miletich JP, Goldhaber SZ, Stampfer MJ, Hennekens CH. Age-specific incidence rates of venous thromboembolism among heterozygous carriers of factor V Leiden mutation. *Ann Intern Med* 1997; **126**: 528–31.

29 Sorensen HT, Mellemkjaer L, Steffensen FH, Olsen JH, Nielsen GL. The risk of a diagnosis of cancer after primary deep venous thrombosis or pulmonary embolism. *N Engl J Med* 1998; **338**: 1169–73.

30 Ridker PM, Hennekens CH, Selhub J, et al. Interrelation of hyperhomocyst(e)inemia, factor V Leiden, and risk of future venous thromboembolism. *Circulation* 1997; **95**: 1777–82.

31 Den Heijer M, Koster T, Blom HJ, et al. Hyperhomocysteinemia as a risk factor for deep-vein thrombosis. *N Engl J Med* 1996; **334**: 759–62.

32 Nygard O, Nordrehaug JE, Refsum H, Ueland PM, Farstad M, Vollset SE. Plasma homocysteine levels and mortality in patients with coronary artery disease. *N Engl J Med* 1997; **337**: 230–6.

33 Graham IM, Daly LE, Refsum HM, et al. Plasma homocysteine as a risk factor for vascular disease. The European Concerted Action Project. *JAMA* 1997; **277**: 1775–81.

34 Boushey CJ, Beresford SAA, Omenn GS, Motulsky AG. A quantitative assessment of plasma homocysteine as a risk factor for vascular disease. Probable benefits of increasing folic acid intake. *JAMA* 1995; **274**: 1049–57.

35 Ridker PM, Hennekens CH, Lindpaintner K, et al. Mutation in the gene coding for coagulation factor V and the risk of myocardial infarction, stroke, and venous thrombosis in apparently healthy men. *N Engl J Med* 1995; **332**: 912–17.

36 Rosendaal FR, Siscovick DS, Schwartz SM, et al. A common prothrombin variant (20210 G to A) increases the risk of myocardial infarction in young women. *Blood* 1997; **90**: 1747–50.

37 Rosendaal FR, Siscovick DS, Schwartz SM, et al. Factor V Leiden (resistance to activated protein C) increases the risk of myocardial infarction in young women. *Blood* 1997; **89**: 2817–21.

38 Amowitz LL, Komaroff AL, Miletich JP, Ridker PM. Factor V Leiden is not a risk factor for myocardial infarction among young women. *Blood* 1999; **93**: 1432 (Letter).

39 Ridker PM, Miletich JP, Stampfer M, Goldhaber SZ, Lindpainter K, Hennekens CH. Factor V Leiden and risks of recurrent idiopathic venous thromboembolism. *Circulation* 1995; **92**: 2800–2.

40 Simioni P, Prandoni P, Lensing AWA, et al. The risk of recurrent venous thromboembolism in patients with an Arg506Gln mutation in the gene for factor V (factor V Leiden). *N Engl J Med* 1997; **336**: 399–403.

41 Thomas DP, Roberts H. Hypercoagulability in venous and arterial thrombosis. *Ann Intern Med* 1997; **126**: 638–44.

42 Jacques PF, Selhub J, Bostom AG, Wilson PW, Rosenberg IH. The effect of folic acid fortification on plasma folate and total homocysteine concentrations. *N Engl J Med* 1999; **340**: 1449–54.

43 Jackson M, Olsen S, Gomez ER, Alving B. Use of antithrombin III concentrates to correct antithrombin III deficiency during vascular surgery. *J Vasc Surg* 1995; **22**: 804–7.

44 Menache D, O'Malley JP, Schorr JB, et al. Evaluation of the safety, recovery, half-life, and clinical efficacy of antithrombin III (human) in patients with hereditary antithrombin III deficiency. *Blood* 1990; **75**: 33–9.

45 Brandjes D, Buller H, Heijboer H, et al. Randomized trial of effect of compression stockings in patients with symptomatic proximal-vein thrombosis. *Lancet* 1997; **349**: 759–62.

46 Schambeck CM, Schwender S, Haubitz I, Geisen UE, Grossman RE, Keller F. Selective screening for the factor V Leiden mutation: is it advisable prior to the prescription of oral contraceptives? *Thromb Haemost* 1997; **78**: 1480–3.

47 Iturbe-Alessio I, Fonesece MC, Mutchinik O, Santos MA, Zajarias A, Salazar E. Risks of anticoagulant therapy in pregnant women with artificial heart valves. *N Engl J Med* 1986; **315**: 1390–3

48 Preston FE, Rosendaal FR, Walker ID, et al. Increased fetal loss in women with heritable thrombophilia. *Lancet* 1996; **348**: 913–16.

49 Ginsberg JS, Hirsh J. Use of antithrombotic agents during pregnancy. *Chest* 1998; **114**: 524S–530S.

50 Conrad J, Hoerllou MH, Dreden PV, Lecompte T, Samama M. Thrombosis and pregnancies in congenitial deficiencies in antithrombin III, protein C or protein S; study of 78 women. *Thromb Haemost* 1990; **63**: 319–20.

51 Orme ML, Lewis PJ, de Swiet M, et al. May mothers given warfarin breast-feed their infants? *Br Med J* 1977; **1**: 1564–5.

52 Douketis JD, Ginsberg JS, Holbrook A, et al. A reevaluation of the risk for venous thromboembolism with the use of oral contraceptives and hormone replacement therapy. *Arch Intern Med* 1997; **157**: 1522–30.

53 Daly E, Vessey MP, Hawkins MM, et al. Risk of venous thromboembolism in users of hormone replacement therapy. *Lancet* 1996; **348**: 977–80.

54 Grodstein F, Stampfer MJ, Colditz GA, et al. Postmenopausal hormone therapy and mortality. *N Engl J Med* 1997; **336**: 1769–75.

55 Rizzoli R, Bonjour J-P. Hormones and bones. *Lancet* 1997; **349**: S120–23.

56 Tang M-X, Jacobs D, Stern Y, et al. Effect of oestrogen during menopause on risk and age at onset of Alzheimer's disease. *Lancet* 1996; **348**: 429–32.

57 Waselenko JK, Nace MC, Alving BM. Women with thrombophilia: assessing the risks for thrombosis with oral contraceptives or hormone replacement therapy. *Semin Thromb Hemost* 1998; **24**(Suppl. 1): 33–9.

4

Acquired hypercoagulable states

ABRAHAM MATTHEWS, BARBARA A KONKLE

INTRODUCTION

A hypercoagulable state, or thrombophilia, refers to a state of increased risk of thrombosis. In general, these states can be divided into two categories. The primary hypercoagulable states include inherited defects involving specific proteins of the coagulation or fibrinolytic systems and are discussed in Chapter 3. The secondary hypercoagulable states encompass a wide spectrum of acquired conditions that predispose to thrombotic events (Table 4.1). In this group, several hemostatic abnormalities have been implicated in the generation of a prothrombotic state, and defects in more than one specific component of the coagulation system probably account for the increased risk of thrombosis. This chapter is limited to an overview of frequently encountered conditions associated with an acquired (secondary) hypercoagulable state. For the purposes of this chapter, an acquired hypercoagulable state is arbitrarily defined as a noninherited disorder, disease, or intervention that is associated with an increased frequency of thrombosis.

ANTIPHOSPHOLIPID ANTIBODIES AND ANTIPHOSPHOLIPID SYNDROME

Antiphospholipid antibodies comprise a heterogeneous family of autoantibodies, usually IgG or IgM but occasionally IgA. These antibodies were originally described

Table 4.1 *Acquired hypercoagulable states*

Antiphospholipid syndrome
    Lupus anticoagulants
    Anticardiolipin antibodies
Malignancy
Hematologic diseases
    Myeloproliferative disorders
    Paroxysmal nocturnal hemoglobinuria
    Thrombotic thrombocytopenic purpura
Hyperviscosity
    Hypergammaglobulinemia
    Sickle cell disease
    Hyperleukocytic leukemias
    Polycythemia vera
Endocrine diseases
    Diabetes mellitus
    Cushing's syndrome
Autoimmune/vasculitic disorders
    Systemic lupus erythematosus
    Behçet's disease
    Giant cell arteritis
    Buerger's disease
    Takayasu's disease
Pregnancy/puerperium
Venous stasis
    Immobilization
    Postoperative state
Hyperlipidemia
Hyperhomocysteinemia
Therapeutic interventions
    Oral contraceptives
    Estrogen replacement therapy
    Warfarin-induced skin necrosis
    Prothrombin complex concentrates
    Artificial surfaces
    Heparin-induced thrombocytopenia
Inflammatory bowel disease

in patients with systemic lupus erythematosus,[1] and have subsequently been identified in patients without systemic lupus erythematosus.[1,2] There are two separate populations of antiphospholipid antibodies detectable by distinct assay methods. Lupus anticoagulants prolong (inhibit) phospholipid-dependent in-vitro coagulation assays. Anticardiolipin and other related antibodies react in a solid phase immunoassay. Although the correlation between the two tests in an individual is significant, many patients who are positive for the lupus anticoagulant do not have elevated levels of anticardiolipin antibodies, and vice versa.[3]

The antiphospholipid syndrome refers to the constellation of antiphospholipid antibodies and clinical symptoms and is characterized primarily by recurrent venous and/or arterial thrombosis and fetal wastage.

Primary antiphospholipid syndrome

An association between elevated levels of antiphospholipid antibodies and clinical symptoms in individuals with no underlying disorders defines the primary antiphospholipid syndrome.[4] Women tend to be affected more than men.[5] Venous or arterial thromboembolic disease or recurrent fetal wastage may, in fact, be the first evidence of a primary antiphospholipid syndrome. Occasionally, low-titer antinuclear antibodies are detected, but patients do not demonstrate any definitive clinical or serological evidence of autoimmune diseases.

Secondary antiphospholipid syndrome

Clinical entities associated with the secondary antiphospholipid syndrome include systemic lupus erythematosus, other chronic systemic autoimmune diseases, recent bacterial or viral infections, human immunodeficiency virus (HIV) infection, and malignancies. This syndrome has also been described in patients receiving procainamide, phenothiazines, hydralazine, quinidine, haloperidol, and fluphenazine. Antiphospholipid antibodies can persist for several months following discontinuation of these drugs.

Mechanisms by which antiphospholipid antibodies produce thrombosis remain a subject of ongoing debate. Perhaps the most important recent information about the pathogenesis of thrombosis has come from the knowledge that antiphospholipid antibodies are not directed against anionic phospholipid, as previously thought, but rather against a variety of phospholipid-binding proteins.[2] These plasma proteins probably become antigenic by forming neoepitopes on complexing with the phospholipid. β-2 glycoprotein 1 (GP1) is one of the best-characterized antigenic targets, and although the physiologic function of β-2 GP1 is not clearly known, in-vitro data suggest that β-2 GP1 may possibly have an anticoagulant role.[5,6] Antibodies directed against β-2 GP1 could therefore potentially play a role in initiating thrombosis. However, no one mechanism has yet explained the multiple clinical manifestations of the antiphospholipid syndrome, and research in these areas continues.

Clinical manifestations

Major clinical features associated with the antiphospholipid syndrome include recurrent thrombosis, thrombocytopenia, fetal wastage, and, rarely, bleeding.[2]

THROMBOSIS

Thrombotic events may be arterial or venous, with the occurrence of thromboembolic complications being nearly equal in both sides of the circulation.[3] The risk for thrombosis appears to be higher in patients with IgG antibodies, systemic lupus erythematosus, and in individuals with high-titer anticardiolipin antibodies.[1,7,8] A significantly lesser risk is seen in patients with drug-induced antiphospholipid antibodies.[9,10] IgA anticardiolipin antibodies are rare and a recent study concluded that their presence alone is not associated with thrombosis or other antiphospho-lipid-related manifestations.[11]

The risk of thrombosis in patients with lupus anticoagulants has been evaluated primarily through retrospective analysis and has varied from 17% to 71%.[1,3,12] By averaging the published data, it appears that approximately 30% of all patients with lupus anticoagulants have experienced at least one thrombotic event. Among patients with systemic lupus erythematosus, 42% of the lupus anticoagulant-positive and 40% of the anticardiolipin antibody-positive individuals had a history of throm-bosis; in contrast, the prevalence of thrombosis in lupus anticoagulant-negative or anticardiolipin antibody-negative systemic lupus erythematosus patients was only 10–18%.

The frequency of thrombotic events in lupus anticoagulant-positive or anticardi-olipin antibody-positive patients with autoimmune disorders other than systemic lupus erythematosus has not been clearly established. In two series of patients with rheumatoid arthritis, the combined prevalence of thrombosis was 10% in anticardi-olipin antibody-positive patients and 6% in anticardiolipin antibody-negative patients.[13,14] The frequency of drug-induced antiphospholipid antibody-associated thrombosis is uncertain, but is probably low. A review of the published data suggests an incidence of thrombosis ranging from 0% to 24%.[9,15] Most of the studies report a very low frequency of thromboembolic events associated with the presence of drug-induced antiphospholipid antibodies. In the study reporting a 24% incidence of thrombosis, it is possible that comorbid conditions were pivotal in initiating thrombosis, rather than antiphospholipid antibodies.

The site of initial thrombosis tends to predict sites of recurrent thrombotic events, i.e., recurrent arterial thrombosis follows an initial arterial event and venous events precede venous thrombosis.[3] Common sites of venous thrombosis include the deep veins of the lower extremities, with or without pulmonary emboli. Thrombo-sis in unusual venous sites, such as mesenteric, hepatic, renal, cerebral, axillary veins, and inferior vena cava has been reported. Arterial thrombotic complications occur primarily in the central nervous system. Principal manifestations include transient ischemic attacks and strokes. Migraine, multi-infarct dementia, chorea, transverse myelopathy, and the Guillain–Barré syndrome have also been documented.

Myocardial infarction, thromboembolic pulmonary hypertension, bowel infarc-tion, and gangrene of the extremities and digits are less frequent, but do occur in patients with antiphospholipid antibodies. Rarely, a fulminant form of the antiphos-pholipid syndrome occurs in some individuals with high-titer antiphospholipid antibodies with catastrophic consequences. Microvascular and macrovascular thromboses occur in multiple organs, including the kidney, lung, central nervous system, heart, and skin, resulting in a very high mortality.

THROMBOCYTOPENIA

Mild to moderate thrombocytopenia has been correlated with the presence of antiphospholipid antibodies, at least in patients with systemic lupus erythematosus.[4] In these patients there is also a strong correlation with the presence of antiplatelet antibodies. The thrombocytopenia may in part be a reflection of the in-vitro activ-ity of these antibodies against platelet phospholipid. The presence of antiphospholipid antibodies in thrombocytopenic individuals without systemic lupus erythematosus has been investigated.[16] Of 149 adults with idiopathic thrombocytopenic purpura, 46% had either positive lupus anticoagulant activity or anticardiolipin antibodies at the time of diagnosis. Elevated platelet-associated IgG was found in 83% of the 127 patients tested, and all cases with elevated anticardiolipin antibodies also had increased levels of platelet-associated IgG. However, no relationship was found between either of these measurements and any clinical parameters, including thrombosis.

FETAL LOSS

Recurrent fetal wastage is a major complication of the antiphospholipid syndrome. Fetal loss can occur at anytime during gestation and occurs in up to 80% of pregnancies in untreated women with antiphospholipid antibodies and a history of recurrent miscarriage.[17] Any woman with a history of two or more first trimester miscarriages or a second or third trimester intrauterine death or intrauterine growth retardation should be screened for lupus anticoagulants and anticardiolipin antibodies. Thrombosis of the placental vasculature and placental infarction are probable mechanisms for fetal loss.[17]

BLEEDING

The majority of patients with isolated antiphospholipid antibodies do not have an abnormal bleeding tendency. Antibodies to prothrombin are present in 50–75% of patients with lupus anticoagulants, and mild hypoprothrombinemia, usually insufficient to prolong the prothrombin time significantly, is present in approximately 25% of these patients.[2,3] A small percentage of patients have severely depressed prothrombin levels and can manifest severe bleeding. Thus, in this patient population, the remote possibility of significant bleeding should be kept in mind. Interestingly, patients with lupus anticoagulants who have concomitant moderate or severe depression of prothrombin levels have a lower than expected risk of thrombosis.[12]

Laboratory evaluation

LUPUS ANTICOAGULANTS

Individuals suspected of having a lupus anticoagulant should be evaluated in a systemic fashion. By international agreement,[18] the minimum laboratory criteria to make a diagnosis of a lupus anticoagulant include: (1) prolongation of at least one phospholipid-dependent coagulation assay; (2) demonstrating that this prolongation is due to an inhibitor and not a factor deficiency; and (3) demonstrating that the inhibitor is directed against phospholipid (and not a coagulation factor).

Tests commonly used for detecting lupus anticoagulants include the activated partial thromboplastin time (aPTT), the tissue thromboplastin inhibition test (TTI), the kaolin clotting time (KCT), the dilute Russell viper venom time (dRVVT), and the dilute aPTT. Except for the standard aPTT, the other tests depend on the use of reduced concentrations of phospholipid reagents for enhanced sensitivity. The prothrombin time (PT) is an insensitive test for lupus anticoagulants; however, it can be prolonged because of concomitant hypoprothrombinemia. Prolongation of any of these tests can be caused by deficiencies of specific clotting factors, by specific inhibitors to clotting factors, or by general inhibitors such as heparin, as well as by lupus anticoagulants. Deficiencies are ruled out by correction of the prolonged tests upon addition of an equal volume of normal plasma, i.e., mixing study. If the prolonged test does not correct to normal, a specific coagulation inhibitor or the presence of heparin must be ruled out before a lupus anticoagulant can be diagnosed. Heparin can be excluded by the history, as well as by the performance of the thrombin time, a test that is prolonged by heparin but is normal in the presence of a lupus anticoagulant.

The dRVVT may be the most specific of the tests for lupus anticoagulants. Additionally, there are some data suggesting that dRVVT positivity may be a better predictor of thrombotic risk than KCT positivity,[19] but this remains to be established. It is important to recognize that, even when using the most sensitive phospholipid reagent, the aPTT is the least sensitive of all the tests, and some patients with low-titer lupus anticoagulants may not exhibit a prolonged aPTT. In this setting, the dRVVT, the dilute aPPT, and the KCT may be positive in those patients with a normal standard aPTT.[19] Several other studies have compared the KCT with other lupus anticoagulant tests and have found it to be somewhat more sensitive.[19,20] On the other hand, the KCT and dilute aPPT are more or less sensitive to abnormalities of the entire intrinsic pathway and are therefore prolonged in the presence of the most common coagulation factor inhibitors. It is also important to recognize that, with the exception of the KCT, the other tests require addition of phospholipid and the results of those tests may therefore vary with the source of phospholipid. Neutralizing the lupus anticoagulant by exogenous phospholipid confirms the specificity of the inhibitor towards phospholipid. This may be achieved by the platelet neutralization procedure. In this procedure, the aPTT is repeated after addition of platelet membranes; prolongations due to the presence of a lupus anticoagulant are generally normalized by the phospholipids of the platelet membranes. Alternatively, lupus anticoagulants may be neutralized by hexagonal phase phospholipids and neutralization of a prolonged aPTT by the addition of hexagonal phosphatidylethanolamine phase may be used as a confirmatory test.[21] As no single test identifies all patients with lupus anticoagulants and several tests identify approximately 90% of this population,[19] recommendations for testing are listed in Table 4.2.

ANTICARDIOLIPIN ANTIBODIES

It is also important to test for the presence of anticardiolipin antibodies in patients suspected of having the antiphospholipid syndrome, because lupus anticoagulants may be absent. Anticardiolipin antibodies are detected on enzyme-linked immunosorbent assay (ELISA) plates coated with cardiolipin and blocked with serum, usually bovine or human. Interestingly, in the majority of patients with the antiphospholipid syndrome, no reactivity is detected in this assay if no serum is present either in the blocking agent or contributed by the patient's sample itself. β-2 glycoprotein 1 is one of the proteins present in the blocking serum or test plasma and is apparently responsible for the large majority of positive anticardiolipin antibody assays.[2] Patients with certain infections, for example syphilis, HIV, malaria,

Table 4.2 *Recommendations for lupus anticoagulant testing*

1 Sensitive screening tests for lupus anticoagulants should be used. The aPTT is the one most routinely used by hospital clinical laboratories, but is probably not the best choice. The dRVVT and KCT are better choices. At least two of these tests should be applied to obtain the maximal yield of lupus anticoagulant positivity.

2 If the lupus anticoagulant screening test is prolonged, a mixing study must be done. If the mixing study is prolonged, a thrombin time should be done to rule out the presence of heparin or other interference with the thrombin–fibrinogen reaction. A prolonged thrombin time casts doubt on the results of lupus anticoagulant screening tests and should be investigated further. In many laboratories, a reptilase time would then be done, because it is normal in the presence of heparin. Abnormalities of both the aPTT and the thrombin time can occur in diffuse intravascular coagulation, because of the presence of fibrin split products or, much less commonly, because of the presence of an abnormal fibrinogen or a circulating antithrombin.

3 If the thrombin time is normal, the diagnosis lies between a specific coagulation inhibitor, such as to factor VIII, or a lupus anticoagulant. Because of the specificity of the dRVVT, most of the more common coagulation factor inhibitors can probably be excluded. A factor V inhibitor would not be eliminated, but these rare inhibitors generally reveal their presence by significant bleeding.

4 As a confirmatory test, the platelet neutralization procedure or the hexagonal phase phosphatidylethanolamine test should be used.

aPTT = activated partial thromboplastin time; dRVVT = dilute Russell viper venom time; KCT = kaolin clotting time.

and Q-fever, often have anticardiolipin antibodies directed against cardiolipin itself, independent of the presence of β-2 GP1. These antibodies are apparently not associated with a thrombotic risk.

It should be noted that levels of antiphospholipid antibodies can fluctuate significantly.[22] During an acute thrombotic episode, antibody titers can actually decline, albeit transiently, to normal levels.[23] Therefore, negative tests for lupus anticoagulants and/or anticardiolipin antibodies do not totally exclude the presence of these antibodies. Repeating the laboratory assays 2–4 months apart is important in confirming a definite abnormality. As mentioned earlier, IgA anticardiolipin antibodies are rare and routine screening for this isotype is no longer recommended.

Currently, a great deal of effort is being directed to an analysis of the relative merits of the measurement of antibodies to β-2 GP1 and prothrombin as indices of thrombotic risk. As described above, anti-β-2 GP1 antibody testing may help exclude patients with infection-related anticardiolipins. Preliminary studies suggest that anti-β-2 GP1 antibodies may be more closely associated with thrombosis then anticardiolipin or antiprothrombin antibodies.[24] However, large prospective studies are still needed to settle this important issue.

Management

The antiphospholipid syndrome has the potential to produce serious morbidity and mortality, and treatment has proven to be difficult. However, a few generalizations can be made.

(a) Treatment is not indicated when the antiphospholipid antibody is detected as an isolated finding, unless there is associated thrombosis or fetal wastage. This generalization also applies to individuals with no evidence of thromboembolic events but with detectable antiphospholipid antibodies for prolonged periods.
(b) Patients who suffer a thromboembolic event and are persistently positive for lupus anticoagulants and/or anticardiolipin antibodies have a recurrence rate close to 50%. These patients will require long-term anticoagulant prophylaxis.
(c) The initial site of thrombosis tends to predict future sites of recurrences – an initial venous event predisposes to recurrent venous thrombosis, and there are arterial recurrences after an initial arterial event.
(d) There are no reliable methods to predict which patients are at risk for thromboembolic complications.

In individuals with the secondary antiphospholipid syndrome, eliminating or treating the underlying disorder frequently results in the reduction or disappearance of the antiphospholipid antibodies. For example, autoimmune diseases such as systemic lupus erythematosus are associated with antiphospholipid antibodies, and thromboembolic events cause significant morbidity and mortality in these patients. Treating the underlying autoimmune disease with steroids and other immunosuppressive therapy often eliminates or reduces the activity of these inhibitory antibodies.[3,22] However, immunosuppression does not necessarily prevent recurrent thrombosis, and long-term anticoagulation is often required, despite normalization of clotting assays or antiphospholipid antibody activity.

Anticoagulation of patients with antiphospholipid syndrome who develop acute venous thrombosis should be similar to that of individuals who do not have antiphospholipid antibodies, as described elsewhere in this text. Oral anticoagulation should be initiated only after effective heparinization has been achieved. If unfractionated heparin (UFH) is used, it may be difficult to monitor the dosage of heparin, as many patients will have a prolonged aPTT prior to treatment, due to the presence of the lupus anticoagulant. Anticoagulation can be monitored in these patients by specific heparin assays (anti-factor Xa, or protamine neutralization) or, alternatively, the thrombin time can be followed. This test is sensitive to heparin but is not prolonged by lupus anticoagulants. Treatment with LMWH obviates the need for monitoring therapy in most incidences. LMWHs appear effective in treating patients with lupus anticoagulants, although studies using these agents in this setting are needed.

Patients with recurrent venous thrombosis associated with antiphospholipid antibodies should receive long-term anticoagulation with warfarin. One study found that low to normal intensity oral anticoagulation (International Normalized Ratio, INR, 1.5–3.0) in patients with antiphospholipid antibody-associated thrombosis may not adequately protect against recurrent thrombosis.[25] Additionally, in this patient population, cessation of warfarin therapy imposes a high risk for recurrent thromboembolic events and hence life-long anticoagulation may be indicated. However, the benefits of long-term anticoagulation should be balanced against the risk of bleeding. Monitoring the INR may be problematic, because some patients have slightly prolonged baseline PTs and, even in an individual with a relatively normal PT, the INR may not reflect the true level of anticoagulation.[26] In such circumstances, the INR can be compared with actual factor assays, particularly factor II, to see if adequate anticoagulation is present. Because factor assays are performed with diluted plasma, they are less affected by lupus anticoagulants than the PT/INR. However, an assay such as chromogenic factor X assay, which is not phospholipid dependent, may be better in this circumstance.

The optimal long-term treatment of patients with antiphospholipid antibody-associated arterial thrombosis is unclear.[14] There is evidence that supports anticoagulating these patients with intermediate to high dose warfarin (INR = 3.0–3.5). The high probability of recurrent arterial thrombosis in these patients justifies long-term anticoagulation.

The utility of aspirin for treating antiphospholipid antibody-positive patients with recurrent thrombosis has not been definitively studied. Nonetheless, it would seem reasonable to use aspirin, or other antiplatelet therapy, in patients who develop recurrent thrombosis while on oral anticoagulation, especially in cases of arterial events, including central nervous system events. However, the combination of aspirin with oral anticoagulants should be employed cautiously, because some antiphospholipid antibody-positive patients with systemic lupus erythematosus, for example, are thrombocytopenic. Alternative options for the treatment of these patients include long-term therapy with heparin. Antiphospholipid antibody-positive patients who develop recurrent thrombosis despite therapeutic anticoagulation represent a difficult and often frustrating challenge.

Pregnant patients with antiphospholipid antibodies should be monitored closely and do not require treatment unless there is a prior history of antiphospholipid-associated thrombosis and/or fetal wastage, or there is evidence of fetal growth retardation. The precise regimen for managing a pregnant patient with antiphospholipid antibodies who has experienced prior thromboembolic events and/or fetal wastage has not been clearly established. At present, treatment options include heparin, aspirin, and perhaps occasionally intravenous gammaglobulin. In the past, pregnant women have been treated with corticosteroids and low-dose aspirin, but maternal complications were frequent,[27] and other regimens are now recommended to manage pregnant patients with antiphospholipid antibodies who have experienced prior thromboembolic events or fetal wastage. These include subcutaneous UFH or LMWH alone or in combination with low-dose aspirin.[28]

Treatment options for the occasional patient who develops the fulminant antiphospholipid syndrome include intravenous heparin, plasmapheresis, intravenous immunoglobulins, high-dose steroids, and/or cyclophosphamide.[3] Despite aggressive measures, the fulminant form of the antiphospholipid syndrome has a very high mortality rate. Patients who develop severe prothrombin deficiency or severe thrombocytopenia (less than 20 000/μL) in association with antiphospholipid antibodies may require high-dose prednisone in addition to other supportive measures.

MALIGNANCY

There is a strong association between cancer and the risk of thromboembolism as described over a century ago by Armand Trousseau. The reported occurrence of thrombosis in patients with malignancies ranges between 5% and 15%, and thrombosis is the second most common cause of death in patients with solid tumors.[29,30] Individuals with carcinoma of the pancreas, lung, stomach, colon, gallbladder, ovaries, primary brain tumors, and acute promyelocytic leukemia have the highest incidence of thromboembolic complications. The pathogenesis of thrombosis in malignancy is complex and multifactorial. Factors that further increase the susceptibility of cancer patients to thromboembolism include surgical intervention, the postoperative state, prolonged immobilization from any cause, anticancer medications (chemotherapeutic agents and hormonal therapy), insertion of indwelling central venous catheters, and infections.[31–3]

Greater emphasis should be placed on the primary prevention of thromboembolic events in patients with malignancies. Low-dose heparin, LMWH at prophylactic doses, or physical measures should be employed in patients with cancer who are confined to bed from any cause or when undergoing low-risk surgical procedures. Individuals with cancer undergoing major abdominal or pelvic surgery have a high risk of developing significant postoperative venous thrombosis. These patients should receive prophylaxis equivalent to that used for patients undergoing major orthopedic surgery. Adjusted-dose heparin or LMWH (average doses being twice as high as doses recommended for general prophylaxis) and physical measures are effective in decreasing the frequency of venous thromboembolic complications in the postoperative period.

Patients with underlying malignancies have a high incidence of upper limb venous thromboembolism associated with indwelling central venous catheters.[33] Warfarin administered at a dose of 1 mg daily has been shown to decrease the prevalence of catheter-related thrombosis.[34] If cost is not an issue or if a catheter-related clot develops while on low-dose warfarin, LMWH (e.g., dalteparin 2500 units administered subcutaneously daily) has been shown to be an effective alternative.[35] It should be noted that the PT is usually not prolonged with low-dose warfarin (see Chapter 17 for more information).

Acute deep venous thrombosis in a cancer patient is a common clinical problem. In the absence of contraindications, acute thromboembolic events should be treated with a standard course of intravenous full-dose unfractionated heparin or therapeutic doses of subcutaneous LMWH. Heparin should be overlapped with and followed by warfarin. Warfarin at a dose that maintains the INR between 2 and 3 should be considered for as long as the cancer is active. Cessation of anticoagulant therapy in these patients is associated with a high risk of recurrent thromboembolism.[36] Unfortunately, despite therapeutic doses of warfarin, many cancer patients develop recurrent thrombosis and represent a difficult therapeutic challenge. For such patients, the acute event can be treated with UFH or LMWH, followed by a higher dose of warfarin (INR 3.0–4.0). However, increasing the intensity of the INR response increases the risk of bleeding complications. If the risk of bleeding is unacceptable with high-dose warfarin or if warfarin has proved to be ineffective, other options to prevent recurrent thrombosis include subcutaneous heparin in adjusted doses or LMWH. In those individuals for whom anticoagulation is contraindicated, inferior vena cava filters may be considered. However, this does not prevent thrombus formation, and clots can develop anywhere within the vascular system.

Anticoagulating patients with either primary or metastatic brain tumors remains a controversial and difficult issue. The literature suggests that many of these patients can be safely managed with anticoagulant therapy, but no conclusive statement can be made.[36] It is emphasized that treatment of this patient population should be individualized. Patients with brain metastases from a renal or melanoma primary and those with hemorrhagic brain tumors should not be anticoagulated.

Recently, there has been some evidence that LMWH may have antineoplastic properties. In two, small, randomized studies comparing the efficacy of LMWH with that of unfractionated heparin in the treatment of deep venous thrombosis, cancer-related mortality rates were lower in patients randomized to LMWH.[37] An ongoing multicenter study is investigating this hypothesis.

HEMATOLOGIC DISORDERS

Hematologic diseases associated with an underlying hypercoagulable state include the myeloproliferative disorders and paroxysmal nocturnal hemoglobinuria. The myeloproliferative disorders are a group of related diseases and include polycythemia vera, essential thrombocythemia, myelofibrosis, and myeloid metaplasia. These diseases are neoplasms of the pluripotent hematopoietic stem cell. Paroxysmal nocturnal hemoglobinuria is an acquired clonal disorder of the hematopoietic stem cell. The disease is characterized by the formation of defective erythrocytes, granulocytes, and platelets that have an impaired ability to anchor protective glycosylphosphotidylinositol-linked proteins (e.g., decay-accelerating factor) to cell membranes.

Patients with these disorders suffer significant morbidity and mortality from arterial and/or venous thrombosis.[38–41] Typically, thrombotic events occur in characteristic sites such as the splenic, hepatic, portal, mesenteric, and renal vessels, and the Budd–Chiari syndrome is most frequently associated with paroxysmal nocturnal hemoglobinuria and the myeloproliferative disorders. Microvascular thrombosis of the digits, typically resulting in painful burning and discoloration of the hands and feet, is a hallmark feature of the myeloproliferative disorders. In addition to thrombotic complications in the unusual sites mentioned above, these diseases also produce cerebral microcirculation infarcts, deep vein thrombosis, pulmonary embolism, and occlusions of the coronary arteries.

The mechanisms of thrombosis in these patients are unclear, and several factors may be involved. For example, in polycythemia vera, an elevated hematocrit and increased blood viscosity may contribute to the increased risk of thrombosis. In the myeloproliferative diseases, thrombocytosis per se may not be an independent risk factor for enhanced thrombogenicity. In polycythemia vera and essential thrombocythemia, platelet counts may be very elevated. Although these conditions are associated with an increased risk of thrombosis, clear correlation between elevated platelet counts and an increased frequency of thrombosis is not evident in the literature.

Management of thrombotic events

Patients with myeloproliferative disorders and paroxysmal nocturnal hemoglobinuria who develop acute thromboembolic complications should be treated in the standard fashion with heparin, usually followed by oral anticoagulation with warfarin. These patients often require warfarin on an indefinite basis as well as therapy to control their myeloproliferative disorder. Patients with polycythemia vera and essential thrombocythemia are at increased risk not only for thrombosis, but also for hemorrhagic events. Anticoagulation should therefore be monitored closely to minimize the risk of bleeding.

Patients with myeloproliferative diseases undergoing surgical procedures are at high risk for developing postoperative thrombosis. During the postoperative period, physical measures, early ambulation, and the judicious use of heparin are important in decreasing the frequency of thrombotic events. Patients with polycythemia vera requiring emergency surgery should be rapidly phlebotomized to a normal hematocrit, and those with essential thrombocythemia often require preoperative lowering of platelet counts to normal ranges.

VASCULITIS

Thromboembolic complications occur frequently in patients with vasculitis.[42] Vasculitis occurs with several diseases and is characterized by inflammation and necrosis of blood vessels. The pathogenic mechanisms involved in thrombus formation may include damage to endothelial surfaces (e.g., immune complex mediated), decreased fibrinolysis, presence of antiphospholipid antibodies, vascular endothelial dysfunction, and diminished plasminogen activator levels. Systemic lupus erythematosus, Behçet disease, Kawasaki disease, giant cell arteritis, Buerger disease (thromboangiitis obliterans), and Takayasu's disease are some examples of diseases with an increased frequency of vasculitis-induced thrombotic events.

NEPHROTIC SYNDROME

The nephrotic syndrome is associated with a systemic hypercoagulable state.[42,43] The precise nature of the thrombotic tendency is not well understood. Postulated mechanisms for enhanced thrombogenicity include a decreased level of natural anticoagulant proteins (antithrombin III, protein S), hyperaggregability of platelets, altered fibrinolysis, and high levels of plasma procoagulants (fibrinogen, factors V, VII, VIII, and X). Renal vein thrombosis is a common complication, although thrombotic manifestations may occur elsewhere. Additionally, patients may have relative heparin resistance due to low antithrombin III levels. In some circumstances, restoration of antithrombin III with antithrombin III concentrate may be needed.[44] Patients may also exhibit relative warfarin resistance, which is due to warfarin being highly albumin bound and excreted with albumin in the urine.[45]

HYPERHOMOCYSTEINEMIA

Hyperhomocysteinemia is characterized by elevated levels of plasma homocysteine and may be caused by genetically based defects in the metabolism of methionine/homocysteine or acquired nutritional deficiencies. It is important to rule out hyperhomocysteinemia as a risk factor for thrombosis because of its easy treatment with vitamin supplementation. Hyperhomocysteinemia and its treatment are discussed further in Chapter 3.

THERAPEUTIC INTERVENTIONS

Oral contraceptives

Oral contraceptives consisting of combinations of estrogen and progesterone were introduced in the 1960s and have since become one of the preferred methods of contraception. Epidemiological studies from the 1960s and 1970s have established a relationship between the use of these drugs and an increased risk of thrombosis, related, in part, to the dose of estrogen used.[46,47] With the introduction of second-generation, low-dose oral contraceptives there has been a significantly decreased risk of thrombotic complications, but the risk is not totally eliminated.[48–50] The third-generation oral contraceptives (containing newer progestins) may be associated with a higher thrombotic risk compared to the second-generation preparations, but further studies are needed to address this issue and are currently underway.[51,52]

Multiple studies have demonstrated a variety of thrombotic events associated with oral contraceptive use. Deep venous thrombophlebitis and pulmonary embolism, cerebrovascular accidents, particularly in patients with a history of migraine, postoperative thrombosis, peripheral artery occlusion, mesenteric vascular insufficiency, aorto-iliac thrombosis, renal artery thrombosis, and Budd–Chiari syndrome have been described. It should be pointed out that most of these studies were done when higher-dose estrogen-containing contraceptives were being used and few studies controlled for other possible confounding factors such as smoking.

The relationship between oral contraceptive use and the risk for myocardial infarction or stroke deserves special mention. The early epidemiological studies showed that the use of oral contraceptives was associated with a twofold to fourfold increase in the risk of myocardial infarction.[52] However, several more recent studies indicate that the risk is less than twofold and is probably related to changes in formulations, more cautious use of oral contraceptives, and lifestyle modifications.[52,53] The current use of contemporary low-dose oral contraceptives by young women (< 40 years of age) in the absence of clinical risk factors and cigarette smoking does not appear to increase the risk of myocardial infarctions. In general, cardiovascular complications occur mainly in smokers and in individuals with predisposing clinical risk factors. Therefore, smokers who choose to use oral contraceptives must be advised to stop smoking.

Several earlier studies have documented a relationship between the use of high-dose oral contraceptives and an increased risk of cerebrovascular events.[50,54,55] Recent data indicate that low-dose oral contraceptives produce little increase in risk for ischemic strokes and it is reasonable to suggest that a large increase in risk can be safely excluded.[46,48,55]

The presence of factor V Leiden mutation (a point mutation in factor V leading to activated protein C resistance) coupled with the use of oral contraceptives substantially increase the risk for thromboembolism.[56,57] Women with a personal and/or family history of multiple thromboembolic events may be considered for screening studies to rule out the factor V Leiden mutation. We recommend avoiding oral contraceptives in individuals with the factor V Leiden mutation if alternative contraception is acceptable to the patient and her partner, as the presence of both factors significantly increases the risk for thrombosis. One must remember, however, that the risk of thrombosis with pregnancy is greater.

Hormone replacement therapy

Postmenopausal hormone replacement therapy (HRT) is associated with amelioration of menopausal subjective symptoms, lowered risks of osteoporosis and cardiovascular disease, and decreased mortality rates.[58,59] The estrogen dose in HRT is significantly less than in oral contraceptives, and the risk of thrombosis attributable to therapy is less.[60] However, HRT is administered in an older population with an overall increased incidence in thrombosis compared to the population taking oral contraceptives. The estimated risk of venous thromboembolism associated with HRT is 2–3/10 000.[61]

A history of thrombosis and/or a family history of thromboembolic complications are not absolute contraindications to HRT. However, we caution that in such situations an assessment of individual risks and potential benefits be made prior to initiating HRT. Further studies in this area are needed.

INFLAMMATORY BOWEL DISEASE

Patients with inflammatory bowel disease have an increased frequency of thrombotic complications, and thromboembolism is an important cause of death in this patient population.[62] The majority of thrombi tend to develop in the venous circulation, although, rarely, arterial thrombi may occur.[62-4] Thrombosis has also been reported to occur in unusual sites, including the hepatic vein, portal vein, cerebral venous circulation, and retinal vessels. The mechanisms of enhanced thrombogenicity are not clearly understood. The development of thrombosis may be related to active inflammatory disease; however, thromboembolic complications also occur in a substantial group of patients who show no evidence of active inflammatory disease.[64,65]

Conditions that increase the risk of thrombosis in patients with inflammatory bowel disease include septicemia, prolonged bed rest, and surgical procedures.[64] There does not appear to be an association between inherited risk factors, including factor V Leiden, and thrombosis in inflammatory bowel disease.[64] Patients with inflammatory bowel disease have been reported to have a higher prevalence of anticardiolipin antibodies than normal controls; however, this was not associated with an increased risk of thrombosis.[66] In hospitalized patients with inflammatory bowel disease it may be appropriate to consider subcutaneous UFH or LMWH for prophylaxis in addition to standard physical measures. Patients with this disease who develop acute venous thrombosis can be successfully managed with intravenous heparin administered in the usual fashion or with subcutaneous LMWH. Oral anticoagulation with warfarin may prevent recurrent complications. However, patients with inflammatory bowel disease may have underlying vitamin K deficiency, recurrent gastrointestinal tract bleeding, etc. Hence, because of the potential for increased hemorrhagic complications, long-term anticoagulation should only be considered after a detailed risk/benefit assessment is made. Therapy needs to be individualized, and patients receiving anticoagulants should be monitored very closely. Patients may develop recurrent thromboembolic events despite adequate medical therapy. Occasionally, surgical resection of diseased bowel may ameliorate the propensity toward thrombosis, and it may be reasonable to consider surgery with patients with acute or intractable inflammatory bowel disease who have severe or recurrent thromboembolic complications.

CONCLUSION

As outlined in this chapter, the secondary hypercoagulable states consist of a diverse group of clinical conditions that have ill-defined complex coagulopathies resulting in an increased thrombotic tendency. The evaluation of any patient with a hypercoagulable state must be individualized and should be based on a thorough clinical assessment. For example, a family history of thrombosis, thrombosis at an early age, or recurrent thrombosis without apparent precipitating factors may suggest a primary hypercoagulable state rather than a secondary one. Similarly, a history of multiple arterial occlusions in a young person may suggest hyperhomocysteinemia; the Budd–Chiari syndrome may indicate a myeloproliferative disorder or paroxysmal nocturnal hemoglobinuria; and a history of systemic lupus erythematosus or other autoimmune diseases is suggestive of antiphospholipid antibodies. In patients suspected of having a secondary hypercoagulable state, identifying and treating the underlying systemic disorder should be pursued, as doing so may decrease the propensity toward thrombosis.

REFERENCES

1 Love PE, Santoro SA. Antiphospholipid antibodies: anticardiolipin and the lupus anticoagulant in systemic lupus erythematous (SLE) and in non-SLE disorders. *Ann Intern Med* 1990; **112**: 682–98.
2 Shapiro SS. The lupus anticoagulant/antiphospholipid syndrome. *Annual Rev Med* 1996; **47**: 533–53.
3 Feinstein DI. Inhibitors of blood coagulation. In: Hoffman R, Benz EJ, Shattil SJ, Furie B, Cohen HJ, Silberstein LD eds *Hematology: basic principles and practice*. New York: Churchill Livingstone, 1995: 1746–53.
4 Asherson RA, Khamashta MA, Gil A, et al. Cerebrovascular disease and antiphospholipid antibodies in systemic lupus erythematous, lupus-like disease, and the primary antiphospholipid syndrome. *Am J Med* 1989; **86**: 391–9.
5 Roubey RAS. Autoantibodies to phospholipid binding plasma proteins: a new view of lupus anticoagulants and other antiphospholipid antibodies. *Blood* 1994; **84**: 2854–67.

6 Guerin J, Feighery C, Sim RB, Jackson J. Antibodies to β2–glycoprotein 1 – a specific marker for the antiphospholipid syndrome. *Clin Exp Immunol* 1997; **109**: 304–9.

7 Shapiro SS, Thiagarajan P. Lupus anticoagulants. *Prog Hemost Thromb* 1982; **6**: 263–85.

8 Harris EN, Chan JKH, Asherson RA. Thrombosis, recurrent fetal loss, and thrombocytopenia: predictive value of the anticardiolipin antibody test. *Arch Intern Med* 1986; **146**: 215–36.

9 Gastineau DA, Kazmier FJ, Nichols WL, Bowie EJ. Lupus anticoagulant: an analysis of the clinical and laboratory features of 219 cases. *Am J Hematol* 1985; **19**: 265–75.

10 Canoso RT, de Oliverra RM. Chlorpromazine-induced anticardiolipin antibodies and lupus anticoagulant: absence of thrombosis. *Am J Hematol* 1988; **27**: 272–5.

11 O'Callaghan AS, Oodi-Ros J, Monegal-Ferran F, et al. IgA anticardiolipin antibodies – relation with other antiphospholipid antibodies and clinical significance. *Thromb Haemost* 1998; **79**: 282–5.

12 Lechner K, Pabinger-Fasching I. Lupus anticoagulants and thrombosis. A study of 25 cases and review of the literature. *Haemostasis* 1982; **15**: 254–62.

13 Fort JG, Cowchock FS, Abruzzo JL, Smith JB. Anticardiolipin antibodies in patients with rheumatic diseases. *Arthritis Rheum* 1987; **30**: 752–60.

14 Keane A, Woods R, Dowding V, Roden D, Barry C. Anticardiolipin antibodies in rheumatoid arthritis. *Br J Rheumatol* 1987; **26**: 346–50.

15 Triplett DA, Brandt JY, Musgrave KA, Orr CA. The relationship between lupus anticoagulants and antibodies to phospholipid. *JAMA* 1988; **259**: 550–4.

16. Stasi R, Stipa E, Masi M, et al. Prevalence and clinical significance of elevated antiphospholipid antibodies in patients with idiopathic thrombocytopenic purpura. *Blood* 1994; **84**: 4203–8.

17 Rai RS, Clifford K, Cohen H, Regan L. High prospective fetal loss in untreated pregnancies of women with recurrent miscarriages and antiphospholipid antibodies. *Hum Reprod* 1995; **10**: 3301–4.

18 Brandt JT, Triplett DA, Alving B, Scharer I. Criteria for the diagnosis of lupus anticoagulants: an update. On behalf of the Subcommittee on Lupus Anticoagulant/Antiphospholipid Antibody of the Scientific and Standardization Committee of the ISTH. *Thromb Haemost* 1995; **74**: 1185–90.

19 Martin BA, Branch DW, Rodgers GM. Sensitivity of the activated partial thromboplastin time, the dilute Russell viper venom time, and the kaolin clotting time for the detection of the lupus anticoagulant: a direct comparison using plasma dilutions. *Blood Coag Fibrinol* 1996; **7**: 31–8.

20 Triplett DA, Brandt JT, Kaczor D, Schaeffer J. Laboratory diagnosis of lupus inhibitors: a comparison of the tissue thromboplastin inhibition procedure with a new platelet neutralization procedure. *Am J Clin Pathol* 1983; **79**: 678–82.

21 Rauch J, Tannenbaum M, Janoff AS. Distinguishing plasma lupus anticoagulants from antifactor antibodies using hexagonal (H) phase phospholipids. *Thromb Haemost* 1989; **62**: 892–6.

22 Alarcon-Segovia D, Deleze M, Oria CV, et al. Antiphospholipid antibodies and the antiphospholipid syndrome in systemic lupus erythematosus and a prospective analysis of 500 consecutive patients. *Medicine* 1989; **68**: 353–65.

23 Drenkard C, Sanchez-Guerroro J, Alarcon-Segovia D. Fall in antiphospholipid antibody at time of thrombocclusive episodes in systemic lupus erythematosus. *J Rheumatol* 1989; **16**: 614–17.

24 Forastiero RR, Martinuzzo ME, Cerrato GS, Kordich LC, Carreras LO. Relationship of anti β_2-glycoprotein I and anti-prothrombin antibodies to thrombosis and pregnancy loss in patients with antiphospholipid antibodies. *Thromb Haemost* 1997; **78**: 1008–14.

25 Khamashta MA, Cuadrado MJ, Mujic F, Taub NA, Hunt BJ, Hughes GR. The management of thrombosis in the antiphospholipid antibody syndrome. *N Engl J Med* 1995; **332**: 993–7.

26 Moll S, Ortel TL. Monitoring warfarin therapy in patients with lupus anticoagulants. *Ann Intern Med* 1997; **127**: 177–85.

27 Laskin CA, Bombardier C, Hannah ME, et al. Prednisone and aspirin in women with autoantibodies and unexplained recurrent fetal loss. *N Engl J Med* 1997; **337**: 148–53.

28 Kutteh WH, Ermel LD. A clinical trial for the treatment of antiphospholipid antibody-associated recurrent pregnancy loss with lower dose heparin and aspirin. *Am J Reprod Immunol* 1996; **35**: 402–7.

29 Agnelli G. Venous thromboembolism and cancer: a two-way clinical association. *Thromb Haemost* 1997; **78**: 117–20.

30 Patterson WP. Coagulation and cancer: an overview. *Semin Oncol* 1990; **17**: 137–9.

31 Pritchard KI, Paterson AH, Paul NA, Zee B, Fine S, Pater J. Increased thromboembolic complications with concurrent Tamoxifen and chemotherapy in a randomized trail of adjuvant therapy for women with breast cancer. *J Clin Oncol* 1996; **14**: 2731–7.

32 Prandoni P. Antithrombotic strategies in patients with cancer. *Thromb Haemost* 1997; **78**: 141–4.

33 Lokich JJ, Becker B. Subclavian vein thrombosis in patients treated with infusion chemotherapy for advanced malignancy cancer. *Cancer* 1983; **52**: 1586–9.

34 Bern MM, Lockich JJ, Wallach SR, et al. Very low doses of warfarin can prevent thrombosis in central venous catheters: a randomized prospective trial. *Ann Intern Med* 1990; **112**: 423–8.

35 Monreal M, Alastrue A, Rull M, et al. Upper extremity deep venous thrombosis in cancer patients with venous access devices – prophylaxis with a low molecular weight heparin (Fragmin). *Thromb Haemost* 1996; **75**: 251–3.

36 Bona RD, Hickey AD, Wallace DM. Efficacy and safety of oral anticoagulants in patients with cancer. *Thromb Haemost* 1997; **78**: 137–40.

37 Green D, Hull RD, Brant R, Pineo GF. Lower mortality in cancer patients treated with low molecular weight versus standard heparin. *Lancet* 1992; **339**: 1476.

38 Rosse WF. Paroxysmal nocturnal hemoglobinuria. In: Hoffman R, Benz EF, Shathil SJ, Furie B, Cohen HJ, Silberstein LE eds *Hematology: basic principles and practice*. New York: Churchill Livingstone, 1995: 370–81.

39 Hoffman R, Boswell HS. Polycythemia vera. In: Hoffman R, Benz EF, Shattil SJ, Furie B, Cohen HJ, Silberstein LE eds *Hematology: basic principles and practice*. New York: Churchill Livingstone, 1995: 1121–41.

40 Hoffman R, Silverstein MN, Hromas R. Primary thrombocythemia. In: Hoffman R, Benz EF, Shathil SJ, Furie B, Cohen HJ, Silberstein LE eds *Hematology: basic principles and practice*. New York: Churchill Livingstone, 1995: 1174–83.

41 Kessler CM, Klein HG, Havlik RJ. Uncontrolled thrombocytosis in chronic myeloproliferative disorders. *Br J Haematol* 1982; **50**: 157–67.

42 Orth SR, Ritz E. The nephrotic syndrome. *N Engl J Med* 1998; **338**: 1202–11.

43 Rabelink TJ, Zwaginga JJ, Koomans HA, Sixma JJ. Thrombosis and hemostasis in renal disease. *Kidney Int* 1994; **46**: 287–96.

44 Lechner K, Kyle PA. Antithrombin III concentrates – are they clinically useful? *Thromb Haemost* 1995; **73**: 340–8.
45 Holbrook AM, Wells PS, Crowther NR. Pharmacokinetics and drug interactions with warfarin. In: Poller L, Hirsch J eds *Oral anticoagulants*. New York: Oxford University Press, 1996: 30–48.
46 Schwartz SM, Siscovick DS, Longstreth WT Jr, et al. Use of low-dose oral contraceptives and stroke in young women. *Ann Intern Med* 1997; **127**(Pt 1): 596–603.
47 Mortality among oral contraceptive users. Royal College of General Practitioners Oral Contraceptive Study. *Lancet* 1997; **2**: 727.
48 Chasan-Taber L, Stampfer MJ. Epidemiology of oral contraceptives and cardiovascular disease. *Ann Intern Med* 1998; **128**: 467–77.
49 Gerstman BB, Piper JM, Tomita DK, Ferguson WJ, Stadel BV, Lundin FE. Oral contraceptive estrogen dose and the risk of deep venous thromboembolic disease. *Am J Epidemiol* 1991; **133**: 32–7.
50 Bottiger LE, Boman G, Eklund G, Westerholm B. Oral contraceptives and thromboembolic disease: effects of lowering oestrogen content. *Lancet* 1980; **1**: 1097–101.
51 Thorogood M. Oral contraceptives and myocardical infarction: new evidence leaves unanswered questions. *Thromb Haemost* 1997; **78**: 334–8.
52 Lewis MA, Spitzer WO, Heinemann LA, MacRae KD, Bruppacher R, Thorogood M. Third generation oral contraceptives and risk of myocardial infarction: an international case-control study. Transnational Research Group on Oral Contraceptives and the Health of Young Women. *Br Med J* 1996; **312**: 88–90.
53 Sidney S, Petitti DB, Quesenberry CP Jr, Klatsky AL, Ziel HK, Wolf S. Myocardial infarction in users of low-dose oral contraceptives. *Obstet Gynecol* 1996; **88**: 939–44.
54 Hannaford PC, Croft PR, Kay CR. Oral contraception and stroke. Evidence from the Royal College of General Practitioners' Oral Contraception Study. *Stroke* 1994; **25**: 935–42.
55 Petitti DB, Sidney S, Bernstein A, Wolf S. Stroke in users of low dose oral contraceptives. *N Engl J Med* 1996; **335**: 8–15.
56 Helmerhorst FM, Bloemenkamp KW, Rosendaal FR, Vandenbroucke JP. Oral contraceptives and thrombotic disease: risk of venous thromboembolism. *Thromb Haemost* 1997; **78**: 327–33.
57 Vandenbroucke JP, Koster T, Briet E, Reitsma PH, Bertina RM, Rosendaal FR. Increased risk of venous thrombosis in oral contraceptive users who are carriers of factor V Leiden mutation. *Lancet* 1994; **344**: 1453–7.
58 Chae CU, Ridker PM, Manson JE. Postmenopausal hormone replacement therapy and cardiovascular disease. *Thromb Haemost* 1997; **78**: 770–80.
59 Douketis JD, Ginsberg JS, Holbrook A, et al. A reevaluation of the risk for venous thromboembolism with the use of oral contraceptives and hormone replacement therapy. *Arch Intern Med* 1997; **157**: 1522–30.
60 Devor M, Barrett-Connor E, Renvall M, Feigal D Jr, Ramsdell J. Estrogen replacement therapy and the risk of venous thrombosis. *Am J Med* 1992; **92**: 275–82.
61 Daly E, Vessey MP, Hawkins MM, et al. Risk of venous thromboembolism in users of hormone replacement therapy. *Lancet* 1996; **348**: 977–80.
62 Talbot RW, Heppell J, Dozois PR, et al. Vascular complications of inflammatory bowel disease. *Mayo Clin Proc* 1986; **61**: 140–5.

63 Braverman D, Bogoch A. Arterial thrombosis in ulcerative colitis. *Am J Dig Dis* 1978; **23**: 1148–50.

64 Jackson LM, O'Gorman PJ, O'Connell J, Cronin CC, Cotter KP, Shanahan F. Thrombosis in inflammatory bowel disease: clinical setting, procoagulant profile and factor V Leiden. *QJM* 1997; **90**: 183–8.

65 Chiarantini E, Valanzano R, Liotta AA, et al. Hemostatic abnormalities in inflammatory bowel disease. *Thromb Res* 1996; **82**: 137–46.

66 Aichbichler BW, Petritsch W, Reicht GA, et al. Anti-cardiolipin antibodies in patients with inflammatory bowel disease. *Dig Dis Sci* 1999; **44**: 852–6.

5

Heparin and low molecular weight heparin

DAWN E HAVRDA

INTRODUCTION

Since its discovery in 1916 and for approximately 75 years, unfractionated heparin (UFH) had been the only agent available in the USA to produce a rapid, immediate anticoagulation response.[1] However, since the Food and Drug Administration's (FDA) approval of a low molecular weight heparin (LMWH), enoxaparin, in 1993 the selection of fast-acting anticoagulants has been broadened. Currently, besides enoxaparin (Lovenox®), there are two other LMWH preparations – dalteparin (Fragmin®) and ardeparin (Normiflo®) – as well as one low molecular weight heparinoid – danaparoid (Organan®) – approved in the USA that have been found to be at least as effective and safe as UFH for selected indications. The LMWHs and danaparoid have several pharmacokinetic and pharmacodynamic advantages over UFH, such as better bioavailability, subcutaneous administration, and a predictable anticoagulant response that does not require monitoring. Other advantages of the LMWHs and danaparoid over UFH include possibly less bleeding risk, a lower incidence of thrombocytopenia, and potentially less risk of developing osteoporosis.

MECHANISM OF ACTION

Unfractionated heparin is a mix of heterogeneous glycosoaminoglycans or polysaccha-rides with an average molecular weight of 15 000 daltons (range 5000–30 000). One-third of molecules of UFH contains a unique pentasacchride complex with a high affinity for antithrombin. UFH interacts with antithrombin to accelerate the inactivation of clotting factors IIa (thrombin), Xa, and IXa, which produces the antithrombotic effect. The inactivation of thrombin by UFH requires the creation of a complex consisting of antithrombin, UFH, and thrombin (Fig. 5.1). This ternary complex is only formed with UFH molecules that are at least 18 saccharides in length. Conversely, any length of UFH is capable of inhibiting factor Xa; therefore, the interaction between antithrombin and UFH alone is sufficient to inactivate factor Xa (Fig. 5.1). Thrombin can also be inhibited through a secondary pathway that involves heparin cofactor II. This property does not contribute significantly to the antithrombotic effect of UFH, because it requires much larger doses of UFH than are usually employed in clinical settings.[2]

The LMWHs are derived by enzymatic or chemical depolymerization of UFH, producing smaller fragments with molecular weights of 4000–8000 daltons. Each LMWH is produced from UFH using a different process, leading to different molec-ular weights and potencies for inactivation of factors IIa and Xa. Therefore the FDA does not consider any of the preparations to be interchangeable or equivalent. Less than 50% of the LMWH compounds contain saccharide chains greater than 18 units, resulting in a reduction in their ability to inhibit thrombin, because the ternary complex cannot be formed (Fig. 5.1). UFH has equal potency for the inactivation of

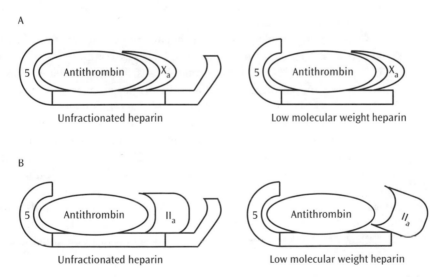

Figure 5.1 *Mechanism of action of unfractionated heparin and low molecular weight heparins. (A) With both unfractionated heparin and the low molecular weight heparins, only binding of the pentasaccharide to antithrombin is required to inactivate factor Xa. (B) Inhibition of factor IIa requires a ternary complex of antithrombin, the heparin, and factor IIa; only heparin molecules > 18 saccharides are large enough to form the complex and inactivate factor IIa.*

Table 5.1 *Characteristics of unfractionated heparin, the low molecular weight heparins and danaparoid*[1,3,5,6–9,58]

	Unfractionated heparin	Ardeparin	Dalteparin	Enoxaparin	Danaparoid
Mean molecular weight (daltons)	15 000	6000	5000	4500	6000
Antifactor Xa : IIa ratio	1:1	2:1	2:1	2.7:1	$\geq$ 20:1
Half-life (hours)	0.4–2.5[a]	3.3	4	4	17–28
Time to peak antifactor Xa activity (hours)		2–3	4	2–4	4–5
Bioavailability after SC injection	29%	92%	87%	91%	100%
Mean cross-reactivity in HIT	100%	~90%	~90%	~90%	< 5%

[a]Half-life dependent on the dose administered and concentration of circulating plasma proteins.
SC = subcutaneous; HIT = heparin-induced thrombocytopenia.

factor Xa and IIa (antifactor Xa : IIa ratio of 1 : 1), whereas the LMWHs favor the inhibition of factor Xa (antifactor Xa : IIa ratios of 2 : 1 to 4 : 1), which leads to less effect on coagulation tests, such as the activated partial thromboplastin time (aPTT) (Table 5.1). An additional property of LMWH is a reduced effect on the suppression of platelet aggregation compared to UFH, and therefore less bleeding and thrombocytopenia. Due to these differences between the compounds, the LMWHs are presumed to have a better risk–benefit profile.[2–4]

Danaparoid is the first low molecular weight heparinoid to be approved in the USA. Unlike UFH or LMWH, danaparoid does not have any components of UFH, but is made of a mixture of other glycosaminoglycans, heparan sulfate (84%), dermatan sulfate (12%), and chondroitin sulfate (4%). It has an average molecular weight similar to that of LMWH, of 6000 daltons. The exact anticoagulant mechanism of danaparoid is not known, but it is hypothesized to include inactivation of factor Xa by antithrombin. Danaparoid has less ability to inhibit thrombin than UFH and LMWH, with an antifactor Xa : IIa ratio of $\geq$ 20 : 1 (Table 5.1). Another possible antithrombotic mechanism of danaparoid is inhibition of thrombin by heparin cofactor II. In addition, when compared to UFH, danaparoid more effectively prevents factor IX activation, which leads to a delay in the activation of factor X and may also contribute to its anticoagulant effect. Similar to LMWH, danaparoid has little or no effect on platelet aggregation, leading to less thrombocytopenia and possibly less bleeding.[5]

PHARMACOKINETICS AND PHARMACODYNAMICS

Some of the limitations of UFH compared to the newer anticoagulant agents can be explained by its pharmacodynamic and pharmacokinetic characteristics (Table 5.1).

UFH has an unpredictable anticoagulant response, variable bioavailability, and an unpredictable dose–response correlation. Some of these properties can be explained by one of the methods of elimination of UFH – a rapid, dose-dependent clearance. After its administration, UFH binds to saturable sites on endothelial cells and macrophages, which results in a rapid clearance of a proportion of the dose, as well as a reduction in the amount available for anticoagulant activity. The second mode of elimination of UFH is a slower, nonsaturable, renal route. The clearance of UFH is also dependent on molecular size, with the lower molecular weight fractions being cleared more slowly.[1,2]

In addition to binding with endothelial cells and macrophages, UFH also binds to other plasma proteins, such as some acute phase reactants, histidine-rich glyco-protein, von Willebrand factor, fibronectin, and vitronectin, which prevents the UFH molecules from being able to interact with antithrombin. The ability to bind these various circulating proteins leads to the unpredictable bioavailability of UFH, disproportional increases in the intensity and duration of the anticoagulation response with escalating doses, inconsistent responses to fixed doses, and the potential for UFH resistance. Due to the variability in anticoagulant response, there is often difficulty in initially achieving therapeutic anticoagulation, and monitoring using the activated partial thromboplastin time (aPTT) is a necessity when treatment doses are administered. In addition, platelets also antagonize the anticoagulant response of UFH by protecting platelet-bound factor Xa from inactivation and secreting platelet factor 4, which neutralizes UFH. Unfractionated heparin, as is also true for LMWH, is unable to inhibit fibrin-bound thrombin, which may lead to inferior outcomes compared to the newer anticoagulant preparations.[1,2]

Unfractionated heparin can be given intravenously or subcutaneously. The initial subcutaneous dose of UFH must be adjusted to compensate for the reduced bioavailability of that route of administration. After a subcutaneous injection, the anticoagulant response is generally delayed 1 to 2 hours; therefore, an intravenous bolus of UFH can be administered if an immediate effect is desired. Intermittent intravenous doses of UFH have been associated with more bleeding compared with continuous infusion; therefore, a continuous intravenous infusion of UFH is preferred. The half-life of UFH varies from 0.4 to 2.5 hours, depending on the dose administered and the amount of circulating plasma proteins (Table 5.1).[1,2]

The LMWHs have superior bioavailability, longer half-lives, and a more predictable anticoagulant response in comparison to UFH. A reason for the advantages of LMWH over UFH is their lack of binding to endothelial cells, macrophages, and plasma proteins. The LMWHs have longer half-lives because they are eliminated renally (Table 5.1). Because they do not bind to plasma proteins, the anticoagulant response is more dependable, with fixed doses producing consistent anticoagulant responses. Therefore, there is no need for monitoring of the anticoagulant effect, except in renal impairment, when the duration of anticoagulant activity may be prolonged, or in some pediatric cases.[2,4]

Because the LMWHs have excellent bioavailability and more predictable antico-agulant responses, they are generally given subcutaneously, but they have been administered intravenously in clinical trials. After subcutaneous administration, enoxaparin, dalteparin, and ardeparin are 86–92% bioavailable, with peak antifactor Xa activity occurring in 2 to 4 hours. The half-life of the three LMWH compounds is approximately 4 hours, which allows for dosing every 12–24 hours (Table 5.1).[6–8]

Like LMWH, danaparoid does not share the characteristics of binding to endothelial cells, macrophages, or plasma proteins with UFH. Danaparoid has been found to exhibit a linear relationship between dose and antifactor Xa activity that allows for a more consistent and predictable anticoagulant effect. It is predominantly given subcutaneously, but can also be administered intravenously. After subcutaneous administration, danaparoid is 100% bioavailable, with the peak antifactor Xa activity occurring in 4–5 hours. Elimination of danaparoid is chiefly renal, with a half-life of 17–28 hours for antifactor Xa activity and 2–4 hours for antifactor IIa activity. Due to the difference in half-lives of factors Xa and IIa, danaparoid is recommended to be given at least twice daily (Table 5.1). Monitoring of the anticoagulant response is not required for danaparoid, except in the presence of renal insufficiency.[5,9]

DOSING

Due to UFH's unpredictable response, the dosing of UFH is dependent on the ability to monitor the anticoagulant effect. In the past, the aPTT ratio was used to monitor UFH therapy, with a usual therapeutic range of 1.5–2.5 times control, which may vary depending on the indication.[2] One problem with the use of the aPTT ratio is the variability in sensitivity of the different reagents used to measure the aPTT. Depending on the sensitivity of the reagent used, a specific aPTT ratio may correspond to a variety of degrees of anticoagulation. Another problem with using the aPTT is that the lower molecular weight fragments of UFH that are cleared more slowly have less effect on the aPTT, while still possessing antithrombotic activity. To overcome these obstacles, it is recommended that therapeutic aPTT ratios be defined for the specific reagent utilized, corresponding to an antifactor Xa activity level of 0.3–0.7 U/mL or a heparin level of 0.2–0.4 U/mL by protamine titration. If the aPTT is not calibrated according to the antifactor Xa activity or the heparin level, it cannot be assured that the value obtained with the specific reagent is therapeutic.[2,10]

Another factor in UFH dosing is the most appropriate intravenous regimen to use when full anticoagulation is indicated to achieve a therapeutic aPTT in a timely manner. The dosing of UFH has been an area of active research, especially with the strong relationship between under-anticoagulation, or a subtherapeutic aPTT, and a higher incidence of 20–25% in recurrent venous thromboembolic events.[1,10–12] The UFH requirement varies among individuals due to fluctuating concentrations in heparin-neutralizing plasma proteins. In acute venous thromboembolism or acute coronary syndromes, the concentrations of the heparin-neutralizing plasma proteins are higher compared with those used for patients receiving UFH for prophylactic reasons. This phenomenon results in a lower bioavailability of UFH and the need for higher doses to achieve a therapeutic aPTT value.[1,10] As a result of these difficulties, various dosing nomograms have been developed.

Standard dosing nomograms generally use an intravenous loading dose of UFH of 5000 units, followed by a continuous infusion, usually starting at 1000–1300 units/hour (approximately 30 000 units/24 hours). The aPTT values are measured 6 hours after the initiation or a dosage change and the infusion rate is adjusted accordingly. If the aPTT value is too low, the infusion rate is increased and a bolus dose of

UFH may be administered; if the aPTT value is too high, the infusion may be discontinued for a specified period of time and the rate reduced. Clinical trials have indicated that the 5000 units intravenous bolus and 30 000 units/24 hours comprise the minimal effective starting dose to achieve therapeutic aPTT values.[2,10] An example of an algorithm using this standard dosing regimen for UFH is shown in Fig. 5.2.

Standard dosing nomograms have been compared to a variety of weight-based nomograms for intravenous UFH dosing. Perhaps the strongest support for the use of a weight-based nomogram, and the most cited comparison study, was reported by Raschke and colleagues in 1993.[13] They found that the use of a weight-based nomogram, based on total body weight, resulted in a significant reduction

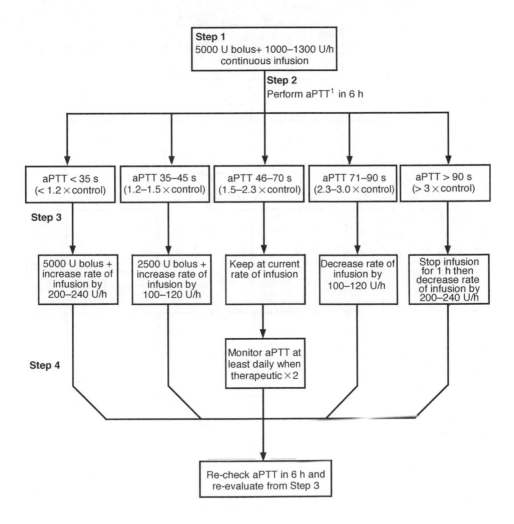

[1]The aPTT range should be correlated to a heparin concentration of 0.2–0.4 U/mL by protamine titration or an antifactor Xa activity of 0.3–0.7 U/mL.

Figure 5.2 *Standard care dosing nomogram.*[10,13] *(aPPT = activated partial thromboplastin time.)*

in the time to achieving therapeutic aPTT values (mean of 14.1 hours with the weight-based nomogram versus 22.3 hours). In addition, the weight-based nomogram achieved a therapeutic aPTT in more patients by the first blood draw (86% with the weight-based nomogram versus 32%, $p < 0.001$) and by 24 hours (97% with the weight-based nomogram versus 77%, $p = 0.002$). The use of the weight-based nomogram also required fewer infusion adjustments. Although there was no difference in bleeding complications between the groups, there was a higher incidence of recurrent venous thromboembolic events with the standard dosing nomogram (25% versus 5% in the weight-based heparin group, $p = 0.02$).[2,10,13] An algorithm of the weight-based nomogram used by Raschke and colleagues is shown Fig. 5.3.

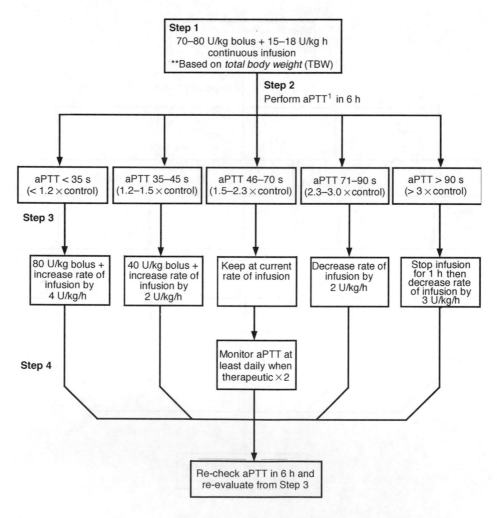

[1]The aPTT range should be correlated to a heparin concentration of 0.2–0.4 U/mL by protamine titration or an antifactor Xa activity of 0.3–0.7 U/mL.

Figure 5.3 *Weight-adjusted heparin dosing.*[2,10,13,17] *(aPPT = activated partial thromboplastin time.)*

To summarize, some of the advantages of using a weight-based versus a standard dosing approach for indications requiring full anticoagulation include easier titration, fewer infusion adjustments, more rapid attainment of therapeutic aPTT values, a greater proportion of patients achieving a therapeutic aPTT within 24 hours, and possibly a reduction in the rate of recurrent thrombotic events. One of the potential problems with the weight-based nomogram is dosing in obese patients. The nomogram is based on total body weight, which may result in large starting doses of UFH in such patients. Some practitioners have found the weight-based method results in excessive aPTT values, whereas others have not, including the trial by Raschke and colleagues.[13–15] Until an appropriate regimen has proven effective in obese patients, the weight-based nomogram should be used, because its efficacy has been proven in nonobese and obese patients, and the risk of recurrent events is greater when a therapeutic aPTT is not reached in a timely manner. The weight-based nomogram is becoming more widely used and is currently recommended for use in unstable angina and acute myocardial infarction by the Agency for Healthy Care Policy and Research (AHCPR) and the American College of Cardiology/American Health Association (ACC/AHA).[16,17]

Unfractionated heparin may also be given subcutaneously to produce therapeutic aPTT ratios and as fixed doses for the prophylaxis of venous thromboembolic events. As long as the aPTT values are therapeutic, the subcutaneous route has been found to be equally as effective as the intravenous route. The American College of Chest Physicians (ACCP) recommends an initial dose of at least 35 000 units/24 hours, given in two daily doses (17 500 units every 12 hours). As discussed previously, the therapeutic effect will be delayed for 1–2 hours; therefore, if an immediate anticoagulant effect is needed, an intravenous bolus of 5000 units should be given with the first subcutaneous dose. With the subcutaneous regimen, the aPTT value should be monitored midway through the dosing interval or 6 hours after the last dose, and dosing adjustments can be made depending on that value.[2,10] Fixed doses of UFH are recommended for patients receiving them for prophylaxis of venous thromboembolism. The doses used are less than those required to produce therapeutic anticoagulation, generally 5000 units subcutaneously two or three times daily. Therefore, the aPTT value is not expected to be prolonged. Because dosage adjustments are not needed and the aPTT value is not effected as much, monitoring of the aPTT values does not need to be as frequent or aggressive. This process of giving low, fixed doses of UFH for the prevention of thrombotic events is referred to in this chapter as low dose heparin therapy. The intramuscular administration of UFH is not recommended because of the potential for the development of painful hematomas.[1,2]

Dosing of the LMWHs is much simpler than UFH because of their pharmacodynamic and pharmacokinetic advantages. Enoxaparin, dalteparin, and ardeparin are administered subcutaneously in weight-adjusted, fixed dosages. Pharmacodynamic studies have shown the peak antifactor Xa activity to be highly correlated with body weight. Therefore, calculating the dose based on body weight would be expected to produce the best anticoagulant response. The exception to this is the use of enoxaparin and dalteparin in the prophylaxis of venous thromboembolism in general and orthopedic surgery, in which they have been effective in fixed subcutaneous doses independent of body weight. To date, no trials have compared fixed standard dosing to fixed weight-adjusted dosing of the LMWHs; therefore, if one method is superior, it has yet to be determined. Regardless, the better bioavailability, predictable anticoagulant response, and longer duration of action of the LMWHs allow for the use of weight-based or fixed dosages, subcutaneous administration, and the elimination of the need for continuous intravenous infusions and frequent monitoring of the anticoagulant effect as seen with UFH. Like UFH, LMWHs should not be given intramuscularly.[4]

Like the LMWHs, danaparoid is administered in fixed weight-based subcutaneous doses and is not recommended for intramuscular administration. The dosage advocated is based on the weight of the patient, and individuals who weigh more than 90 kg will need a higher dose for select indications. The pharmacokinetic advantages of danaparoid over UFH allow for the ease in administration and dosing.[5,9]

INDICATIONS

Prophylaxis of venous thromboembolism

Unfractionated heparin and the LMWHs are recommended by the ACCP for the prophylaxis of venous thromboembolism in a variety of clinical situations. This section discusses the role of UFH in either fixed subcutaneous low doses or adjusted subcutaneous doses to obtain an aPTT value in the upper range of normal, and LMWH and danaparoid in the prevention of venous thromboembolic events (see Chapter 9).[18]

GENERAL SURGERY

In individuals undergoing major general surgery, such as urologic, gynecologic, thoracic, or vascular procedures, the risk of total deep vein thrombosis without prophylaxis is 19–25% and up to 29% in patients with an underlying malignancy. Proximal deep vein thrombosis occurs in 6–7% of patients, and symptomatic pulmonary embolism in 1.6%. The use of low-dose heparin started 2 hours prior to surgery has been shown to reduce the risk of deep vein thrombosis by 68%. Low-dose heparin has also proven efficacious in patients with malignancy, and has not been found to increase the frequency of hemorrhagic events. Trials with enoxaparin and dalteparin in general surgery patients have begun therapy 1–2 hours preoperatively and have found these LMWHs to be at least as effective as low-dose heparin, with similar bleeding complications and perhaps fewer wound hematomas. In higher-risk individuals undergoing general surgery, such as patients with a history of venous thromboembolic events, malignancy, ischemic stroke, or spinal cord injury, enoxaparin 30 mg subcutaneously twice daily and dalteparin 5000 units subcutaneously daily were effective at reducing the complication of venous thromboembolism to a degree similar to low-dose heparin without increasing hemorrhagic events. Therapy with low-dose heparin or LMWH should continue for at least 7–14 days postoperatively or until the patient is ambulatory. If the patient is to undergo spinal anesthesia, there is an increased risk of spinal hematomas with anticoagulant use that can lead to significant morbidity and mortality; therefore, the risk–benefit profile should be considered before initiating anticoagulant prophy-laxis.[6,7,18] Dosages for UFH, enoxaparin, and dalteparin in general surgery patients are listed in Table 5.2. (For more information, see Chapter 9.)

ORTHOPEDIC SURGERY

Individuals undergoing orthopedic surgery of the lower extremities or hip or knee replacement have a very high risk of developing postoperative deep vein thrombosis and pulmonary embolism, with incidences of 36–84% and 0.7–30%, respectively.[18] Thus, the primary prevention of thrombotic complications is cost effective and recommended in all patients.

In hip replacement surgery, low-dose heparin has been shown to reduce the risk of developing postoperative deep vein thrombosis by 39%; however, deep vein throm-bosis still occurs in 31% of patients. Another regimen of UFH, utilizing preoperative low-dose heparin followed by adjusted-dose UFH after surgery to maintain the aPTT ratio in the upper range of normal, has been effective, with a total incidence of deep vein thrombosis of 11%, a reduction of 78%.[18] Enoxaparin, dalteparin, and danaparoid are FDA-approved for the prevention of deep vein thrombosis and pulmonary embolism after total hip replacement.[19] Enoxaparin has been shown to be efficacious in subcutaneous doses of 40 mg daily, started prior to surgery, and 30 mg subcutaneously twice daily, begun after surgery. However, when the two dosages were compared, both given postoperatively, the 30 mg subcutaneously twice daily dose was superior and is currently recommended in the USA by the FDA. Enoxaparin has also been shown in clinical trials to be superior to low-dose heparin and equally or more efficacious than adjusted-dose UFH, with no difference in bleeding events.[6,18] Trials have also demonstrated enoxaparin to be more effective than adjusted-dose warfarin; however, the risk of bleeding is greater with the LMWH.[18] Dalteparin, 5000 units subcutaneously daily initiated prior to surgery, has been evaluated and found to be equivalent in efficacy and safety to low-dose heparin and adjusted-dose heparin.[4,7] Compared to adjusted-dose warfarin, dalteparin has been found to be more effica-cious in preventing a deep vein thrombosis. Two different subcutaneous dosage regimens of ardeparin, 50 units/kg twice daily and 90 units/kg once daily, initiated postoperatively have been compared to warfarin, with no difference in venous throm-boembolic or hemorrhagic events between the groups.[20] However, due to the limited data on the effectiveness of ardeparin in preventing postoperative deep vein throm-bosis in total hip replacement, it is not approved by the FDA for this indication. Danaparoid, started preoperatively at a subcutaneous dose of 750 units twice daily, has been found to be superior to adjusted-dose warfarin, with no difference in bleed-ing rates. To date, it has not been compared to any of the LMWHs, low-dose heparin or adjusted-dose heparin.[9] In summary, the LMWHs or adjusted-dose UFH are recommended by the ACCP for the prevention of deep vein thrombosis or pulmonary embolism after total hip replacement surgery. The use of LMWH or danaparoid offers the advantages of once-daily or twice-daily dosing, lack of monitor-ing for dose titration, and a predictable anticoagulant response.

After total knee replacement surgery, the LMWHs have been shown to be the most efficacious agents in preventing venous thromboembolism. With the use of

Table 5.2 *Dosages of UFH and LMWHs in the prevention and treatment of venous thromboembolism*[2,4–7,9,18,19,21]

Indication	Agent and dose
General surgery	
Moderate[a] or high[b] risk	UFH 5000 U SC Q 8–12 hours, start 2 hours preop. × 7 days[c]
	Enoxaparin 40 mg SC Q 24 hours, start 2 hours preop. × 7–10 days[c,d,e]
	Dalteparin 2500 U SC Q 24 hours, start 2 hours preop. × 5–10 days[c,d,e]
Highest risk[f]	Adjusted-dose UFH SC Q 12 hours to maintain aPTT at high-normal[c,g]
	UFH 5000 U SC Q 8–12 hours, start 2 hours preop. × 7–10 days + IPC[c,e]
	Enoxaparin 30 mg SC Q 12 hours, start 12–24 hours postop. × 7–10 days[c,e]
	Dalteparin 5000 U SC Q 24 hours, start the evening prior to surgery × 7–10 days[c,d,e]
HIT[h]	≤ 90 kg: danaparoid 750 U SC Q 8–12 hours, start 1–4 hours preop.
	> 90 kg: danaparoid 1250 U SC Q 8–12 hours, start 1–4 hours preop.
Total hip replacement	Adjusted-dose SC UFH to a therapeutic aPTT[c,g]
	Enoxaparin 30 mg SC Q 12 hours, start 12–24 hours postop until discharge,[c,d,e] consider 40 mg SC Q 24 hours, for 21 days in high-risk patients[d]
	Dalteparin 2500 U SC 2 hours preop. and the day of surgery, then 5000 U SC Q 24 hours until discharge, [c,d,e] consider 5000 U SC Q 24 hours for 21–28 days in high-risk patients[d]
	Danaparoid 750 U SC Q 12 hours, start 2 hours pre-op.[d]
HIT[h]	≤ 90 kg: danaparoid 750 U SC Q 8–12 hours, start 2 hours preop.
	> 90 kg: danaparoid 1250 U SC Q 8–12 hours, start 2 hours preop.
Total knee replacement	Ardeparin 50 U/kg SC Q 12 hours, start 12–24 hours postop. until discharge[c,d,e]
	Enoxaparin 30 mg SC Q 12 hours, start 12–24 hours postop. until discharge[c,d,e]
HIT[h]	≤ 90 kg: danaparoid 750 U SC Q 8–12 hours, start 1–4 hours preop.
	> 90 kg: danaparoid 1250 U SC Q 8–12 hours, start 1–4 hours preop.
Acute spinal cord injury	Adjusted-dose SC UFH to a therapeutic aPTT[g] × 3 months[c]
	Enoxaparin 30 mg SC Q 12 hours × 3 months[c,e]
Multiple trauma	Enoxaparin 30 mg SC Q 12 hours until ambulatory[c,e]
Medical conditions	
Myocardial infarction	Adjusted-dose CI UFH to a therapeutic aPTT[c,g]
	UFH 7500 U SC Q 12 hours[c]
Ischemic stroke	UFH 5000 U SC Q 8–12 hours[c]
	Dalteparin 2500 U SC Q 12 hours[c,e]
	Danaparoid 750 U SC Q 12 hrs
Other conditions	UFH 5000 U SC Q 8–12 hours[c]
	Enoxaparin 30 mg SC Q 12 hours until ambulatory[c,e]
Acute treatment of DVT	Adjusted-dose CI or SC UFH to a therapeutic aPTT[g] × 5–10 days[c]
	Enoxaparin 1.5 mg/kg SC Q 24 hours × 5–10 days (inpatient)[c,d,e]
	Enoxaparin 1 mg/kg SC Q 12 hours × 5–10 days (outpatient)[c,d,e]
	Dalteparin 200 U/kg SC Q 24 hours or 100 U/kg SC Q 12 hours × 5–10 days[c,e]

Indication	Agent and dose
Acute treatment of PE	Adjusted-dose CI or SC UFH to a therapeutic aPTT[g] $\times$ 5–10 days[c] Enoxaparin 1 mg/kg SC Q 12 hours $\times$ 5–10 days[c,d,e] Dalteparin 200 U/kg SC Q 24 hours or 100 U/kg SC Q 12 hours $\times$ 5–10 days[c,e]
Acute treatment of DVT/PE with HIT[h]	*< 5 days* Danaparoid bolus IV[i], then 400 U/hour $\times$ 4 hours, 300 U/hour $\times$ 4 hours, then 150–200 U/hour[j] $\geqslant$ *5 days* Continue danaparoid IV at 150–200 U/hour[j] OR $\leqslant$ 90 kg: danaparoid 750 U SC Q 8–12 hours > 90 kg: danaparoid 750 U SC Q 8 hours or 1250 U SC Q 8–12 hours
Secondary prevention of VTE[k]	Adjusted-dose subcutaneous to a therapeutic aPTT[c,g] Enoxaparin 40 mg SC Q 24 hours[c,e] Dalteparin 5000 U SC Q 12–24 hours[c,e]

[a]Moderate risk: 40–60 years with major or minor surgery and no risk factors; > 40 years with major surgery and no risk factors; or minor surgery with risk factors.
[b]High risk: > 40 years with major surgery with risk factors; > 60 years with major surgery with no risk factors; 40–60 years with major surgery with risk factors; patients with a myocardial infarction; or medical patients with risk factors.
[c]Recommended in the 1998 American College of Chest Physicians (ACCP) supplement.
[d]FDA-approved indication for LMWH or danaparoid.
[e]No specific LMWH is recommended by the 1998 ACCP Conference.
[f]Highest risk: > 40 years with major surgery and prior venous thromboembolic event or malignancy or hypercoagulable disorder; elective major orthopedic surgery of the lower extremity, hip fracture, stroke, multiple trauma, or spinal cord injury.
[g]aPTT value = heparin level of 0.2–0.4 U/mL or antifactor Xa activity of 0.3–0.7 U/mL.
[h]For more information, please see Chapter 14.
[i]Danaparoid bolus: < 60 kg, 1500 U; 60–75 kg, 2250 U; 76–90 kg, 3000 U; > 90 kg, 3750 U.
[j]To maintain anti-Xa levels of 0.5–0.8 U/mL.
[k]If warfarin therapy is contraindicated.
UFH = unfractionated heparin; LMWHs = low molecular weight heparins; U = units; SC = subcutaneous; Q = every; preop. = preoperatively; aPTT = activated partial thromboplastin time; IPC = intermittent pneumatic compression; postop. = postoperatively; HIT = heparin-induced thrombocytopenia; CI = continuous infusion; DVT = deep vein thrombosis; PE = pulmonary embolism; IV = intravenous; VTE = venous thromboembolism.

low-dose heparin, deep vein thrombosis still occurs postoperatively in 42% of patients, with a risk reduction of 31%. Enoxaparin 30 mg subcutaneous twice daily, initiated 12 hours after surgery, has been proven to be more effective than low-dose heparin and adjusted-dose warfarin, with similar bleeding rates.[4,6,18] Ardeparin 50 units/kg subcutaneous twice daily, started 12 hours after surgery, has also been effective in preventing postoperative venous thromboembolic events in knee replacement patients, and has been found to be significantly superior to adjusted-dose warfarin. Hemorrhagic events were higher with ardeparin compared to warfarin, which may be explained by the onset of anticoagulant action of the two agents. To date, ardeparin has not been compared to low-dose heparin or adjusted-dose heparin therapy.[4,8,21] The LMWHs are recommended by the ACCP in the prophylaxis of venous thromboembolism after total knee replacement. Dosages of the agents used in orthopedic surgery are listed in Table 5.2. (For more information see Chapter 9.)

Despite the evidence that the LMWHs are efficacious and safe in the prevention of venous thromboembolism in orthopedic surgery patients, some controversies do exist. The optimal time of initiation – preoperative versus postoperative – is one area of debate. The more extensive the surgery and the longer the duration, the greater the risk of blood loss and venous thromboembolism. Preoperative initiation may possibly be more effective at preventing deep vein thrombosis and pulmonary embolism, but may result in increased intraoperative bleeding. Conversely, initiating therapy postoperatively may reduce the incidence of bleeding during surgery, but may not prevent the thrombi formed intraoperatively. Currently, there are no trials evaluating preoperative versus postoperative initiation in the prophylaxis of orthopedic patients. A preoperative regimen is widely used in Europe, whereas the postoperative initiation is favored in the USA and recommended by the ACCP.[4,18,22]

Another area of debate in the prevention of venous thromboembolism in orthopedic surgery is the optimal duration of prophylaxis postoperatively. Traditionally, prophylaxis has been continued for the duration of the hospital stay, usually from 7 to 14 days, and discontinued when the patient is discharged. Unfortunately, the risk of developing a deep vein thrombosis or pulmonary embolism may persist beyond this period.[23,24] Recent trials have evaluated enoxaparin 40 mg and dalteparin 5000 units subcutaneously daily, continued for 21–28 days after discharge, in patients undergoing hip replacement surgery. The extended prophylaxis regimens have shown a significant reduction in venous thromboembolism after discharge, with minimal bleeding events. However, in the trials, most of the venous thromboembolic events were asymptomatic, and the rate of symptomatic events was low. For instance, in one trial, symptomatic deep vein thrombosis occurred in 2% of patients treated with LMWH versus 9% in those receiving placebo, in contrast to the total incidence of 18% with LMWH and 39% with placebo.[25] Enoxaparin has been cleared by the FDA for prolonged prophylaxis after hip replacement patients at a subcutaneous dose of 40 mg daily.[24-7]

Some issues that remain to be clarified with extended prophylaxis are if it is cost effective to continue prophylaxis after discharge; what the benefit is in preventing an asymptomatic deep vein thrombosis; if the use of extended prophylaxis prevents symptomatic deep vein thrombosis and pulmonary embolism, and if there is a select group of patients for whom extended prophylaxis may be indicated. The ACCP recommends that the prophylaxis duration in total hip and total knee replacement patients should be 7–10 days. However, in patients with ongoing risk factors, extended prophylaxis beyond discharge may be considered (for more information see Chapter 9).[18]

ACUTE SPINAL CORD INJURY

Patients with acute spinal cord injury are at increased risk of developing venous thromboembolic events, with an incidence of deep vein thrombosis ranging from 15% to 81%. The risk continues until approximately 3 months after the injury, with the greatest risk being in the first 2 weeks. The optimal prophylaxis regimen in patients with acute spinal cord injury has yet to be determined. Small trials have found that low-dose heparin did not substantially impact the risk of deep vein thrombosis following an acute spinal cord injury. Adjusted-dose UFH does confer adequate prevention of venous thromboembolic events, with a reported incidence of 7%, but at the expense of an increase in bleeding rates.[4,18] Small trials evaluating a LMWH not available in the USA, tinzaparin, showed it to be efficacious in the prophylaxis of deep vein thrombosis and pulmonary embolism, with lower bleeding complications than adjusted-dose UFH. A small retrospective review of the use of enoxaparin 30 mg subcutaneously twice daily in acute spinal cord injury patients demonstrated it to be effective in preventing venous thromboembolism.[18,28] Because the period of risk of venous thromboembolic events is highest initially following the injury, prophylaxis is recommended for a minimum of 3 months with either LMWH or adjusted-dose UFH.[18] Well-designed clinical trials are needed to evaluate further the most effective means of prophylaxis. Table 5.2 lists the doses of UFH and LMWH used in acute spinal cord injury. (For more information see Chapter 9.)

MAJOR TRAUMA

Trauma patients represent a heterogeneous group of individuals, and the disparity between the patients and the type of trauma makes it difficult to determine the true incidence of venous thromboembolic events. However, in patients with major trauma, the risk of deep vein thrombosis has been reported to exceed 50%.[18] Clinical trials evaluating the use of prophylactic regimens are also limited because of this heterogeneity. A big concern with using anticoagulants as prophylaxis is the risk of bleeding associated with the injuries, and it is estimated that approximately 14% of patients have contraindications for anticoagulants due to the extent and degree of their injuries. Low-dose heparin has not been shown to be effective at reducing the risk of venous thromboembolism. In one clinical trial, enoxaparin 30 mg subcutaneously twice daily, starting within 36 hours of the trauma, was found to be significantly superior to low-dose heparin in reducing the rate of total deep vein thrombosis, and proximal deep vein thrombosis with no difference in major bleeding events. However, 31% of patients receiving enoxaparin still suffered a deep vein thrombosis. Therefore, although enoxaparin is superior to low-dose heparin in this respect, it does not eliminate the risk of venous thromboembolism.[18,29] At this time, the ACCP recommends prophylaxis based on the individual patient and his or her risk factors. Low molecular weight heparin (see Table 5.2) may be used if anticoagulant prophylaxis is indicated, and low-dose heparin should not be considered (see Chapter 9).

MEDICAL CONDITIONS

The use of anticoagulation prophylaxis in hospitalized medical patients has not been evaluated to a significant degree. The risk of developing a venous thromboembolism is dependent on a variety of factors, such as disease states and patient risk factors. Patients with myocardial infarction and those with ischemic stroke have been the two populations most frequently studied. In patients with an acute myocardial infarction who are not treated with anticoagulants, deep vein thrombosis has been reported to occur in 17–38% within 72 hours and in 50–60% within 5–7 days. Low-dose and adjusted-dose UFH to prolong the aPTT ratio to 1.5–2.5 have both been associated with reductions in the incidence of deep vein thrombosis after an acute myocardial infarction with similar efficacy. Therefore, if a patient with an acute myocardial infarction does not receive full anticoagulation with UFH, low-dose heparin should be considered (see Table 5.2).[18,30] Patients suffering from ischemic stroke have a 63% incidence of deep vein thrombosis, which most commonly originates in the paralytic extremity. Low-dose heparin and dalteparin 2500 units subcutaneously twice daily have been found to reduce the risk of deep vein thrombosis, without an increase in bleeding episodes. Danaparoid 750 units subcutaneously twice daily has similar or superior efficacy to low-dose heparin with no difference in the rate of hemorrhagic transformation of the stroke. Therefore, prophylaxis with low-dose heparin, LMWH, or danaparoid can be considered in patients with lower extremity paralysis.[18,31] Trials in individuals with medical conditions other than myocardial infarction or ischemic stroke are limited. In patients with congestive heart failure, low-dose heparin was efficacious and reduced the incidence of deep vein thrombosis. Other trials have compared LMWH to low-dose heparin and found they were similar in efficacy and safety. Enoxaparin has been effective in doses of 20–60 mg subcutaneously daily, without an increased risk of bleeding events. Due to the lack of evidence, the ACCP recommends assessing the patient risk factors for developing venous thromboembolism and treating accordingly. Adequate treatment options would include low-dose heparin or LMWH (see Table 5.2).[18,32] (For more information, see Chapter 9.)

Treatment of venous thromboembolism (see Chapter 10)

Unfractionated heparin has been used in the treatment of acute venous thromboembolism since its efficacy was established in 1960. It has been effective in the treatment of calf and proximal deep vein thrombosis, and pulmonary embolism. In 1972, the relationship between achieving a therapeutic aPTT value and the risk of recurrent venous thromboembolic events was established. This was confirmed in a trial in 1992 that found that, if the minimum therapeutic APPT ratio was not achieved, symptomatic venous thromboembolic events recurred in 20–25% of the patients. However, in patients achieving at least an aPTT ratio of 1.5, the recurrence rate was reduced to 5%.[1,10–12] The goals of initial anticoagulation in patients with acute deep vein thrombosis and pulmonary embolism are to prevent extension of the thrombus, pulmonary embolism, recurrent venous thromboembolic events, and long-term complications. The ACCP recommends that patients with an acute deep vein thrombosis or pulmonary embolism be treated with intravenous or adjusted-dose subcutaneous UFH to prolong the aPTT to a value that corresponds to a heparin level of 0.2–0.4 U/mL by protamine titration or an antifactor Xa activity of 0.3–0.6 U/mL.[10] Generally, a continuous infusion of UFH is easier to administer and titrate and is usually the route employed, although, regardless of the route of administration, the patient will need to be hospitalized for UFH therapy due to the monitoring involved to assure an optimal degree of anticoagulation. Dosages of UFH are discussed above, and Figs 5.1 and 5.2 contain algorithms for adjusting and monitoring continuous intravenous infusions of UFH. The advantage the weight-based algorithm has over standard dosing is a higher proportion of patients achieving therapeutic aPTT values within 24 hours of initiating therapy, which leads to fewer recurrent venous thromboembolic events.[2,10,13] The optimal duration of UFH therapy has been previously evaluated, and it was found that short courses of UFH for 4–5 days had an effect on the recurrence rate similar to that of longer durations of 9–10 days. Currently, it is recommended by the ACCP that UFH therapy be continued for at least 5 days, followed by oral anticoagulant therapy.[1,10–12] Oral anticoagulants can be started with the initiation of UFH therapy, and should overlap with UFH for 4–5 days and at least 2 days when the International Normalized Ratio (INR) is in the therapeutic range.[10]

The LMWHs, enoxaparin and dalteparin, and danaparoid have been evaluated for the initial treatment of acute deep vein thrombosis. The LMWHs have been evaluated as subcutaneous regimens that are dosed according to weight and administered every 12–24 hours. Enoxaparin at a subcutaneous dose of 1 mg/kg every 12 hours has been found to be equally efficacious and safe compared to adjusted-dose continuous infusions of UFH. Dosage regimens of dalteparin from 100 units/kg subcutaneously every 12 hours to 200 units/kg subcutaneously once daily have shown similar clinical efficacy in direct comparisons and both have been comparable to UFH therapy.[7,33] Danaparoid, 2000 units intravenous bolus followed by 2000 units subcutaneously twice daily, was superior to adjusted-dose UFH as a continuous infusion in reducing the recurrence or extension of venous thromboembolism. However, only 5 of the 209 patients enrolled in the trial actually had a recurrent event; therefore, due to the low incidence, no comparison was made between danaparoid and UFH. More trials evaluating the use of danaparoid in acute deep vein thrombosis or pulmonary embolism are needed before definite recommendations can be made.[34] At this time, enoxaparin is the only LMWH recommended by the FDA for the treatment of these conditions. Dosage recommendations are listed in Table 5.2.

Due to the advantages of a predictable anticoagulant response with no monitoring of the anticoagulant effect, subcutaneous administration, and dosing every 12–24 hours, the LMWHs have been evaluated for the outpatient treatment of proximal deep vein thrombosis. The only LMWH available in the USA that has been studied in an outpatient setting is enoxaparin. At a subcutaneous dose of 1 mg/kg every 12 hours administered at home, it was found to be as efficacious and safe as a continuous infusion of UFH in hospitalized patients.[35] Patients who receive outpatient LMWHs are started on oral anticoagulants at the same time as the LMWH or on the second day of treatment with the INR monitored daily. When the patient has received at least 5 days of therapy and the INR is therapeutic (INR 2.0–3.0) for at least 2 consecutive days, treatment with the LMWH is discontinued.[33,35–7]

The utility of LMWH in the acute treatment of pulmonary embolism is less well established. Enoxaparin has been evaluated in noncomparative trials for the treatment of patients with acute pulmonary embolism in a wide range of dosage regimens. Dalteparin has been shown in small trials to be as effective and safe as an adjusted-dose, continuous infusion of UFH. Both enoxaparin and dalteparin have been evaluated intravenously and subcutaneously, as well as with adjusted doses according to antifactor Xa activity or in fixed doses. The ACCP only recommends the use of LMWH in stable patients with a pulmonary embolism, whereas adjusted-dose UFH is recommended in all patients with a pulmonary embolism.[10,38]

Typically, after initial anticoagulation with UFH or LMWH, a patient with a deep vein thrombosis or pulmonary embolism is continued on oral anticoagulants, warfarin adjusted to an INR of 2.0–3.0, for at least 3–6 months. Occasionally, a patient may have a contraindication to warfarin and an alternative agent is needed for secondary prevention of recurrent deep vein thrombosis or pulmonary embolism. Trials evaluating the use of UFH for secondary prophylaxis of recurrent thrombotic events have found that low-dose heparin is inferior to adjusted-dose warfarin. However, UFH given subcutaneously every 12 hours and adjusted to an aPTT ratio of at least 1.5 at 6 hours after the dose has been shown to be as efficacious at preventing recurrent events as warfarin therapy.[39] Due to the difficulties with monitoring adjusted-dose subcutaneous UFH and to evaluate another alternative to warfarin, LMWHs have also been studied in comparative trials in the secondary prevention of recurrent venous thromboembolism. Enoxaparin 40 mg subcutaneously daily and dalteparin 5000 units subcutaneously daily were found to be as effective as warfarin at preventing recurrent venous thromboembolic events, with fewer or similar bleeding complications.[40,41] Dalteparin 5000 units subcutaneously twice daily was also found to be as efficacious at preventing recurrences as UFH 10 000 units subcutaneously twice daily, with a trend toward a lower incidence of vertebral fractures in the dalteparin group ($p = 0.054$).[42] Therefore, in patients in whom warfarin is contraindicated and secondary prophylaxis is needed after an acute venous thromboembolic event, reasonable alternatives include adjusted-dose subcutaneous UFH, enoxaparin, or dalteparin.[10] Dosages of these agents are listed in Table 5.2.

To summarize, for the treatment of acute deep vein thrombosis, the LMWHs are a reasonable alternative to UFH, with the potential for outpatient therapy in selected patients. If UFH is employed, a reasonable bolus dose and infusion (Figs. 5.1 and 5.2) should be used due to the importance of achieving an adequate aPTT value within a 24-hour period. Patients should also have aPTT measurements performed at least daily to ensure a therapeutic level throughout treatment with UFH. After acute treatment with either UFH or LMWH, patients should receive oral anticoagulants for at least 3–6 months. If warfarin is contraindicated, adjusted-dose subcutaneous UFH or LMWH may be substituted (see Table 5.2).

Acute coronary syndromes (see Chapter 20)

Anticoagulants have been used for acute coronary syndromes, unstable angina, non-Q-wave (NQW) myocardial infarction, and Q-wave myocardial infarction for approximately 50 years. In unstable angina and NQW myocardial infarction, UFH helps prevent myocardial infarction and recurrent angina. Compared to aspirin alone, UFH more effectively controls recurrent refactory angina in unstable angina and NQW myocardial infarction, but if the patient is not on concurrent aspirin therapy, rebound angina may result when UFH is discontinued. Trials have shown that the combination of UFH and aspirin conveys an additive benefit and is superior to either agent alone. The ACCP and AHCPR recommend an intravenous infusion of UFH adjusted to an aPTT ratio of 1.5–2.5 in patients presenting with unstable angina or NQW myocardial infarction, as well as initiation of long-term aspirin therapy (Table 5.3).[16,30]

Table 5.3 *Dosages in acute coronary syndromes*[4,16,17,29,45]

Indication	Agent and dose
Unstable angina or NQWMI	Adjusted-dose CI UFH to a therapeutic aPTT[a] × 3–5 days[b] Enoxaparin 1 mg/kg SC BID[b,c] Dalteparin 120 U/kg SC BID[b,c]

Myocardial infarction rt-PA or reteplase	Adjusted-dose CI UFH to a therapeutic aPTT[a] × 48 hours then re-evaluate:[b,d]
	  high risk:[e] continue CI UFH, change to adjusted-dose SC UFH, or warfarin[b,f]
	  others: discontinue or UFH 7500 U SC Q 12 hours[b]

SK or APSAC	High risk:[e] adjusted-dose CI UFH[g] to a therapeutic aPTT[a] × 48 hours then change to adjusted-dose subcutaneousUFH or warfarin[b,f] others: UFH 7500 U SC Q 12 hours[b]
No thrombolytics	High risk:[e] adjusted-dose CI UFH to a therapeutic aPTT[a] × 48 hours then change to warfarin[f] for 3 months[b] others: UFH 7500 U SC Q 12 hours[b]

[a]aPTT value = heparin level of 0.2–0.4 U/mL or antifactor Xa activity of 0.3–0.7 U/mL.
[b]Recommended in the 1998 American College of Chest Physicians (ACCP) supplement.
[c]FDA-approved indication for LMWH or danaparoid.
[d]Start at the same time as the rt-PA or reteplase infusion.
[e]High risk: large or anterior myocardial infarction, atrial fibrillation, previous systemic embolus, known left ventricular thrombus, left ventricular dysfunction, or congestive heart failure.
[f]Adjusted to an INR of 2.0–3.0.
[g]Start at least 4 hours after the infusion and when aPTT ratio < 2.0 (or heparin level < 0.2 U/mL).

NQWMI = non-Q-wave myocardial infarction; CI = continuous infusion; UFH = unfractionated heparin; aPTT = activated partial thromboplastin time; SC = subcutaneous; BID = twice daily; U = units; rt-PA = alteplase; Q = every; SK = streptokinase; APSAC = anisoylated plasminogen streptokinase activator complex; LMWH = low molecular weight heparin; INR = International Normalized Ratio.

Dalteparin and enoxaparin have been evaluated in the treatment of unstable angina and NQW myocardial infarction as potential alternatives to UFH. Dalteparin 120 units/kg subcutaneously twice daily plus aspirin have been shown to be more effective than aspirin alone and equally efficacious to a continuous infusion of UFH (adjusted to an aPTT ratio of 1.5), without an increase in bleeding complicatons.[43,44] Additionally, enoxaparin 1 mg/kg subcutaneously every 12 hours plus aspirin have been proven to be superior to UFH (adjusted to an aPTT value of 55–85 seconds) plus aspirin in the treatment of unstable angina or NQW myocardial infarction. Total bleeding episodes were significantly higher in the enoxaparin group compared to UFH, mainly due to more injection site hematomas.[45] Additional comparison trials of enoxaparin and UFH are currently underway. Enoxaparin and dalteparin have been approved by the FDA for the treatment of unstable angina and NQW myocardial infarction.[19,46] Trials have also evaluated prolonged therapy for 45 days after unstable angina or NQW myocardial infarction with dalteparin 7500 units subcutaneously daily plus aspirin versus aspirin alone. The results have been conflicting in terms of the added benefit and the bleeding risk of prolonged LMWH therapy, and additional trials are needed before extending therapy with LMWH can be advocated.[43,44] The doses of LMWH studied in unstable angina and NQW myocardial infarction are listed in Table 5.3. (For more information, see Chapter 20.)

Unfractionated heparin is one of the standard therapies in the management of myocardial infarction. In patients with an acute Q-wave myocardial infarction who do not receive thrombolytic agents, UFH has been shown to reduce mortality by 35% and reinfarction by 15%.[30] In addition, the risk of stroke is increased in Q-wave myocardial infarction patients due to the potential for systemic embolism from the formation of a left ventricular thrombus. Risk factors for systemic embolism include a large or anterior Q-wave myocardial infarction, atrial fibrillation, left ventricular dysfunction, congestive heart failure, a prior history of systemic embolism, and evidence of a left ventricular thrombus. Trials with UFH have suggested that early therapy can reduce the incidence of systemic embolism and perhaps the formation of a mural thrombus. The ACC/AHA and the ACCP recommend the use of a continuous infusion of UFH (Fig. 5.3) adjusted to an aPTT ratio of 1.5–2.0 in patients who are considered at high risk for the development of a mural thrombus or systemic embolism and do not receive thrombolytic agents. In other patients not considered at high risk, the AHA/ACC and ACCP recommend UFH therapy at no less that 7500 units subcutaneously every 12 hours (Table 5.3).[17,30]

The other area of study with UFH in Q-wave myocardial infarction has been the use of UFH with thrombolytic agents. Clinical trials with streptokinase and anisoylated plasminogen streptokinase activator complex (APSAC) have not shown an additional benefit with the concurrent administration of UFH, but have shown increased bleeding events. However, studies with rt-PA (alteplase) and UFH have found increased patency rates after successful thrombolysis of occluded vessels, with no effect on clinical outcomes. Therefore, the recommendations of the ACCP and ACC/AHA for streptokinase and APSAC administration is to use weight-based UFH (Fig. 5.3) as a continuous infusion to an aPTT ratio of 1.5–2.0 in patients who are at high risk of a systemic embolism (Table 5.3). UFH should not be started until at least 4 hours after the thrombolytic infusion ends and when an aPTT ratio is documented to be less than 2.0, and UFH therapy should continue for at least 48 hours. For rt-PA and reteplase, weight-based UFH (Fig. 5.3) as a continuous infusion adjusted to an aPTT ratio of 1.5–2.0 should be used in all patients (Table 5.3). It is recommended that UFH be started at the same time as rt-PA or reteplase and should continue for at least 48 hours. At the end of 48 hours, adjusted-dose UFH, subcutaneously or intravenously, to an aPTT ratio of 1.5–2.0 or conversion to warfarin (INR 2.0–3.0) should be continued in patients who are at high risk for systemic embolism. In patients who are not at high risk of systemic embolism, the UFH can be discontinued or switched to low-dose heparin (Table 5. 3).[17,30,47]

The LMWHs have not been studied as extensively in Q-wave myocardial infarction as they have been in unstable angina and NQW myocardial infarction. One trial in patients with an acute anterior myocardial infarction found that treatment with dalteparin, 150 units/kg subcutaneously every 12 hours, resulted in a significant reduction in left ventricular thrombus formation compared to placebo. However, there was no difference in arterial embolism, reinfarction, or mortality, and patients treated with dalteparin also had significantly more major and minor bleeding events.[48] Prolonged therapy for 25 days after a myocardial infarction with enoxaparin 40 mg subcutaneously once daily after acute treatment with streptokinase, aspirin, and intravenous UFH has been evaluated in one trial. At 6 months, the patients assigned to enoxaparin therapy had a significant reduction in reinfarction rates compared to the placebo group, and bleeding events were similar between the two groups.[49] The few trials evaluating LMWH in acute myocardial infarction indicate they may be as efficacious as UFH; however, more trials are needed before a recommendation can be made.

Acute ischemic stroke

Low-dose UFH and LMWH are widely used following acute ischemic stroke for the prophylaxis of deep vein thrombosis and pulmonary embolism with a reduction in risk of approximately 60%. The risks involved with full anticoagulation in stroke patients include hemorrhagic transformation of the infarct and hemorrhagic stroke that can result in increased morbidity and mortality. However, there are specific indications for which the use of full anticoagulation is suggested to prevent the progression or recurrence of ischemic stroke. The ACCP recommends the consideration of intravenous UFH for 3–5 days for the treatment of acute cardioembolic stroke, large artery atherosclerotic ischemic stroke, or progressive deterioration of acute ischemic stroke (due to ongoing thromboembolism). A brain imaging study should be completed prior to initiation of UFH to exclude intracranial hemorrhage or a hemorrhagic transformation of the ischemic stroke and to estimate the infarct size. In patients with a large infarct, uncontrolled hypertension, or bleeding disorders, UFH should be avoided.[50]

Clinical trials evaluating LMWH in the treatment of acute ischemic stroke are limited. Nadroparin (not currently available in the USA), given as two subcutaneous doses daily within 48 hours of the onset of stroke symptoms, was shown to be significantly more effective at reducing death and dependency at 6 months compared to placebo, without an increase in bleeding events or hemorrhagic transformation of the infarct. However, a larger trial did not confirm these findings. Before the use of LMWH in the acute treatment of ischemic stroke can be recommended, more clinical studies are needed to confirm the benefit.[50,51] Danaparoid has been evaluated in the acute treatment of ischemic stroke started within 24 hours of stroke onset. It was given as an intravenous bolus followed by a continuous infusion adjusted to an anti-factor Xa activity of 0.6–0.8 U/mL. A benefit with danaparoid was initially witnessed at 7 days in patients classified as having a very favorable outcome; however, no difference was subsequently seen at 3 months. More episodes of major bleeding and more serious brain bleeding occurred in the danaparoid group compared to placebo. Nonetheless, no significant difference in symptomatic hemorrhagic transformations of the infarct was witnessed.[52] More trials are needed to evaluate danaparoid's utility in acute ischemic stroke before it can be recommended.

Anticoagulation in pregnancy

Various indications necessitate the use of anticoagulants in pregnancy, including the treatment and prophylaxis of venous thromboembolic events, the prevention of systemic embolism with prosthetic heart valves, the prevention of pregnancy loss and fetal complications with antiphospholipid syndrome, and inherited and acquired hypercoagulable states (e.g., activated protein C resistance, protein C deficiency, protein S deficiency). Currently, the recommended anticoagulant in pregnant women is UFH. It does not cross the placenta and has not been associated with fetal defects or bleeding. Adjusted-dose subcutaneous UFH is generally used and is administered every 12 hours, with a goal mid-interval aPTT ratio of 1.5–2.0 for venous thromboembolism and at least 2.0 for mechanical heart valves, as recommended by the ACCP. The risk of major bleeding to the mother with UFH is 2%, which is similar to that of non-pregnant individuals. At the time of delivery, adjusted-dose subcutaneous UFH has been associated with a persistent anticoagulant effect lasting up to 28 hours after the last injection, due to an unknown mechanism. The ACCP recommends either discontinuing UFH 24 hours prior to an elective delivery or monitoring the aPTT and using protamine as needed if spontaneous labor occurs. Additional concerns with the use of UFH during pregnancy are the risks to the mother of developing thrombocytopenia or osteoporosis. Experience with UFH in pregnancy has been associated with a vertebral fracture rate of approximately 2%, and a partially reversible reduction in bone density in 33% of women with treatment for more than 1 month. After delivery, either warfarin or UFH may be used and both are safe if breast-feeding (see Chapter 16).[53]

Low molecular weight heparins have been used in place of UFH in some pregnant women due to the fact that it is associated with reduced likelihood of developing thrombocytopenia, possibly less osteoporosis, there is no need to monitor the anticoagulant effect, and it can be given in daily doses. Like UFH, LMWH does not cross the placenta and has not been associated with fetal defects or bleeding. Evidence supporting the use of LMWH in pregnancy is limited to small trials and retrospective reports. Enoxaparin 40 mg subcutaneously daily and dalteparin 5000 units subcutaneously once to twice daily have been efficacious in the prevention of thrombotic events and have not produced an additional bleeding risk to the mother or fetus. From the available data, no cases of thrombocytopenia and one report of a symptomatic fracture with prolonged LMWH use have been reported. The incidence of asymptomatic osteopenia or osteoporosis was not assessed in all studies. Therefore, LMWHs may be an alternative to UFH in pregnant women and offer advantages of daily dosing and no monitoring of the anticoagulant effect; however, the risk of osteoporosis with LMWH remains to be defined. More trials are needed to establish dosages for the LMWHs and to compare their efficacy and safety to those of UFH before they can be considered as a first-line anticoagulant in pregnant women (see Chapter 16).[53–6]

MONITORING

When anticoagulating with UFH, a baseline aPTT, PT, INR, and complete blood count (including hematocrit and platelets) should be measured. The aPTT is recommended to be monitored every 6 hours after starting an infusion of UFH or changing the dosage, until it is within the desired therapeutic range. Once optimal anticoagulation is achieved, the aPTT should be measured at least daily. In patients receiving adjusted-dose subcutaneous UFH, the aPTT should be measured at the midpoint of the dosing interval, which is usually 6 hours after the injection is given. A complete blood count, urinalysis, and stool occult blood tests should be monitored periodically throughout therapy. Periodic assessments of the aPTT value should be done with low-dose heparin therapy, in addition to complete blood counts, urinalysis, and stool occult blood tests.[2,10] Signs and symptoms of bleeding should also be monitored throughout therapy and, if bleeding should occur, UFH should be discontinued and protamine administration should be considered.

With the LMWHs and danaparoid, monitoring of coagulation parameters is not necessary due to their predictable anticoagulant response and the lack of prolongation of the aPTT ratio at therapeutic doses. However, when used in patients with renal insufficiency, monitoring of plasma antifactor Xa levels (goal 0.5–0.8 U/mL) for dose adjustment is recommended due to a reduction in their renal elimination and more prolonged anticoagulant activity.[4] Besides monitoring antifactor Xa levels in renal insufficiency, the manufacturer of danaparoid also recommends monitoring in patients weighing more than 90 kg. In addition, a baseline and periodic assessments of a complete blood count (including hematocrit and platelets), urinalysis, and stool occult blood tests are recommended throughout therapy with LMWH or danaparoid.[5,6–9] Patients should also be monitored for signs and symptoms of bleeding.

ADVERSE EFFECTS

Bleeding

Because all of the agents inhibit blood coagulation, hemorrhagic events are one of the potential side-effects of UFH, LMWH, and danaparoid. UFH also has the property of impairing platelet function, which has the potential further to increase the risk of bleeding. The incidence of hemorrhage with treatment with UFH is influenced by different factors, such as the patient's anticoagulant response, the route of administration, patient factors, and the concurrent use of aspirin or thrombolytics. In general, bleeding is more likely to occur when UFH is given in therapeutic doses versus low prophylactic doses. Based on indirect evidence, the risk of hemorrhage may be greater with escalating doses and with increasing and excessively prolonged aPTT values. However, the link between higher doses and more intense anticoagulation response is not conclusive, and bleeding can occur with low doses of UFH and therapeutic aPTTs. Meta-analyses have shown a lower incidence of hemorrhagic events with continuous infusion UFH (6.8%) compared to intermittent intravenous UFH (14.2%, odds ratio, OR, 0.4, $p = 0.01$). However, a higher 24-hour dose of UFH was administered to the patients receiving intermittent intravenous injections, which may contribute to the findings. When the bleeding rates of subcutaneous versus continuous infusion were compared, a similar incidence of bleeding was reported (4.3% and 4.4%, respectively). Patient characteristics, such as recent surgery or trauma, renal failure, and age over 70 years, are also believed to contribute to the risk of bleeding with UFH administration. The concurrent use of aspirin has been shown to increase the risk of perioperative and postoperative bleeding in patients undergoing open heart surgery; however, the combination of aspirin and UFH for acute coronary syndromes has not been shown to be associated with a higher rate of hemorrhagic complications. When UFH is administered with thrombolytic therapy, there is an increased risk of bleeding, but not a higher incidence of fatal hemorrhage. In the thrombolytic trials in which UFH was used, subgroup analyses have suggested that the risk of intracranial bleed is related to the aPTT value, especially values exceeding 80 seconds. When UFH is given without thrombolytics in acute coronary syndromes, there is not a higher risk of hemorrhage. In venous thromboembolic events, the rate of major bleeding with either continuous infusion or adjusted-dose UFH is similar and reported as less than 5%. Low-dose heparin regimens have not been associated with fatal hemorrhagic events, and no difference in terms of bleeding events has been found between dosing UFH every 8 or 12 hours. The more common bleeding event with low-dose heparin is injection site hematomas.[1,57]

In summary, when UFH is used, it is important that patients are evaluated for risk factors predisposing them to bleeding, monitored for signs and symptoms of hemorrhage, and have the aPTT value evaluated routinely to avoid excessive anticoagulation. If bleeding should occur, UFH should be discontinued and the anticoagulant effects can be reversed with the administration of protamine. The dose of protamine is based on the quantity of UFH received in the preceding 4 hours, with 1 mg of protamine given for every 100 units of UFH.[1,58]

When the LMWHs and danaparoid were first introduced, they were postulated to cause less bleeding than UFH due to their greater specificity for inhibition of factor Xa and lack of impairment of platelet function. However, clinical trials have not conclusively confirmed this. Comparative trials have shown that LMWHs have an incidence of bleeding events that is similar or slightly lower than that of UFH, and the limited trials with danaparoid have shown comparable rates with UFH and the LMWHs. The risk of bleeding is dose related with the LMWHs and danaparoid and is increased with concomitant therapy with aspirin and nonsteroidal anti-inflammatory agents. Because the LMWHs and danaparoid are currently marketed for subcutaneous administration, it is not surprising that one of the more frequent side-effects is injection-site hematomas, which are reported to occur in up to 7% of patients.[5-9] Therefore, like to UFH, patients treated with LMWH or danaparoid should be screened for risk factors placing them at higher risk of bleeding events and monitored for signs or symptoms of hemorrhage. If bleeding should occur, the anticoagulant agent should be stopped immediately. Currently, there are no antidotes to neutralize the anticoagulant effect of danaparoid.[5] For the LMWHs, the antifactor IIa effects are neutralized by protamine, but some of the antifactor Xa activity still persists. Protamine is recommended in patients with bleeding who are receiving LMWH, but other supportive measures such as fresh frozen plasma should be readily available.[3]

Recently, the LMWHs have been reported to cause epidural or spinal hematomas in patients undergoing epidural or spinal anesthesia or spinal puncture. Recommendations have been suggested for patients receiving preoperative LMWH to avert this side-effect:

• avoid regional anesthesia in patients with an abnormal bleeding history or receiving medications known to affect hemostasis;

- delay insertion of the spinal needle for 10–12 hours after the LMWH dose;
- avoid regional anesthesia in patients with a hemorrhagic aspirate during placement of the spinal needle;
- consider the use of a single-dose anesthetic rather than continuous epidural anesthesia;
- leave the epidural catheter indwelling overnight and remove it the next day;
- delay subsequent doses of LMWH for at least 2 hours after spinal needle placement or catheter removal (postoperative LMWH should be also delayed at least 2 hours after catheter removal);
- be cautious with the initiation of LMWH in a patient with an indwelling catheter.

All patients who receive LMWH with regional anesthesia or undergoing a spinal puncture should have their neurologic status monitored, particularly for signs of cord compression.[18]

Thrombocytopenia

Two different forms of thrombocytopenia can occur with the use of UFH. Heparin-induced thrombocytopenia type 1 occurs within 1–5 days after the initiation of UFH, resolves within 4 days without the discontinuation UFH, and is not associated with any adverse clinical events. Conversely, heparin-induced thrombocytopenia type 2 (HIT) is a more serious occurrence that can be associated with arterial or venous thrombotic events in up to 60% of patients. HIT occurs in approximately 3% of patients treated with UFH and is an IgG-immune-mediated phenomenon. The IgG antibodies form a complex with UFH and platelet factor 4 that can bind to platelets, leading to platelet aggregation and thrombocytopenia. Typically, platelet values begin to fall 5–15 days after the initiation of UFH, but may be witnessed within hours if the patient has previously received UFH. Platelet counts are usually reduced to $20–150 \times 10^9/L$, but a reduction in the platelet count of greater than 40% from baseline is also suspicious for HIT. In addition, there have been cases of HIT presenting as thrombotic events with minimal reduction in platelet counts but the demonstration of heparin-induced antibodies. The treatment for HIT is the immediate discontinuation of UFH. With discontinuation, platelet counts return to normal in 90% of patients within 1 week. If the patient requires further anticoagulation, an agent with low cross-reactivity with heparin-induced antibodies should be used, such as danaparoid, argotroban, or lepirudin.[2,3,5] Warfarin should not be used alone to treat HIT due to the risk of venous limb gangrene. The ACCP recommends waiting to initiate warfarin until the platelet count is greater than $100 \times 10^9/L$ and the patient is adequately anticoagulated with danaparoid or lepirudin.[2] (For more information, see Chapter 14.)

Low molecular weight heparins can also cause thrombocytopenia, but the incidence is much lower than with UFH. The early, transient, benign thrombocytopenia is seen in approximately 5% of patients treated with LMWH, and the immune-mediated thrombocytopenia has been reported in less than 1% of patients. However, when LMWHs are used in patients with active or prior HIT, the thrombocytopenia may be reproduced. The LMWHs have a reported cross-reactivity in HIT of more than 90% (see Table 5.1).[2,3,6,7] The cross-reactivity with danaparoid in patients with HIT is much lower, at less than 5%, and danaparoid has been used successfully to anticoagulate patients with HIT without further bleeding or thrombotic events and an increase in platelet counts in 80% of patients (see Table 5.1). Other anticoagulants that can be used in patients with HIT are lepirudin and argatroban; however, only lepirudin is available in the USA at the time of writing.[5] The recommended dosages of danaparoid in HIT are listed in Table 5.2.

Osteoporosis (see Chapter 14)

Another side-effect of UFH is osteoporosis. The mechanism by which UFH causes osteoporosis is not known, but may be related to the dose and duration of therapy. Manifestations of heparin-induced osteoporosis range from bone pain with or without radiologic findings (e.g., rib fractures, vertebral collapse) to asymptomatic osteopenia and low bone densities.[2] Symptomatic fractures have been reported in 2% of patients and an asymptomatic reduction in bone density has been found in one-third of patients receiving UFH for more than 1 month.[53] The incidence of osteoporosis with LMWH appears to be lower than with UFH, but there is not sufficient evidence to confirm the effect of LMWH on bone density. One trial compared dalteparin 5000 units subcutaneously twice daily and UFH 10 000 units subcutaneously twice daily for 3–6 months and found a trend toward fewer spinal fractures in the dalteparin group (2.6% versus 17.6% with UFH, $p = 0.054$). A trial involving enoxaparin 40 mg subcutaneously daily demonstrated a reduction in bone density of greater than one standard deviation with prolonged treatment during pregnancy in 29% of the women. However, this finding is flawed, because no baseline measurement of bone density was completed and 78% of patients had previously received UFH therapy.[55] Despite these findings, there are data demonstrating the safety of the use of LMWH in patients with heparin-induced osteoporosis.[4,7] Information on the use of danaparoid has not shown any cases of osteoporosis with use for 3 or more months.[5] In summary, individuals who receive prolonged UFH therapy have a significant risk for developing osteoporosis, and the incidence with LMWH and danaparoid needs to be evaluated further.

Other adverse reactions

Dermatologic reactions are possible with the administration of UFH, LMWH, and danaparoid. Unfractionated heparin has been associated with urticaria, erythematous papules and plaques, and skin necrosis, which are usually located at the site of the injection. The most serious of the dermatologic reactions with UFH is skin necrosis, which is believed to be immune related due to the delayed onset of 5 days after the injection. Patients experiencing delayed skin necrosis are also at risk of more serious adverse events, such as HIT.[2] Enoxaparin, dalteparin, and ardeparin have also been reported to cause skin reactions that are generally at the site of injection, and danaparoid has been associated with skin rash in 0.9% of patients.[1,2,5–8] UFH, LMWHs, and danaparoid have been reported to cause hypersensitivity reactions consisting of a variety of symptoms including urticaria, rash, pruritis, edema, asthma, and tachypnea.[1,2,5,6,8]

Other adverse events that have been associated with UFH therapy include alopecia and hypoaldosteronism. Heparin-induced hypoaldosteronism has been reported rarely, and usually patients have presented with hyperkalemia and metabolic changes.[1,2]

The LMWHs and, rarely, UFH have been associated with asymptomatic, transient increases in liver transaminases – alanine aminotransferase (ALT) and aspartate aminotransferase (AST). With discontinuation of the LMWH, the elevations have returned to normal values, without any further hepatic damage. The transient increases in the liver transaminases have been reported to occur in 2–9% of patients receiving enoxaparin, dalteparin, or ardeparin.[6–8] Thus far, no such reports of elevations in liver function tests have been reported with the use of danaparoid.[5] The other side-effect associated with the LMWH and danaparoid has been pain at the site of injection.[6,8,9]

CONTRAINDICATIONS

Unfractionated heparin and the LMWHs are contraindicated in patients with evidence of heparin-induced thrombocytopenia.[5,6,8,58] In patients with severe renal or liver disease, the LMWHs should be used with caution, due to potential changes in the pharmacokinetic and pharmacodynamic parameters of the drugs.[8,58] No anticoagulant agent is recommended in patients with hemorrhagic diathesis, active major bleeding, or hypersensitivity to the product or sulfite or pork products. They should be used cautiously in diseases with increased risk of bleeding, such as severe uncontrolled hypertension, acute bacterial endocarditis, congenital or acquired bleeding disorders, active ulcerative gastrointestinal disease, hemorrhagic stroke, diabetic retinopathy, postcerebral, spinal, or ophthalmological surgery, or following epidural or spinal anesthesia or lumbar puncture.[5,8] The use of UFH or LMWH with platelet inhibitors, such as aspirin and nonsteroidal anti-inflammatory agents, should be done with caution due to an increased potential for bleeding complications.

CONCLUSION

Unfractionated heparin remains the treatment of choice for many indications due to its proven efficacy and experience with its use. With the introduction of the LMWHs and low molecular weight heparinoids, alternatives to UFH are now available. The use of UFH is limited by the need for monitoring when full anticoagulation is required, the lack of a predictable anticoagulant response, and side-effects such as bleeding, thrombocytopenia, and osteoporosis. The LMWHs and danaparoid offer many advantages over UFH, such as no monitoring of the anticoagulant effect, superior bioavailability, a predictable anticoagulant response, and less risk of developing thrombocytopenia and possibly osteoporosis.

REFERENCES

1 Hirsh J, Fuster V. Guide to anticoagulant therapy, Part 1: Heparin. *Circulation* 1994; **89**: 1449–68.

2 Hirsh J, Warkentin TE, Raschke R, et al. Heparin and low-molecular weight heparin: mechanism of action, pharmacokinetics, dosing considerations, monitoring, efficacy, and safety. *Chest* 1998 **114**: 489S–510S.

3 Nurmohamed MT, ten Cate H, ten Cate JW. Low molecular weight heparin(oid)s: clinical investigations and practical recommendations. *Drugs* 1997; **53**: 736–51.

4 Weitz JI. Low-molecular weight heparins. *N Engl J Med* 1997; **337**: 688–98.

5 Wilde MI, Markham A. Danaparoid: a review of its pharmacology and clinical use in the management of heparin-induced thrombocytopenia. Drugs 1997; **54**: 903–24.

6 Noble S, Peters DH, Goa KL. Enoxaparin: a reappraisal of its pharmacology and clinical applications in the prevention and treatment of thromboembolic disease. *Drugs* 1995; **119**: 388–410.

7 Howard PA. Dalteparin: a low-molecular weight heparin. *Ann Pharmacother* 1997; **31**: 192–203.

8 Package insert. Normiflo (ardeparin sodium). Philadelphia, PA: Wyeth Laboratories Inc., May 23, 1997.

9 Skoutakis VA. Danaparoid in the prevention of thromboembolic complications. *Ann Pharmacother* 1997; **31**: 876–87.

10 Hyers TM, Agnelli G, Hull RD, et al. Antithrombotic therapy for venous thromboembolic disease. *Chest* 1998; **114**: 561S-78S.

11 Kearon C. Drug trials that have influenced our practice in the treatment of venous thromboembolism. *Thromb Haemost* 1997; **78**: 553–7.

12 Valentine KA, Hull RD, Pineo GF. Low-molecular-weight heparin therapy and mortality. *Semin Thromb Hemost* 1997; **23**: 173–8.

13 Raschke RA, Reilly BM, Guidry JR, et al. The weight-based heparin dosing nomogram compared with a 'standard care' nomogram. *Ann Intern Med* 1993; **119**: 874–81.

14 Holliday DM, Watling SM, Yanos J. Heparin dosing in the morbidly obese patient. *Ann Pharmacother* 1994; **28**: 1110–11.

15 Nemeth JS, Marxen TL, Piltz GW. Weight-based protocol for improving heparin therapy. *Am J Health-Syst Pharm* 1996; **53**: 1164–6.

16 Braunwald E, Mark DB, Jones RH, et al. Unstable angina: diagnosis and management. Clinical Practice Guideline No. 10 (amended). Rockville, MD: Public Health Service, Agency for Health Care Policy and Research, National Heart, Lung, and Blood Institute. AHCPR Publication No. 94–0602; 1994.

17 Ryan TR, Anderson JL, Antman EM, et al. ACC/AHA guidelines for the management of patients with acute myocardial infarction. *J Am Coll Cardiol* 1996; **28**: 1328–428.

18 Clagett GP, Anderson FA, Geerts WH, et al. Prevention of venous thromboembolism. *Chest* 1998; **114**: 531S–60S.

19 Package insert. Fragmin (dalteparin sodium). Kalamazoo, MI: Pharmacia Upjohn Company, May 1999.

20 The RD Heparin Arthroplasty Group. RD heparin compared with warfarin for prevention of venous thromboembolic disease following total hip or knee arthroplasty. *J Bone Joint Surg [Am]* 1994; **76**: 1174–85.

21 Heit JA, Berkowitz SD, Bona R, et al. Efficacy and safety of low molecular weight heparin (ardeparin sodium) compared to warfarin for the prevention of venous thromboembolism after total knee replacement surgery: a double-blind, dose-ranging study. *Thromb Haemost* 1997; **77**: 32–8.

22 Kearon C, Hirsh J. Starting prophylaxis for venous thromboembolism postoperatively. *Arch Intern Med* 1995; **155**: 366–72.

23 Arcelus JI, Caprini JA, Traverso CI. Venous thromboembolism after hospital discharge. *Semin Thromb Hemost* 1993; **19(Suppl. 1)**: 142–6.

24 Planes A, Vochelle N, Darmon JY, et al. Risk of deep-venous thrombosis after hospital discharge in patients having undergone total hip replacement: double-blind randomised comparison of enoxaparin versus placebo. *Lancet* 1996; **348**: 224–8.

25 Bergqvist D, Benoni G, Björgell O, et al. Low-molecular weight heparin (enoxaparin) as prophylaxis against venous thromboembolism after total hip replacement. *N Engl J Med* 1996; **335**: 696–700.

26 Dahl OE, Andreassen G, Aspelin T, et al. Prolonged thromboprophylaxis following hip replacement surgery: results of a double-blind, prospective, randomised, placebo-controlled study with dalteparin (Fragmin®). *Thromb Haemost* 1997; **77**: 26–31.

27 Bergqvist D. Prolonged prophylaxis in postoperative medicine. *Semin Thromb Hemost* 1997; **23**: 149–54.

28 Harris S, Chen D, Green D. Enoxaparin for thromboembolism prophylaxis in spinal injury: preliminary report on experience with 105 patients. *Am J Phys Med Rehabil* 1996; **75**: 326–7.

29 Geerts WH, Jay RM, Code KI, et al. A comparison of low-dose heparin with low-molecular-weight heparin as prophylaxis against venous thromboembolism after major trauma. *N Engl J Med* 1996; **335**: 701–7.

30 Cairns JA, Theroux P, Lewis HD, et al. Antithrombotic agents in coronary heart disease. *Chest* 1998; **114**: 611S–33S.

31 Turpie AGG. Prophylaxis of venous thromboembolism in stroke patients. *Semin Thromb Hemost* 1997; **23**: 155–7.

32 Bergman JF, Neuhart E. A multicenter randomized double-blind study of enoxaparin compared with unfractionated heparin in the prevention of venous thromboembolic disease in elderly in-patients: the Enoxaparin in Medicine Study Group. *Thromb Haemost* 1996; **76**: 529–34.

33 Tuskstra F, Koopman MMW, Büller HR. The treatment of deep vein thrombosis and pulmonary embolism. *Thromb Haemost* 1997; **78**: 489–96.

34 de Valk HW, Banga JD, Wester JWJ, et al. Comparing subcutaneous danaparoid with intravenous unfractionated heparin for the treatment of venous thromboembolism: a randomized controlled trial. *Ann Intern Med* 1995; **123**: 1–9.

35 Levine M, Gent M, Hirsh J, et al. A comparison of low-molecular-weight heparin administered primarily at home with unfractionated heparin administered in the hospital for proximal deep-vein thrombosis. *N Engl J Med* 1996; **334**: 677–81.

36. Chaffee BJ. Low-molecular-weight heparins for treatment of deep vein thrombosis. *Am J Health-Syst Pharm* 1997; **54**: 1995–9.

37 Dedden P, Chang B, Nagel D. Pharmacy-managed program for home treatment of deep vein thrombosis with enoxaparin. *Am J Health-Syst Pharm* 1997; **54**: 1968–72.

38 Charland SL, Klinter DEJ. Low-molecular-weight heparins in the treatment of pulmonary embolism. *Ann Pharmacother* 1998; **32**: 258–64.

39 Pini M. Prevention of recurrences after deep venous thrombosis: role of low-molecular-weight heparins. *Semin Thromb Hemost* 1997; **23**: 51–4.

40 Pini M, Aiello S, Manotti C, et al. Low molecular weight heparin versus warfarin in the prevention of recurrences after deep vein thrombosis. *Thromb Haemost* 1994; **72**: 191–7.

41 Das SK, Cohen AT, Edmondson RA, et al. Low-molecular-weight heparin versus warfarin for prevention of recurrent venous thromboembolism: a randomized trial. *World J Surg* 1996; **20**: 521–7.

42 Monreal M, Lafoz E, Olive A, et al. Comparison of subcutaneous unfractionated heparin with a low molecular weight heparin (Fragmin®) in patients with venous thromboembolism and contraindications to coumarin. *Thromb Haemost* 1994; **71**: 7–11.

43 Fragmin During Instability in Coronary Artery Disease Study Group. Low-molecular-weight heparin during instability in coronary artery disease. *Lancet* 1996; **347**: 561–8.

44 Klein W, Buchwald A, Hillis SE, et al. Comparison of low-molecular-weight heparin with unfractionated heparin acutely and with placebo for 6 weeks in the management of unstable coronary artery disease. *Circulation* 1997; **96**: 61–8.

45 Cohen M, Demers C, Gurfinkel EP, et al. A comparison of low-molecular-weight heparin with unfractionated heparin for unstable coronary artery disease. *N Engl J Med* 1997; **337**: 447–52.

46 Spinler SA, Nawarskas JJ. Low-molecular-weight heparins for acute coronary syndromes. *Ann Pharmacother* 1998; **32**: 103–10.

47 Cairns JA, Kennedy JW, Fuster V. Coronary thrombolysis. *Chest* 1998; **114**: 634S–57S.

48 Kontny F, Dale J, Abildgaard U, Pedersen TR. Randomized trial of low molecular weight heparin (dalteparin) in prevention of left ventricular thrombus formation and arterial embolism after acute anterior myocardial infarction: the Fragmin in Acute Myocardial Infarction (FRAMI) study. *J Am Coll Cardiol* 1997; **30**: 962–9.

49. Glick A, Kornowski R, Michowich Y, et al. Reduction of reinfarction and angina with use of low-molecular-weight heparin after streptokinase (and heparin) in acute myocardial infarction. *Am J Cardiol* 1996; **77**: 1145–8.

50 Albers GW, Easton D, Sacco RL, Teal P. Antithrombotic and thrombolytic therapy for ischemic stroke. *Chest* 1998; **114**: 683S–98S.

51 Kay R, Wong KS, Yu YL, et al. Low-molecular-weight heparin for the treatment of acute ischemic stroke. *N Engl J Med* 1995; **333**: 1588–93.

52 The Publications Committee for the Trial of ORG 10172 in Acute Stroke Treatment (TOAST) Investigators. Low molecular weight heparinoid, ORG 10172 (danaparoid), and outcome after acute ischemic stroke: a randomized controlled trial. *JAMA* 1998; **279**: 1265–72.

53 Ginsberg JS, Hirsh J. Use of antithrombotic agents during pregnancy. *Chest* 1998; **114**: 524S–30S.

54 Hunt BJ, Doughty HA, Majumdar G, et al. Thromboprophylaxis with low molecular weight heparin (Fragmin) in high risk pregnancies. *Thromb Haemost* 1997; **77**: 39–43.

55 Nelson-Piercy C, Letsky EA, de Swiet M. Low-molecular weight heparin for obstetric thromboprophylaxis: experience of sixty-nine pregnancies in sixty-one women at high risk. *Am J Obstet Gynecol* 1997; **176**: 1062–8.

56 Dulitzki M, Pauzner R, Langevitz P, et al. Low-molecular-weight heparin during pregnancy and delivery: preliminary experience with 41 pregnancies. *Obstet Gynecol* 1996; **87**: 380–3.

57 Levine M, Raskob GE, Landefeld CS, Kearon C. Hemorrhagic complications of anticoagulant treatment. *Chest* 1998; **114**: 511S–23S.

58 Havrda DE, Anderson JR, Talbert RL. Thrombosis. In: Carter BL, Angaran DM, Lake KD, et al., eds *Pharmacotherapy Self-Assessment Program*, 3rd edn. Kansas City, MO: American College of Clinical Pharmacy, 1998: 207–60.

6

Antiplatelet therapy

JOSÉ A LÓPEZ, PERUMAL THIAGARAJAN

INTRODUCTION

The hemostatic system consists of platelets, the endothelial cells lining the vasculature, and the coagulation factors. The platelets arise from cytoplasmic fragmentation of megakaryocytes in the bone marrow and circulate in blood as disc-shaped, anucleate particles. The platelet membrane, which consists of a typical bilayer of phospholipids, contains membrane glycoproteins that interact with various ligands, either soluble ligands that activate the platelets, or fixed ligands within the vessel wall or on other cells through which the platelets adhere to these structures. One unique feature of the platelet is that its plasma membrane contains numerous invaginations into the platelet interior, connected to the exterior through small pores. This feature imparts upon the platelet a much greater surface area than would normally be found on such a small cell. Platelets also contain three types of granules, two of which are unique, the α granules and the dense granules. The α granules contain hemostatic proteins (e.g., fibrinogen, von Willebrand factor (vWf), and factor V) and growth factors (e.g., platelet-derived growth factor and transforming growth factor β). The dense granules are rich in adenosine diphosphate (ADP), Ca^{2+}, and serotonin. The contents of both types of granules are released when platelets become activated, and function to amplify the response to blood vessel injury, both by activating other platelets and by stimulating cells in the vessel wall to proliferate.

PLATELETS IN HEMOSTASIS AND THROMBOSIS

Under normal circumstances, thrombosis is prevented by the resistance of the lining endothelial cell layer to interaction with platelets. When the continuity of the endothelial layer is disrupted and the underlying matrix is exposed, a coordinated series of events is set in motion to seal the defect. Platelets play the primary role in this process. They first adhere to the exposed matrix through an interaction between the glycoprotein Ib-IX-V complex on their surface and vWf in the subendothelium. This first interaction, often called platelet adhesion, sets the stage for other adhesive reactions that allow the platelets essentially to plaster-over the vessel-wall defect. These other adhesive reactions involve platelet integrins such as the platelet glyco-protein IIb–IIIa complex ($\alpha_{IIb}\beta_3$), $\alpha_2\beta_1$, and $\alpha_1\beta_5$, which bind subendothelial matrix components such as fibrinogen, vWf, collagen, and fibronectin. The high fluid shear stresses brought about by vascular constriction favor the interaction of plasma vWf with glycoprotein Ib–IX–V on the circulating platelet, providing yet another mecha-nism for activating the platelet. This interaction and the interactions of other platelet agonists released from the granules or otherwise generated at the site of vascular injury activate platelets by transducing signals across their plasma membranes, thus increasing the cytoplasmic calcium concentration. This increased intraplatelet free calcium concentration, in turn, leads to a number of structural and functional changes of the platelet. Morphologically, the platelets change dramatically from discs to spiny spheres (a process called shape change). The granules are centralized and their contents discharged into the lumen of the open canalicular system, from which they are then released to the exterior (the release reaction). The long membrane projections put forth during the shape-change reaction allow the platelets to inter-act with one another to form an aggregate. This platelet–platelet interaction (platelet aggregation) is mediated by the glycoprotein IIb–IIIa complex, which bind plasma fibrinogen, a divalent protein capable of cross-linking platelets. On resting platelets, glycoprotein IIb–IIIa complexes are densely concentrated on the membrane, but unable to bind soluble fibrinogen until platelet activation converts them to compe-tent fibrinogen receptors.

Platelets, at the site of vascular injury, also have three major mechanisms to recruit additional platelets to the growing hemostatic plug. They release hemostatic proteins and platelet agonists, they synthesize proaggregatory prostaglandins, and they provide a negatively charged surface to catalyze coagulation reactions that ultimately generate thrombin, itself a potent platelet agonist. The release reaction discharges platelet granule contents to the exterior, thus increasing the local concen-trations of the hemostatic factors. ADP and other factors released from the dense granules activate nearby platelets and recruit them to the growing hemostatic plug. In addition, the increase in intraplatelet calcium stimulates membrane phospholi-pase A2 activity, which liberates arachidonic acid from membrane phospholipids. The arachidonic acid is then converted to cyclic endoperoxides by cyclo-oxygenase, and these are converted to thromboxane A2 by thromboxane synthase. Thrombox-ane A2 is a very potent platelet agonist. Thus, the release reaction and the prostaglandin synthesis act to consolidate the initial hemostatic plug by promoting the participation of other platelets in the reaction. When platelets are activated, negatively charged phospholipids move from the inner leaflet of the membrane bilayer to the outer leaflet. This negative surface provides a binding site for enzymes and cofactors of the coagulation system, which then efficiently generate thrombin.

Most stimuli activate platelets by binding to specific receptors on the platelet surface. Occupancy of these receptors leads a series of downstream events that ultimately increases the intracytoplasmic concentration of calcium ions. The receptors for strong agonists such as thrombin, thromboxane A2, and collagen are coupled to activation of phospholipase C. Phospholipase C converts phosphatidylinositol bisphosphate (PIP2) into diacylglycerol (DAG) and inositol triphosphate (IP3). The DAG activates protein kinase C while the IP3 liberates calcium from intracellular storage granules. Many weaker agonists such as ADP and epinephrine transduce signals predominantly by activating phospholipase A2, which leads to the production and secretion of thromboxane A2. Thromboxane A2 then binds its receptor on the surface of the same platelet or on a nearby platelet, activating phospholipase C. Thus, the activation of platelets by weak stimuli such as ADP and epinephrine depends on the prostaglandin synthesis, whereas stronger stimuli such as thrombin and thromboxane can activate platelets independently of prostaglandin synthesis (Fig. 6.1). This accounts for the susceptibility of activation by weak agonists to inhibition by aspirin (discussed below).

In the normal circulation, platelet activation is prevented by several endogenous inhibitors of platelets elaborated by the vessel wall. The primary inhibitors include

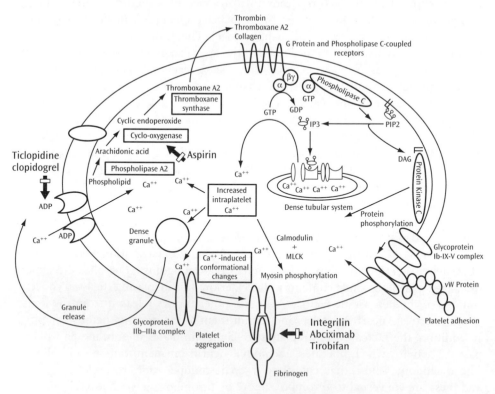

Figure 6.1 *Platelet activation by various ligands and its inhibition by commonly used antiplatelet drugs. (ADP, adenosine diphosphate; GTP, guanine triphosphate; GDP, guanine diphosphate; MLCK, myosin light chain kinase; DAG, diacylglycerol; IP3, inositol triphosphate; PIP2, phosphatidyl inositol biphosphate; vW, von Willebrand.)*

prostacyclin (a product of endothelial arachidonic acid metabolism) and nitric oxide. Prostacyclin binds to a specific receptor on the platelet surface and activates adenylyl cyclase, which converts adenosine triphosphate (ATP) to cyclic adenosine monophosphate (cAMP). Among its potent effects is the activation of protein kinase A, which phosphorylates several vital proteins on serine or threonine residues and alters their functions. Protein kinase A phosphorylates a calcium-dependent ATPase, an enzyme that sequesters calcium in the dense tubular system. Phosphorylation of phospholipase C prevents PIP2 hydrolysis and IP3 generation, further depressing cytoplasmic calcium levels. As intraplatelet free calcium mediates many of the activation responses, its sequestration leads to a quiescent state (Fig. 6.2). In addition, cAMP-dependent phosphorylation of the β chain of glycoprotein Ib prevents collagen-induced actin polymerization. A number of other proteins are also phosphorylated by protein kinase A, including myosin light chain kinase, actin-binding protein, and Ras-related protein Ib (Rap Ib). These changes undoubtedly affect platelet function.

Nitric oxide, which is formed in endothelial cells, diffuses into the platelets and activates soluble guanylyl cyclase, which converts guanosine triphosphate (GTP) to cyclic guanosine monophosphate (cGMP). Cyclic GMP acts synergistically with cAMP to inhibit calcium mobilization from stored granules and phosphatidylinositol hydrolysis. Both prostacyclin and nitric oxide inhibit platelet procoagulant activity.

Arterial thrombosis occurs at high flow rates and at sites of underlying arterial wall disease. Thrombi may be initiated by the rupture of arterial plaque and exposure of thrombogenic materials or by the turbulent flow and high shear force caused by the narrowed arteries. Thus, the predisposing factors for arterial thrombosis are primarily vessel wall disease processes, in which platelets may play an

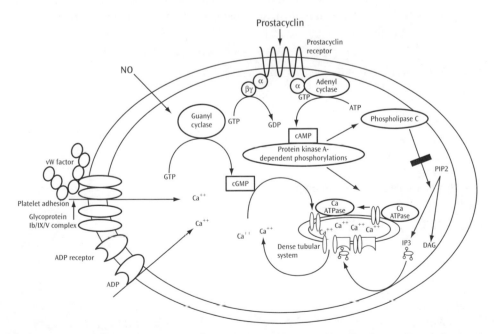

Figure 6.2 *Inhibition of platelet activation by prostacyclin and nitric oxide. (NO, nitric oxide; cGMP, cyclic guanine monophosphate. Other abbreviations as Fig. 6.1.)*

important primary role. In contrast, the most important predisposing factor for venous thrombosis is stasis, which favors the fluid-phase coagulation reactions in regions of low flow (e.g., the valve pockets in the lower extremities of patients during bed rest). The risk of venous thrombosis is increased with systemic hypercoagulability, due either to the presence of activated coagulation factors (e.g., the postoperative state) or deficiency of physiological inhibitors of coagulation (e.g., antithrombin III deficiency). While venous thrombosis may occur at the site of injury, underlying vessel wall damage is not thought to be required. Platelets are only secondarily involved in the formation of venous thrombi.

INHIBITION OF PLATELET FUNCTION

The ideal antiplatelet agent should block intravascular platelet-dependent thrombosis without interfering with hemostasis or wound healing. It should be effective immediately and should be safe and effective orally. Theoretically, one can inhibit various aspects of platelet function, namely, initial adhesion to the subendothelium, the release reaction, agonist-induced prostaglandin synthesis, platelet–platelet cohesion, or the platelet procoagulant activity.

Antiplatelet drugs are used in two distinct clinical conditions. They are used either as a long-term therapy to prevent the complications of atherosclerosis or acutely during unstable angina, myocardial infarction, stroke, or to prevent the immediate recurrence of thrombosis after an arterial thrombotic event. In the former situation, an orally effective and safe drug is preferred, whereas, in the latter, a potent, immediately acting parenteral drug is optimal.

This review discusses in detail some of the compounds used therapeutically in clinical practice as well as some of the promising experimental drugs being tested in clinical trials (Table 6.1).

Table 6.1 *Clinically tested antiplatelet drugs*

Inhibitors of platelet prostaglandin synthesis
    Cyclo-oxygenase inhibitors
        Aspirin[a]
        Indomethacin[a]
        Sulfinpyrazone[a]
        Indobufen
    Thromboxane synthase inhibitors
        Dazoxiben
    Thromboxane A2 receptor antagonist
        Ridogrel
ADP receptor inhibitors
    Ticlopidine[a]
    Clopidogrel[a]
Inhibitors of platelet glycoprotein IIb–IIIa
    Abciximab[a]
    Integrilin[a]
    Tirobifan, fradafiban, lamifiban

[a]Drugs approved by the Food and Drug Administration.

CYCLO-OXYGENASE INHIBITORS

Aspirin

Aspirin is the oldest and the most commonly used antiplatelet drug and is the standard against which all other antiplatelet drugs are compared.[1,2] Aspirin was initially introduced in the beginning of the twentieth century as an antipyretic and analgesic. Its antithrombotic action was not appreciated until five decades later, when it was reported to decrease the incidence of myocardial infarction. Subsequently, it was shown that aspirin prevents the synthesis of prostaglandin in platelets and other tissues by covalent modification of a serine residue in the enzyme cyclo-oxygenase.[2] This modification is irreversible. Because platelets do not have the messenger RNA to synthesize new enzymes, the inhibition lasts for their 7–10 day lifespan. Platelets carrying this inactive enzyme are hemostatically defective, as agonist-induced prostaglandin synthesis plays a major role in recruiting additional platelets to the growing hemostatic plug. In all other cells, including endothelial cells, the cyclo-oxygenase inhibitory effect of aspirin is transient, because they are able to synthesize new proteins. The inhibitory effect of aspirin on platelet aggregation can be shown in doses as low as 20 mg a day given over several days; maximal inhibition occurs at doses of 80–100 mg a day. Higher doses of aspirin have other effects on the hemostatic system, such as acetylation of fibrinogen. Acetylated fibrinogen has a diminished capacity to form fibrin, and the fibrin that does form is more susceptible to lysis.[3] How these non-platelet effects of aspirin contribute to its overall antithrombotic properties is not known.

Following its oral ingestion, aspirin is slowly absorbed from the gastrointestinal tract within 0.5–1 hour. Most of its pharmacological effects (modification of platelet cyclo-oxygenase) occur in the portal circulation during transit from the gastrointestinal tract to the liver.

INDICATIONS FOR ASPIRIN

Recently, the Antiplatelet Trialist Collaborative Group reviewed all clinical trials of long-term antiplatelet therapy in the prevention of arterial thrombotic diseases.[4–6] Their analyses showed that aspirin in doses of 75–325 mg per day is as effective as higher doses in secondary prevention in high-risk patients. It reduced the risk of myocardial infarction, stroke, and death by more than 30% in patients with unstable and stable angina, transient ischemic attacks, myocardial infarction, peripheral vascular disease, and in those having vascular procedures. Among low-risk patients (primary prevention), a significant reduction in myocardial infarction (approximately 30%) was accompanied by a nonsignificant increase in stroke.

Aspirin has a dramatic beneficial effect in the treatment of erythromelalgia, a burning pain in the digits that complicates myeloproliferative disorders such as polycythemia vera and essential thrombocytosis. It has been suggested that the symptoms are caused by the aggregation of platelets in the microcirculation, a consequence of functional platelet abnormality associated with the disorder. Aspirin usually produces immediate and complete relief. Aspirin is also effective in preventing abortions in patients with antiphospholipid antibody syndrome, complications of pregnancy-induced hypertension, and progression of glomerulonephritis in some clinical studies. In addition, the use of aspirin is also being advised in the maintenance therapy of thrombotic thrombocytopenic purpura, and in Kawasaki disease.

THE EFFECT OF ASPIRIN ON THE BLEEDING TIME

Despite the marked inhibition of platelet aggregation by even small doses of aspirin in vitro, the effect of aspirin on the bleeding time is modest and unpredictable. Following ingestion of two to three tablets of aspirin, the bleeding time generally increases, an increase lasting for 3–4 days. Nevertheless, it is often difficult to show a prolongation of the bleeding time beyond the normal range in many normal individuals. The aspirin-induced prolongation of the bleeding time can be demonstrated only when using the template bleeding time, a procedure in which a transverse skin incision is made and the capillary pressure is raised by inflating a blood pressure cuff. Smaller doses of aspirin (< 150 mg), which can be shown consistently to inhibit platelet aggregation, do not prolong the bleeding time. However, in the presence of an underlying hemostatic defect, the effect of aspirin on bleeding time can be very dramatic. For example, aspirin will significantly prolong the bleeding time in patients with mild von Willebrand disease, who may have bleeding times within the normal range in the absence of aspirin. This phenomenon can be exploited to diagnose mild von Willebrand disease and is known as the aspirin challenge test. Aspirin also exaggerates the prolonged bleeding time seen in patients with chronic renal failure and other qualitative platelet disorders. Alcohol can potentiate the prolonged bleeding time seen with aspirin.

GASTROINTESTINAL SIDE-EFFECTS

The most common side-effects of aspirin are gastrointestinal upset and bleeding. These effects are dose related and more likely to occur at doses of over 325 mg per day. It is not widely appreciated that even though lower doses of aspirin do not generally cause gastrointestinal symptoms, they can still cause significant gastrointestinal blood loss.[7] Some studies indicate that patients who have received aspirin are also more likely to have increased postoperative bleeding and an increased blood requirement following major cardiovascular surgery. However, other studies have not found a correlation between aspirin ingestion and postoperative bleeding. These conflicting studies show the difficulty in assessing the mild hemostatic defect induced by aspirin.

FUTURE DIRECTIONS

In efforts to decrease the side-effects and increase the platelet specificity of aspirin, time-release preparations have been devised that are absorbed slowly from the gastrointestinal tract into the portal circulation, where they react with platelet cyclo-oxygenase. The small amount of aspirin reaching the liver at any one time can then be metabolized completely, preventing any active drug from entering the systemic circulation. Thus, the cyclo-oxygenase in the endothelial cells of the systemic vasculature will not be modified and prostacyclin production by the endothelium will not be impaired.

Other cyclo-oxygenase inhibitors

Other cyclo-oxygenase inhibitors such as sulfinpyrazone and indobufen have also been shown to be effective antithrombotic drugs in certain clinical situations.[8] Unlike aspirin, these drugs inhibit cyclo-oxygenase in a reversible, dose-dependent manner and the effect depends upon the half-life of the drug. There is no clear advantage of these drugs over aspirin, which is safe and inexpensive.

THROMBOXANE A2 INHIBITORS

Thromboxane synthesis inhibitors prevent the formation of thromboxane A2 specifically and do not reduce vascular prostacyclin formation, but may actually increase its synthesis by shunting cyclic endoperoxides from the platelets to the endothelial cells. Several of these compounds have been studied in clinical trials. Despite the theoretical advantages of selective inhibition of thromboxane synthesis, the clinical trials have not been very promising. The cyclic endoperoxides by themselves are potent agonists of the thromboxane A2 receptor, which may account for the failure of these compounds. Thromboxane receptor antagonists have also been developed. A new drug, ridogrel (a selective thromboxane synthase inhibitor and thromboxane A2 receptor blocker), has been shown to improve the outcome for patients with acute myocardial infarction who were also treated with tissue plasminogen activator and heparin.[9] The short-term effect was similar to that of aspirin, but with a slightly lower incidence of new ischemic events.

PROSTACYCLIN MIMETICS

Prostacyclin is the most potent endogenous inhibitor of platelet functions. Many prostacyclin mimetics that are orally active have been tried in clinical trials, but none has been shown to be superior to aspirin. One of the major side-effects of these drugs is hypotension. More clinical trials are necessary before these agents can be recommended for use in clinical practice.

AGENTS INTERFERING WITH THE ADP RECEPTOR

Ticlopidine

Ticlopidine is a thienopyridine that interferes with ADP-induced platelet activation. It also inhibits the stimulatory effect of other agents that activate platelets secondarily by releasing ADP from dense granules.[10,11] Thus, ticlopidine, unlike aspirin, inhibits shear-induced platelet aggregation. The full antiplatelet effect of ticlopidine in vivo requires 3–5 days of oral administration and persists for up to 10 days after the withdrawal of the drug, paralleling the platelet lifespan. Ticlopidine does not affect arachidonic acid metabolism in platelets and is inactive in vitro. No antiplatelet activity of ticlopidine can be demonstrated in plasma in vivo, suggesting that ticlopidine is converted to an active metabolite which is bound to platelets.

Ticlopidine has been studied in several clinical trials, in which it was given at a dose of 250 mg orally twice a day. It was shown to be effective in the prevention of stroke, myocardial infarction, and peripheral arterial disease and was slightly more effective than aspirin in the Ticlopidine Aspirin Stroke Study (TASS).[12] In a 5-year follow-up period, significantly fewer patients on ticlopidine were found to have strokes or to die (13.8 per 100 patients) than patients on aspirin (18.1 per 100 patients). Ticlopidine has also been shown to be effective in decreasing ischemic heart disease and peripheral vascular disease, but its superiority over aspirin remains to be established.

SIDE-EFFECTS OF TICLOPIDINE

The most frequent side-effects of ticlopidine are diarrhea and rash, which occur in about 20% of patients treated. In about 2% of the patients, the complications are severe enough to cause discontinuation of the medication. Another potentially serious side-effect is neutropenia, which occurs in 2.4% of the treated patients. This complication generally occurs within 3 months of beginning therapy and usually, but not always, is reversible when the drug is discontinued. Close monitoring of the white blood cell count every 2 weeks in the first 3 months of ticlopidine therapy is essential. Several reports appeared recently describing the rare occurrence of thrombotic thrombocytopenic purpura or aplastic anemia in patients treated with ticlopidine. Thus, the advantages of ticlopidine over aspirin are that it is slightly more effective as an antiplatelet agent and does not cause serious gastrointestinal bleeding. Nevertheless, one has to weigh these advantages against the rare, but potentially serious, other side-effects when choosing between aspirin and ticlopidine.

Recently, ticlopidine (250 mg twice a day for 4 weeks) in conjunction with aspirin (100 mg twice a day) has been compared with conventional anticoagulant therapy (heparin, phenprocoumoron, and aspirin) in a prospective, randomized trial in patients undergoing coronary artery stenting.[13] Ticlopidine and aspirin combination was found to be more effective (82% lower risk of myocardial infarction and 78% lower need for repeated interventions) than conventional anticoagulant therapy with aspirin. Occlusion of the stents occurred in 0.8% of those receiving combination and in 5.4% of those on conventional anticoagulant therapy. This combination of aspirin and ticlopidine caused less bleeding and has become standard treatment following angioplasty and stent placement.

Clopidogrel

Clopidogrel, another thienopyridine derivative, has recently been studied in clinical settings at a dose of 75 mg a day. In the CAPRIE (Clopidogrel versus Aspirin in Patients at Risk of Ischemic Events) trial, patients treated with clopidogrel had an annual 5.32% risk of ischemic stoke, myocardial infarction, or vascular death, compared with 5.83% with aspirin. The mean duration of treatment was about 2 years.[14] In this study, the incidence of neutropenia in clopidogrel-treated patients was not different from that in aspirin-treated patients, providing a potential rationale for its use instead of ticlopidine.

GLYCOPROTEIN IIb–IIIa COMPLEX INHIBITORS

In the past few years, a new class of antiplatelet agents has been developed that inhibit platelet aggregation by blocking the glycoprotein IIb–IIIa complex. As discussed earlier, the glycoprotein IIb–IIIa complex undergoes activation-induced conformational changes that render it capable of binding to fibrinogen and other adhesive proteins and thus of mediating the cohesion of platelets. Occupation of the ligand-binding site by inhibitors prevents platelet aggregation induced by even the most powerful agonists. Thus, glycoprotein IIb–IIIa inhibitors have a clear advantage over conventional agonists such as aspirin and ticlopidine, whose inhibitory effects can be bypassed by agents coupled to receptors that directly activate phospholipase C. Nevertheless, these therapeutic advantages come at a price. The incidence of major bleeding complications is much greater in patients treated with these agents than in those treated with conventional agents. For the present, the use of these potent agents should be reserved for certain well-defined conditions and limited to brief time periods surrounding the vascular event or intervention. The glycoprotein IIb–IIIa inhibitors include a modified monoclonal antibody (abciximab), and peptide (integrilin) and synthetic nonpeptide inhibitors (lamifiban, tirobifan, and fradafiban).

Abciximab

Abciximab is derived from a mouse monoclonal antibody (7E3) that binds glycoprotein IIb–IIIa and prevents adhesive ligands binding to the activated receptor. For clinical use, it was modified to decrease its antigenicity by replacement of mouse amino acid sequences with human sequences. This chimeric Fab fragment has been studied in several clinical trials in recent years.[15,16] A multicenter, randomized, placebo-controlled study (EPIC) was conducted to examine its efficacy in treating patients at risk for recurrent ischemia, such as those undergoing coronary atherectomy or angioplasty. The antibody was given as an initial bolus (0.25 mg/kg) followed by a 12-hour infusion (10 µg/min). Abciximab was effective in reducing subsequent myocardial infarction, urgent interventions (coronary angioplasty or coronary artery bypass surgery, stent placement, intraortic balloon pump placement), and death (35% reduction in composite endpoint). This benefit was apparent on the first day of the randomization and continued throughout the entire 30 days of the initial study. A subsequent systematic follow-up also showed that the rates of urgent revascularization and NQW myocardial infarction were decreased for more than 6 months. However, at 6 months there was no reduction in elective revascularization or death.

SIDE-EFFECTS

In initial trials, approximately two-thirds of the patients receiving abciximab experienced major bleeding. Thrombocytopenia, presumably due to an immune response to the antibody, has also been observed. The majority of the bleeding episodes were from the vascular access sites in patients receiving standard doses of heparin. However, retroperitoneal hematomas and gastrointestinal bleeding were also seen. The bleeding complications were reduced in subsequent trials that used lower doses of heparin.

Since its commercial release, abciximab has been utilized in a variety of clinical circumstances such as saphenous vein grafting, after stent placement, and as an adjunct to intracoronary thrombolysis. Although of clear benefit, its high cost will limit its widespread use.

INTEGRILIN

Integrilin, a disulfide-linked cyclic peptide, is a short-acting and reversible inhibitor of platelet aggregation. Integrilin contains a KGD (lysine–glycine–aspartic acid) sequence similar to that found in the snake venom barbourin.[16–18] This sequence is purported to selectively block the platelet glycoprotein IIb–IIIa complex without affecting the functions of other integrins. The potential benefits of integrilin include its ability to bind reversibly, an advantage in treating patients at high risk for bleeding. Integrilin has been evaluated in acute coronary syndromes, extracorporeal bypass, and in normal human volunteers at doses of 75–150 µg/kg as a bolus followed by infusions of 0.75–1 µg/kg per minute. A recently conducted phase III angioplasty trial with integrilin demonstrated a favorable trend for the reduction in the incidence of death, myocardial infarction, and urgent intervention in patients treated with integrilin. It has also been used as an antiplatelet agent in a patient with essential thrombocytosis and acute thrombotic stroke.

Nonpeptide antagonists of glycoprotein IIb–IIIa

Tirofiban, lamifiban, and fradafiban are nonantibody antagonists to platelet glycoprotein IIb–IIIa. Administration of these compounds results in inhibition of platelet aggregation and prolongation of the bleeding time. Early studies show that lamifiban compared favorably with aspirin and heparin in preventing thrombosis.[19] In the RESTORE (Randomized Efficacy Study of Tirofiban for Outcomes and Restenosis) trial, tirofiban reduced adverse cardiac events early after interventions, but no difference between the tirofiban and placebo groups was observed at 30 days. The larger trials of several orally effective drugs of this type will soon be published.

CONCLUSION

Until a decade ago, aspirin was the only effective antiplatelet agent available. Recent advances in our understanding of platelet physiology have stimulated the development of newer antiplatelet drugs such as the glycoprotein IIb–IIIa inhibitors. Undoubtedly, new drugs will soon be developed that are more specific, more potent, and produce fewer side-effects.

REFERENCES

1 Harker LA. Platelets and vascular thrombosis. *N Eng J Med* 1994; **330**: 1006–7.

2 Roth GJ, Calverley DC. Aspirin, platelets, and thrombosis: theory and practice. *Blood* 1994; **83**: 885–98.

3 Bjornsson TD, Schneider DE, Berger, H. Aspirin acetylates fibrinogen and enhances fibrinolysis. Fibrinolytic effect is independent of changes in plasminogen activator levels. *J Pharmcol Exp Ther* 1989; **250**: 154–61.

4 Anonymous. Collaborative overview of randomised trials of antiplatelet therapy – I: Prevention of death, myocardial infarction, and stroke by prolonged antiplatelet therapy in various categories of patients. Antiplatelet Trialists' Collaboration. *BMJ* 1994; **308**: 81–106.

5 Anonymous. Collaborative overview of randomised trials of antiplatelet therapy – II: Maintenance of vascular graft or arterial patency by antiplatelet therapy. Antiplatelet Trialists' Collaboration *BMJ* 1994; **308**: 159–68.

6 Anonymous. Collaborative overview of randomised trials of antiplatelet therapy – III: Reduction in venous thrombosis and pulmonary embolism by antiplatelet prophylaxis among surgical and medical patients. Antiplatelet Trialists' Collaboration *BMJ* 1994; **308**: 235–46.

7 Guslandi M. Gastric toxicity of antiplatelet therapy with low-dose aspirin. *Drugs* 1997; **53**: 1–5.

8 Rajah SM, Nair U, Rees M, et al. Effects of antiplatelet therapy with indobufen or aspirin-dipyridamole on graft patency one year after coronary artery bypass grafting. *J Thorac Cardiovasc Surg* 1994; **107**: 1146–53.

9 The RAPT Investigators. Randomized trial of ridogrel, a combined thromboxane A2 synthase inhibitor and thromboxane A2/prostaglandin endoperoxide receptor antagonist, versus aspirin as adjunct to thrombolysis in patients with acute myocardial infarction. *Circulation* 1994; **89**: 588–95.

10 Schror K. Antiplatelet drugs. A comparative review. *Drugs* 1995; **50**: 7–28.

11 Murray JC, Kelly MA, Gorelick PB. Ticlopidine: a new antiplatelet agent for the secondary prevention of stroke. *Clin Neuropharmacol* 1994; **17**: 23–31.

12 Hass WK, Easton JD, Adams HP, et al. A randomized trial comparing ticlopidine hydrochloride with aspirin for the prevention of stroke in high-risk patients. Ticlopidine Aspirin Stroke Study. *N Engl J Med* 1989; **321**: 501–7.

13 Schomig A, Neumann FJ, Kastrati A, et al. A randomized comparison of antiplatelet and anticoagulant therapy after the placement of coronary-artery stents *N Engl J Med* 1996; **334**: 1084–9.

14 Gent M. CAPRIE steering committee: a randomized, blinded trial of clopidogrel versus aspirin in patients at risk of ischemic events. *Lancet* 1996; **348**: 1329–39.

15 Lincoff AM, Califf RM, Anderson KM, et al. Evidence for prevention of death and myocardial infarction with platelet membrane glycoprotein IIb/IIIa receptor blockade by abciximab (c7E3 Fab) among patients with unstable angina undergoing percutaneous coronary revascularization. EPIC Investigators. Evaluation of 7E3 in preventing ischemic complications. *J Am Coll Cardiol* 1997; **30**: 149–56.

16 The EPILOG Investigators. Platelet glycoprotein IIb/IIIa receptor blockade and low-dose heparin during percutaneous coronary revascularization. *N Eng J Med* 1997; **336**: 1689–96.

17 Tcheng JF, Harrington RA, Kottke-Marchant K, et al. Multicenter, randomized, double-blind, placebo-controlled trial of the platelet integrin glycoprotein IIb/IIIa blocker Integrilin in elective coronary intervention. IMPACT Investigators. *Circulation* 1995; **91**: 2151–7.

18 Tcheng JE. Glycoprotein IIb/IIIa receptor inhibitors: putting the EPIC, IMPACT II, RESTORE, and EPILOG trials into perspective. *Am J Cardiol* 1996; **78**: 35–40.
19 Theroux P, Kouz S, Roy L, et al. Platelet membrane receptor glycoprotein IIb/IIIa antagonism in unstable angina. The Canadian Lamifiban Study. *Circulation* 1996; **94**: 899–905.

7

An overview of warfarin therapy

LYNDA THOMSON, WILLIAM O'HARA

THE DISCOVERY OF WARFARIN

The first step toward the discovery of warfarin began in the 1920s during an outbreak of hemorrhagic disease in cattle in the midwestern USA and Canada. A veterinarian pathologist (Schofield) linked the hemorrhagic occurrences to the ingestion of decaying sweet clover.[1] Another veterinary pathologist (Roderick) determined that the affected cattle had a decrease in prothrombin activity, however; the responsible chemical entity was unknown at that time.[2] Link, a biochemist at the University of Wisconsin, became involved in the investigation of this mysterious hemorrhagic disease in 1933.[3] He was studying the role of coumarin compounds in grasses. Link managed to isolate the causative agent in 1939. The entity was bishydroxycoumarin, or dicumarol.[3] Link's discovery sparked interest in this novel agent, and trials with dicumarol were begun in animals and humans in 1941.[4] Link subsequently synthesized another agent structurally related to dicumarol, which was named warfarin, an acronym for the Wisconsin Alumni Research Foundation (Fig. 7.1).[3] Warfarin sodium was employed worldwide as a rodenticide, causing hemorrhagic death in rodents. Interestingly, warfarin, which possesses superior pharmacokinetic properties in comparison to dicumarol, was not investigated for human use in the treatment of thromboembolic diseases until the 1950s when used to treat President Eisenhower.[3] Since then, warfarin's role has evolved as an important

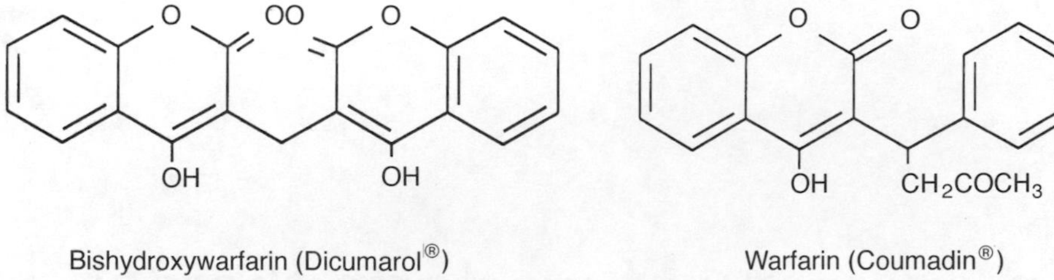

Bishydroxywarfarin (Dicumarol®) Warfarin (Coumadin®)

Figure 7.1 *Chemical structures of bishydroxywarfarin and warfarin.*

therapeutic agent in the management and prevention of thromboembolic disease. It is used extensively for the treatment of deep vein thromboses and pulmonary embolism. Warfarin is also widely used for the prevention of thromboembolic events and associated mortality in individuals with hypercoagulable disorders, a history of recurrent thromboses, cerebrovascular disease, and a wide array of cardiac diseases, including atrial fibrillation, coronary artery disease, cardiomyopathy, unstable angina, myocardial infarction, valvular disease, and in patients with prosthetic valves.

PHARMACOLOGY

Warfarin and other structurally related oral anticoagulants derive their pharmacologic activity from the 4-hydroxycoumarin nucleus, which contains a substituent in the number 3 position. Warfarin is a racemic mixture of two optically active stereoisomers, R and S (Fig. 7.2).[5] The pharmacologic activity of warfarin is due to interference with the production of the vitamin K-dependent clotting factors in the liver, specifically factors II, VII, IX, and X. The S isomer exerts a five-fold greater suppressive effect on the activation of the vitamin K-dependent clotting factors than the R isomer.[5] Warfarin's anticoagulant effect is a result of interference with cyclic interconversion of inactive vitamin K 2,3-epoxide to active vitamin KH_2 (Fig. 7.3).[5-9] This prevents recycling of vitamin K. The vitamin K-dependent clotting factors require carboxylation of gamma-glutamyl residues on N-terminal regions in order to be active.[5-9] The carboxylation reaction requires reduced vitamin K, vitamin KH_2, as a cofactor along with carbon dioxide and oxygen.[5-8] During this reaction, vitamin KH_2 is oxidized to vitamin K 2,3-epoxide. Vitamin K is recycled by the enzymes vitamin K epoxide reductase and vitamin K reductase. Warfarin specifically interferes with these reductase enzymes, leading to a depletion in the vitamin KH_2 stores and subsequent formation of partially carboxylated or decarboxylated clotting factors with minimal coagulant activity.[5-9] Partial carboxylation significantly decreases the ability of the affected clotting factors to become activated and bind to target proteins on phospholipid membranes and endothelial cells.[5-9] Normal clotting factors typically contain 10–13 gamma-carboxyglutamate residues for full coagulant activity.[5] Warfarin-affected clotting factors can contain as little as two to six gamma-carboxyglutamate residues, resulting in only 2–70% of the normal coagulant activity of fully carboxylated clotting factors.[5]

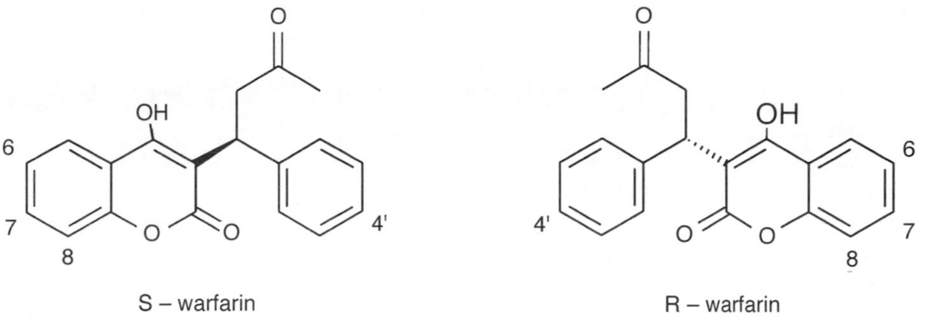

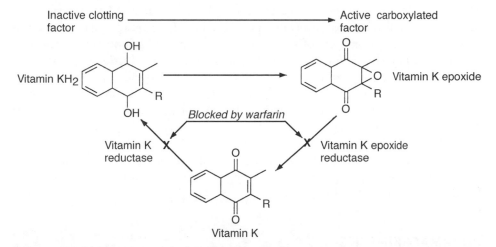

Figure 7.2 *Chemical structure of the stereoisomers of warfarin.*

Figure 7.3 *The vitamin K cycle and the effect of warfarin.*

Onset of pharmacologic effect

An increase in the prothrombin time (PT) and International Normalized Ratio (INR) value can typically be seen within 36 hours after initiation of warfarin therapy. This early increase is a reflection of the inhibition of factor VII, which has the shortest half-life of the vitamin K-dependent clotting factors (Table 7.1). Warfarin also inhibits the activity of two anticoagulant vitamin K-dependent proteins, protein C and protein S. The levels of active protein C and S decline within 24–48 hours after initiation of warfarin.[6,7] The decline in levels of protein C and S before a full anticoagulant affect has occurred can lead to a potential hypercoagulable state and the risk of development of a thrombus or other adverse effects, such as warfarin-induced skin necrosis.[7] For this reason, unfractionated or a low molecular weight heparin is typically given for the first 5 days of warfarin therapy, until warfarin's full pharmacologic effect is achieved, to provide adequate anticoagulation and prevent development of a hypercoagulable state.[8]

Table 7.1 *Normal half-lives of the vitamin K-dependent clotting factors and proteins C and S*[17,56]

Activity	Vitamin K-dependent protein	Half-life (hours)
Anticoagulant	Protein C	9
Anticoagulant	Protein S	60
Coagulant	Factor II	72
Coagulant	Factor VII	4–6
Coagulant	Factor IX	18–24
Coagulant	Factor X	48

Reversal of pharmacologic effect

The administration or ingestion of significant amounts of vitamin K can antagonize the anticoagulant activity of warfarin. The correction of the anticoagulant activity is dependent upon the half-life of the vitamin K-dependent clotting factors and the time required for circulating clotting factors to be cleared. A reduction in the PT and INR values can be seen within 24 hours of administration of phytonadione. Therefore, administration of small doses of phytonadione in conjunction with withholding one to two warfarin doses is usually sufficient for the management of elevated INR values up to 10 in the absence of bleeding.[10] However, in more emergent situations involving life-threatening hemorrhage, the administration of fresh frozen plasma is necessary to provide the patient with active clotting factors, due to the delay in response to phytonadione.[7] For more information on the management of bleeding, please refer to Chapter 13.

PHARMACOKINETICS

Absorption

Warfarin is essentially completely absorbed when administered orally, with a bioavailability approaching 100%.[11] It is primarily absorbed from the stomach and small intestine.[12,13] Food has no effect on the area under the concentration time curve, but may, however, delay the rate of absorption.[11] Malabsorption disease states such as short bowel syndrome do not appear to affect the bioavailability of warfarin.[11,14] Warfarin does not undergo a 'first-pass' effect.[11] Peak plasma concentrations occur between 0.3 and 4.0 hours after oral administration.[11]

Distribution

Warfarin exhibits very high protein binding, mainly to albumin.[11] Approximately 98% of warfarin is protein bound; the remaining 2% of free drug is responsible for exerting the pharmacologic effect.[11] Warfarin distributes to a single compartment with a volume of distribution in the range of 0.11–0.19 L/kg, reflective of the albumin compartment.[11] The volume of distribution is similar for the R and S isomers.[11]

Metabolism

The R and S isomers undergo two distinct metabolic pathways. Both undergo metabolism via the cytochrome p450 oxidative system in the liver's endoplasmic reticulum.[11] Approximately 60% of the R isomer undergoes reduction of the acetonyl side chain to form several warfarin alcohols, mainly 6-hydroxywarfarin and smaller amounts of 4'-, 7-, 8-, and 10-hyrodoxywarfarin.[11,15,16,18] The R isomer metabolites are excreted in the urine.[15] Ninety percent of the S isomer undergoes oxidation, largely to 7-hydroxywarfarin, which is excreted in the bile, and to a lesser extent to 6-hydroxywarfarin.[11,15,18] There is extensive interpatient variability in the metabolism of warfarin, necessitating the need for patient-specific dosing.[15]

Elimination

Stereospecific clearance occurs, with the R isomer cleared half as quickly as the S isomer, resulting in an average racemic half-life of 36–42 hours.[11,15,18] The average half-life of the S isomer is 29 hours (range of 18–52 hours). The average half-life of the R isomer is significantly longer at 45 hours, with a range of 20–70 hours.[18] Average clearance rates are 0.015–0.132 ml/min per kg for S and 0.009–0.121 ml/min per kg for R metabolites.[18] Although the half-life of the R isomer is longer, changes in the metabolism of the S isomer are more clinically significant due to a five-fold greater pharmacologic potency than the R isomer.[13] Clearance of warfarin is dependent upon protein binding; however, alterations in protein binding do not appear to have a significant lasting effect.[11] Displacement of warfarin from albumin-binding sites allows more drug to be metabolized and cleared. Although protein-binding displacement initially increases the amount of free 'pharmacologically active drug,' increased clearance compensates and the free concentration decreases to the normal range. This is why most drug interactions involving displacement of warfarin from protein-binding sites do not appear to be severe in nature. As with the metabolism of warfarin, there is wide variability in the rate of clearance, necessitating patient-specific dosing.[11,18]

Dose/response effect

Steady-state plasma levels of warfarin are reached in approximately 7 days.[11] However, the degree of warfarin's pharmacologic effect is mainly dependent upon depletion of factors II, VII, IX, and X. The rate-limiting step for fully achieving antithrombotic activity is depletion of factor II, which possesses the longest half-life at 42–72 hours.[18] Although there is a correlation between the dose of warfarin and the anticoagulant effect, there is a significant variability in response between patients and over time in a course of therapy.[13] The plasma concentration of warfarin required to maintain an INR value in the therapeutic range can vary considerably and necessitates frequent monitoring of the INR with dosage adjustment, if necessary.[13] Patient response to warfarin therapy is influenced by multiple pharmacokinetic and pharmacodynamic factors, which are discussed in the following sections. Other potential causes for fluctuations in INR values that should be considered include laboratory testing variability and errors, patient noncompliance or nonadherence to therapy, or miscommunication between the patient and healthcare provider.[13]

PHARMACODYNAMIC CONSIDERATIONS

Variability in the pharmacokinetic and pharmacodynamic parameters of warfarin plays an equally important role in determining warfarin dosage requirements and it is often difficult to distinguish between these parameters. Dose–response relationships depend upon diet, age, disease states, and drug interactions and affect how warfarin is absorbed, metabolized, and eliminated.[7,11,15] The liver's ability to produce clotting factors, the effect of other drug and disease states on hemostasis, and vitamin K reductase receptor affinity are other important factors in determining responsiveness.[7,11,15] Pharmacodynamic factors must be considered when determining warfarin dosage requirements, because they can either potentiate or decrease the response to warfarin therapy. Some common causes of a potentiated warfarin response include hypermetabolic states, such as hyperthyroidism or febrile episodes, or administration of the influenza vaccine.[7,11,15] Hypermetabolic states probably increase warfarin responsiveness by increasing the catabolic rate of vitamin K-dependent clotting factors in the liver.[11] Hepatic disease, vitamin K deficiency states, and short-term alcohol bingeing can increase sensitivity to warfarin.[7,11,15] Hepatic disease and short-term alcohol use can depress the production of vitamin K-dependent clotting factors. Fat malabsorption states or acute bouts of diarrhea can cause a decrease in dietary vitamin K absorption and lead to a potentiated warfarin response. Elderly individuals appear to be more sensitive to warfarin's effects, probably because of alteration in pharmacodynamic parameters. Conversely, pregnancy can decrease responsiveness to warfarin and is associated with an elevation in circulating levels of factors VII, VIII, IX, X, and fibrinogen.[7,11,15]

Although rare, warfarin resistance is another pharmacodynamic cause of decreased warfarin responsiveness. Warfarin resistance appears to be a hereditary, autosomal dominant trait resulting in extremely high warfarin dosage requirements, in the range of 5–20 times higher than usual.[7,15] The mechanism of warfarin resistance appears to be due to a decreased sensitivity of tissue receptors to warfarin. Patients with suspected warfarin resistance should have a plasma warfarin level determined to assist with the differentiation between true resistance and other causes such as therapeutic nonadherence, drug or food interactions, or absorption problems. Individualization of warfarin dosing is necessary due to the highly variable and unpredictable nature of the pharmacokinetic and pharmacodynamic factors. These factors can change significantly during a treatment course, which necessitates frequent monitoring of the INR in patients receiving warfarin therapy.

POTENTIAL DRUG INTERACTIONS WITH WARFARIN

In addition to pharmacokinetic and pharmacodynamic considerations, drug interactions are another significant factor complicating the management of warfarin therapy. The list of drugs that reportedly interact with warfarin is extensive; however, much of the data is limited to case reports or small studies. The recent popularity of herbal products has further complicated management, with even less available information. Additionally, patients do not often perceive herbal products to be drugs and may not mention that they a taking them, unless specifically asked by their healthcare provider.

The potential mechanisms of drug interactions with warfarin include alterations in absorption, enhanced or decreased hepatic clearance, and alteration in protein binding of warfarin.[11,19–21] Other interactions include potentiation of anticoagulant effects, either by direct pharmacologic effects of concomitant medications on the PT or inhibition of platelet function.[11,19–21] Table 7.2 lists the drugs that commonly interact with warfarin, and Table 7.3 lists the potential interactions between warfarin and herbal products based upon the limited data currently available.

Table 7.2 *Potential drug interactions*[22]

Drug type	Potentiation of warfarin's effect	Inhibition of warfarin's effect
Antibiotics	Chloramphenicol, ciprofloxacin, cotrimoxazole, erythromycin, fluconazole, isoniazid, itraconazole, ketoconazole, metronidazole, miconazole, tetracycline	Dicloxacillin, griseofulvin, nafcillin, rifampin
Cardiac	Amiodarone, propafenone, propranolol, quinidine, sulfinpyrazone	
Analgesic/anti-inflammatory	Acetaminophen, aspirin, phenylbutazone, piroxicam	
Central nervous system	Alcohol (with liver disease), chloral hydrate, phenytoin	Barbiturates, carbamazepine, chlordiazepoxide
Gastrointestinal	Cimetidine, omeprazole	Sucralfate
Lipid lowering	Clofibrate, lovastatin, gemfibrazole, simvastatin	Cholestyramine
Miscellaneous	Anabolic steroids, disulfiram, influenza vaccine, tamoxifen, vitamin E (high dose)	Enteral feeds (with high vitamin K), thyroxine

THE IMPACT OF DIETARY VITAMIN K ON WARFARIN

Vitamin K, a fat-soluble vitamin, is a necessary cofactor for activation of the vitamin K-dependent clotting factors, II, VII, IX, and X. Vitamin K carboxylates glutamate residues on the N-terminals of factors II, VII, IX, and X. Carboxylation allows the clotting factors to undergo a conformational change in the presence of calcium and subsequently to bind to their target proteins on endothelial cells and phospholipids, a necessary step in the activation of the clotting cascade.[28,29] The importance of

Table 7.3 *Potential interactions of warfarin with herbal products*[23]

Product	Potential effect	Potential mechanism	Reference
Angelica	↑ Bleeding risk	Contains coumarin[a]	25
Celery seed	↑ Bleeding risk	Contains coumarin[a]	25
Chamomile	↑ Bleeding risk	Contains coumarin[a]	25
Feverfew	↑ Bleeding risk	Platelet inhibition, inhibits release of arachidonic acid	24,25
Garlic	↑ Bleeding risk	Platelet inhibition, inhibition of thromboxane synthesis	24,25,27
Ginger	↑ Bleeding risk	Platelet inhibition	24,25,27
Gingko Biloba	↑ Bleeding risk	Platelet inhibition	24,25
Ginseng	↓ INR value	Unknown	23,25
Horse chestnut	↑ Bleeding risk	Contains coumarin[a]	25
Licorice	↑ Bleeding risk	Contains coumarin,[a] platelet inhibition	25
Vitamin E	↑ Bleeding risk	Platelet inhibition	24
Yarrow	↑ Risk of thrombosis	Coagulant effect	25

[a]Coumarin is a naturally ocurring benzopyrone that is structurally similar to warfarin. Coumarin has some anticoagulant pharmacologic properties; however, it is significantly less potent than warfarin and the clinical relevance is unknown.

vitamin K in the synthesis of active clotting factors was first discovered by Henrik Dam in the 1920s. Dam, who was studying the role of sterols in chicks, found that hemorrhagic disease in chicks receiving a lipid-free diet could be prevented with administration of alfalfa.[30] Dam, Almquist, and Doisy isolated and synthesized the active entity in alfalfa, 2-ME-3-phytyl-1,4-naphthoquinone, or phylloquinone.[31] Phylloquinone, or vitamin K_1, is the most common form of vitamin K ingested and is found in many dark-green, leafy vegetables.[32] Menaquinone, or vitamin K_2, is a less common source of dietary vitamin K, which is synthesized by intestinal bacteria and is found in fermented cheeses and liver.

Dietary vitamin K plays a significant role in determining a patient's warfarin dosing requirements and INR stability. The relationship of dietary vitamin K intake and its effect on warfarin dosage requirements was studied in 50 patients initiated on warfarin therapy.[33] The amount of daily vitamin K consumption varied widely from 17 µg/day to 974 µg/day. The investigators correlated a higher warfarin maintenance dosage requirement to maintain an INR > 2.0 in those individuals consuming more than 250 µg/day of vitamin K versus those ingesting less than that amount (warfarin dose requirement 5.7 ± 1.7 mg/day versus 3.5 ± 1.0 mg/day, respectively $p < 0.001$).[33] In order to maintain a stable INR and achieve an optimal therapeutic outcome, patients must be educated about the importance of maintaining a stable ingestion of vitamin K-containing foods. They should receive education regarding those foods containing large quantities of vitamin K and those that should be avoided altogether or ingested in limited amounts. A detailed dietary history should be conducted for any patients with widely fluctuating INR values or those who cannot achieve a therapeutic INR value. All patients should be questioned about

Table 7.4 *Vitamin K content of selected foods*[34,35]

Food	Amount of vitamin K in µg per 100 g portion
Abalone	23
Asparagus, raw	40
Avocado, raw	40
Broccoli, raw	205
Brussel sprouts, raw	177
Cabbage, raw	145
Canola oil	141
Chinese green tea (dry)	1428
Coleslaw	57
Coriander leaf, cooked	1510
Cucumber peel, raw	360
Endive, raw	231
Green beans, snap	47
Kale, raw	817
Lettuce, raw	210
Margarine, stick[a]	51
Mayonnaise	81
Mustard greens, raw	170
Nightshade leaf, raw	620
Parsley, raw	540
Purslane, raw	381
Seaweed, purple	1385
Soybean oil	193
Soybeans, raw	47
Spinach leaf, raw	400
Swiss chard, raw	830
Tofu, raw	2
Turnip greens, raw	251
Watercress, raw	250

[a]1 stick of margarine is equivalent to 113 g.

their vitamin K intake with each office visit, because seasonal variations in diet are a common occurrence. Table 7.4 lists foods that contain high quantities of vitamin K. In addition to the foods listed, other potential sources of vitamin K include multivitamin supplements and enteral nutrition products. Teaching should be reinforced with each office visit to remind patients to maintain a consistent intake of vitamin K-containing foods, to avoid any drastic changes in diet, and to notify their healthcare provider of any dietary changes.

MONITORING

The PT is the most common test used to measure the extent of anticoagulation produced by warfarin. The test is sensitive to a decrease in the levels of three vitamin K-dependent clotting factors (II, VII, and X). The PT is measured by adding calcium and tissue thromboplastin to citrated plasma and recording the time it takes for the sample to clot. The prothrombin ratio (PTR) can then be calculated by dividing the PT by the control PT for the laboratory. A potential problem with the PT is that the tissue thromboplastin used may vary in its sensitivity to warfarin depending upon its origin and method of preparation.[36] This variability has resulted in significant errors in managing patients on warfarin therapy.[37]

To resolve this problem, the World Health Organization (WHO) designated a single batch of human brain thromboplastin as the first international reference preparation in 1977.[38] A calibration model was then developed based upon the assumption that there is a linear relationship between the logarithm of the PTR obtained with the reference and test preparations.[39] The WHO adopted this model in 1982. The results are reported as the INR. The INR is equal to the PT ratio that would have been obtained if the WHO reference thromboplastin had been used. The formula for calculating the INR is:

$$INR = \left(\frac{Patient\ PT^{ISI}}{Mean\ normal\ PT} \right)$$

where the International Sensitivity Index (ISI) is a measure of the responsiveness of a thromboplastin compared to the WHO reference thromboplastin (ISI = 1.0). The lower numbers indicate a more sensitive reagent. The manufacturer of the reagent provides the ISI. Although the INR system is the preferred method of monitoring warfarin therapy, it does have some problems. These are listed in Table 7.5.

Table 7.5 *Problems with the INR system*[5,6,40]

Lack of reliability when beginning warfarin therapy
Loss of precision when high ISI thromboplastins are used
Loss of accuracy with automated clot detectors
Lack of reliability of the ISI provided by the manufacturer
Use of inappropriate control plasma to calculate INR
Interference of lupus anticoagulant with low ISI thromboplastins

ISI = International Sensitivity Index; INR = International Normalized Ratio.

ADULT DOSING

Because warfarin has no effect on circulating coagulation factors, its anticoagulant effect does not begin until the functional factors already in circulation have been cleared. This may take several days because of the long half-life of factor II (72 hours). If the need for anticoagulation therapy is urgent, such as treatment of a deep vein thrombosis or pulmonary embolism, then the patient should be started on an immediate-acting anticoagulant such as intravenous heparin. A baseline PT/INR should be obtained and warfarin started on day 1 of heparin therapy. Heparin should be continued until a therapeutic INR has been achieved and a minimum of 4 days of concomitant therapy with warfarin has been administered.

To predict the required maintenance dose, some investigators have used equations or mathematical models. These are based on an INR determined after the patient has received 10 mg daily for 2–3 days.[41–6] Although effective in predicting the optimal maintenance dose, these methods have some drawbacks. For example, many use a target PT ratio instead of an INR or target the INR at 2–4 instead of the currently accepted range of 2–3. Computer programs have also been used to dose warfarin.[47,48] These programs have demonstrated themselves to be more accurate than experienced personnel in randomized trials.[49,50] Another method to dose warfarin is to begin with 5 mg and adjust the dose based upon a daily INR using a nomogram such as in Table 7.6. A study comparing initial warfarin doses of 5 mg versus 10 mg showed the 5 mg dose to be as effective in obtaining a therapeutic INR by day 5, with less chance of overshooting and increasing the risk of bleeding.[51]

Table 7.6 *Initial warfarin dosing nomogram for adults*

INR	Day 1 (mg)	Day 2 (mg)	Day 3 (mg)	Day 4 (mg)	Day 5 (mg)
< 1.5	5	5	7.5	10	10
1.5–1.99	2.5	2.5	5	7.5	7.5
2.0–2.49		1	2.5	5	5
2.5–2.99		0	1	2.5	2.5
3.0–3.5		0	0	1	1
> 3.5		0	0	0	0

INR = International Normalized Ratio.

If rapid anticoagulation is not necessary, such as in the treatment of chronic atrial fibrillation in a patient without an underlying prothrombotic state, then warfarin therapy may be started as outpatient treatment. An initial dose of 2.5–5 mg daily should be adjusted based upon an INR obtained every 2–3 days. Patients who are elderly, malnourished, have hepatic insufficiency, or are at high risk for bleeding should be started at doses of 2–4 mg, and increased gradually to avoid over-anticoagulation.

Chronic dosing

Once a patient has been receiving a consistent dose of warfarin that maintains him or her within the therapeutic range, INR monitoring should continue at intervals of every 4–6 weeks. Patients who experience changes in their INR outside of the therapeutic range should be questioned regarding compliance or changes in other medications, diet, or activity level. If a change in dose is required, then the weekly dose should be increased or decreased by 5–10% and a repeat INR obtained in 1–2 weeks. It is recommended that the patient receives the same strength warfarin tablet and that the amount taken each day is changed to accommodate different dosing schedules. Table 7.7 is an example of different weekly doses of warfarin using 5-mg tablets.

PEDIATRIC DOSING

Dosing warfarin in pediatric patients presents a unique set of challenges. Newborns have about one-half of the vitamin K-dependent clotting factors of adults.[53] These

Table 7.7 *Various warfarin schedules using fractions of 5-mg tablets*

Mon	Tue	Wed	Thu	Fri	Sat	Sun	Weekly dose (mg)
0.5	1	0.5	0.5	1	0.5	0.5	22.5
0.5	1	0.5	1	0.5	1	0.5	25
0.5	1	0.5	1	0.5	1	1	27.5
0.5	1	1	0.5	1	1	1	30
0.5	1	1	1	1	1	1	32.5
1	1	1	1	1	1	1	35
1.5	1	1	1	1	1	1	37.5
1.5	1	1	1.5	1	1	1	40
1.5	1	1.5	1	1.5	1	1	42.5
1.5	1	1.5	1.5	1	1.5	1.5	45

levels increase to the adult range by 6 months. In addition, pediatric patients have alterations in protein binding and hepatic metabolism.[54] Because of this, close monitoring and more frequent INRs are required. Dosing guidelines are derived from the Fifth ACCP Consensus Conference on Antithrombotic Therapy.[55] If the baseline INR is between 1.0 and 1.3 on day 1, therapy should be started at a dose of 0.2 mg/kg.

The dosages for days 2–4 are shown in Table 7.8 and maintenance dosing guidelines are described in Table 7.9.

Table 7.8 *Warfarin dosing protocol for days 2 through 4 of therapy in pediatric patients*[52]

INR	Dose (mg/kg)
1.1–1.3	0.2
1.4–1.9	0.1
2.0–3.0	0.1
3.1–3.5	0.05
> 3.5	Hold until INR < 3.5, then restart at 50% less than the previous dose

INR = International Normalized ratio.

Table 7.9 *Warfarin maintenance guidelines for pediatric patients*

INR	Action
1.1–1.4	Increase dose by 20%
1.5–1.9	Increase dose by 10%
2.0–3.0	No change
3.1–3.5	Decrease dose by 10%
> 3.5	Hold dose until INR < 3.5, then restart at 20% less than the previous dose

INR = International Normlized Ratio.

PATIENT EDUCATION

The importance of patient education cannot be overemphasized. Patients should have a clear understanding of the reason for their warfarin therapy and potential drug and food interactions in order to encourage adherence to therapy, optimize therapeutic outcomes, minimize fluctuations in the INR, and decrease the risk of adverse events. A comprehensive educational program should be provided to all patients initiating warfarin therapy. The educational program should include the following:

1. A review of warfarin's effect on the clotting factors.
2. The effect of vitamin K on warfarin therapy.
3. Foods which contain high quantities of vitamin K.
4. The importance of a consistent diet.
5. Prescription, nonprescription, and herbal medications to avoid.
6. Nonprescription medications which can be used safely for common ailments.
7. Exercise instructions.
8. Signs and symptoms of thrombosis and hemorrhage.
9. Management of minor bleeding.
10. Instructions for emergency situations.
11. Instructions for missed doses of warfarin.
12. The importance of notifying all healthcare providers about their warfarin therapy.
13. The importance of close follow-up monitoring.

Patients should be able to identify their warfarin tablet strength and dosage. Dosage calendars and pill boxes are useful aids for patients receiving varying daily dosages. Useful information provided to patients will allow them to have a better understanding of their disease state and empower them with information to assist in its management.

REFERENCES

1 Schofield FW. Damaged sweet clover: the cause of new disease in cattle simulating hemorrhagic septicemia and blackleg. *J Am Vet Assoc* 1924; **64**: 553–75.
2 Roderick LM. Problems in the coagulation of the blood. *Am J Physiol* 1931; **96**: 413–25.
3 Link KP. The discovery of dicumarol and its sequels. *Circulation* 1959; **19**: 97–107.
4 Butt HR, Allen EV, Bollman JL. A preparation from spoiled sweet clover which prolongs coagulation and prothrombin time of the blood; preliminary reports of experimental and clinical studies. *Mayo Clin Proc* 1941; **16**: 388–95.
5 Hirsch J, Dalen JE, Anderson DR, et al. Oral anticoagulants. Mechanism of action, clinical effectiveness, and optimal therapeutic range. *Chest* 1998; **114**(Suppl. 5): 445S–69S.
6 Suttie JW. Vitamin K antagonists. In: Colman RW, Hirsh J, Marder VJ, Salzman EW eds *Hemostasis and thrombosis*, 3rd edn. Philadelphia: JB Lippincott, 1994: 1562–6.

7 Hirsh J, Ginsberg JS, Marder VJ. Anticoagulant therapy with coumarin agents. In: Colman RW, Hirsh J, Marder VJ, Salzman EW eds *Hemostasis and thrombosis*, 3rd edn. Philadelphia: JB Lippincott, 1994: 1567–83.

8 Becker RC, Ansell J. Antithrombotic therapy. An abbreviated reference for clinicians. *Arch Intern Med* 1995; **155**: 149–61.

9 Haines ST, Bussey HI. Thrombosis and the pharmacology of antithrombotic agents. *Ann Pharmacother* 1995; **29**: 892–905.

10 Weibert RT, Dzung TE, Kayser SR, Rapaport SI. Correction of excessive anticoagulation with low dose oral vitamin K_1. *Ann Intern Med* 1997; **126**: 959–62.

11 Shetty HGM, Fennerty AG, Routledge PA. Clinical pharmacokinetic considerations in the control of oral anticoagulant therapy. *Clin Pharmacokinet* 1989; **16**: 238–53.

12 Pyoralak K, Jussila J, Mustala O, Siurala M. Absorption of warfarin from stomach and small intestine. *Scand J Gastroenterol* 1971; **6**(Suppl. 9): 95–103.

13 Hirsch J, Dalen JE, Deykin D, Anderson DR, Poller L, Bussey H. Oral anticoagulants. Mechanism of action, clinical effectiveness, and optimal therapeutic range. *Chest* 1995; **108**(Suppl. 4): 231S–46S.

14 Lutomski DM, LaFrance RJ, Bower RH, Fischer JE. Warfarin absorption after massive bowel resection. *Am J Gastroenterol* 1985; **80**: 99–102.

15 Hirsch J. Oral anticoagulant drugs. *N Engl J Med* 1991; **324**: 1865–75.

16 Becker RC, Ansell J. Antithrombotic therapy. An abbreviated reference for clinicians. *Arch Intern Med* 1995; **155**: 149–61.

17 Keller C, Matzdorff AC, Kemkes-Matthes B. Pharmacology of warfarin and clinical implications. *Semin Thromb Hemost* 1999; **25**: 13–16.

18 Wittkowsky AK. Warfarin pharmacology. In: Ansell JE, Oertel LB, Whittkowsky A eds *Managing oral anticoagulant therapy: clinical and operational guidelines*. Gaithersburg, MD: Aspen Publishing Co., 1997; 4B–1:1–1:12.

19 Wells PS, Holbrook AM, Crowther NR, Hirsh J. Interactions of warfarin with drugs and food. *Ann Intern Med* 1994; **121**: 676–82.

20 Harder S, Thurmann P. Clinically important drug interactions with anticoagulants. An update. *Clin Pharmacokinet* 1996; **30**: 416–44.

21 Buckley NA, Dawson AH. Drug interactions with warfarin. *Med J Aust* 1992; **157**: 479–83.

22 Hylek EM, Heiman H, Skates SJ, Sheehan MA, Singer DE. Acetaminophen and other risk factors for excessive warfarin anticoagulation. *JAMA* 1998; **279**: 657–62.

23 Janetzky K, Morreale AP. Probable interaction between warfarin and ginseng. *Am J Health-Syst Pharm* 1997; **54**: 692–3.

24 Gianni L, Dreitlein WB. Some popular otc herbals can interact with anticoagulant therapy. *U S Pharmacist* 1998; May: 80–6.

25 Newall CA, Anderson, LA, Phillipson JD. *Herbal medicines: a guide for health care professionals*. London: The Pharmaceutical Press, 1996: 21, 45, 63, 282.

26 Ridker PM. Toxic effects of herbal teas. *Arch Environ Health* 1987; **42**: 133–6.

27 Srivastava KC. Aqueous extracts of onion, garlic, and ginger inhibit platelet aggregation and alter arachidonic acid metabolism. *Biomed Biochim Acta* 1984; **43**: S335–46.

28 Nelsestuen GL. Role of gamma-carboxyglutamic acid. An unusual transition required for calcium dependent binding of prothrombin to phospholipid. *J Biol Chem* 1976; **251**: 5648–56.

29 Borowski M, Furie BC, Bauminger S, Furie B. Prothrombin requires two sequential metal-dependent conformational transitions to bind phospholipid. Confirmation-specific antibodies directed against the phospholipid binding site on prothrombin. *J Biol Chem* 1986; **261**: 14969–75.

30 Dam H. Antihemorrhagic vitamin of the chick; occurrence and chemical nature. *Nature* 1935; **135**: 652–3.

31 Almquist JH, Stohstad ELR. Dietary hemorrhagic disease in chicks. *Nature* 1935; **136**: 31.

32 Udall JA. Human sources and absorption of vitamin K in relation to anticoagulation stability. *JAMA* 1965; **19**: 127–9.

33 Lubetsky A, Dekel-Stern E, Chetrit A, Lubin F, Halkin H. Vitamin K intake and sensitivity to warfarin in patients consuming regular diets. *Thromb Haemost* 1999; **81**: 396–9.

34 Harris JE. Interaction of dietary factors with oral anticoagulants: review and applications. *J Am Diet Assoc* 1995; **95**: 580–4.

35 Weihrauch JL, Chatra AS. *Provisional table of the vitamin K content of foods*. Washington, DC: Department of Agriculture. Human Nutrition Information Service. February 1994. HNIS/PT-104.

36 Poller L. The effect of the use of different tissue extracts on one-stage prothrombin times. *Acta Haematol* 1964; **32**: 292–8.

37 Bussey HI, Force RW, Bianco TM, Leonard AD. Reliance on prothrombin time ratios causes significant errors in anticoagulation therapy. *Arch Intern Med* 1992; **152**: 278–82.

38 Poller L. Progress in standardization in anticoagulant control. *Hematol Rev* 1987; **1**: 225–41.

39 Kirkwood TBL. Calibration of reference thromboplastins and standardization of the prothrombin time ratio. *Thromb Haemost* 1983; **49**: 238–44.

40 Hirsh J, Poller L. The international normalized ratio. A guide to understanding and correcting its problems. *Arch Intern Med* 1994; **154**: 282–8.

41 Carter BL, Reinders TP, Hamilton RA. Prediction of maintenance dosage from initial patient response. *Drug Intell Clin Pharm* 1983; **17**: 23–6.

42 Williams DB, Karl RC. A simple technique for predicting daily maintenance dose of warfarin. *Am J Surg* 1979; **137**: 572–6.

43 Sharma NK, Routledge PA, Rawlins MD, Davies DM. Predicting the dose of warfarin for therapeutic anticoagulation. *Thromb Haemost* 1982; **47**: 2330–1.

44 Cosh DG, Moritz CK, Ashman KJ, Dally RJ, Gallus AS. Prospective evaluation of a flexible protocol for starting treatment with warfarin and predicting its maintenance dose. *Aust NZ J Med* 1989; **19**: 191–7.

45 Miller DR, Brown MA. Predicting warfarin maintenance dosage based on initial response. *Am J Hosp Pharm* 1979; **36**: 1351–5.

46 Fennerty A, Dolben J, Thomas P, et al. Flexible induction dose regimen for warfarin and prediction of maintenance dose. *BMJ* 1984; **288**: 1268–70.

47 Wilson R, James AH. Computer assisted management of warfarin treatment. *BMJ* 1984; **289**: 422–4.

48 Ryan PJ, Gilbert M, Rose PE. Computer control of anticoagulant dose for therapeutic management. *BMJ* 1989; **299**: 1207–9.

49 Poller L, Wright D, Rowlands M. Prospective comparative study of computer programs used for management of warfarin. *J Clin Pathol* 1993; **46**: 299–303.

50 Ageno W, Turpie AG. A randomized comparison of a computer-based dosing program with a manual system to monitor oral anticoagulant therapy. *J Thromb Thrombolysis* 1998; **5**(Suppl. 1): S69.

51 Harrison L, Johnston M, Massicotte MP, Crowther M, Moffat K, Hirsh J. Comparison of 5-mg and 10-mg loading doses in initiation of warfarin therapy. *Ann Intern Med* 1997; **126**: 133–6.

52 Dalen JE, Hirsh J, eds. Fifth ACCP Consensus Conference on Antithrombotic Therapy. *Chest* 1998; **114**: 439S–769S.

53 Hathaway W, Corrigan J. Report of Scientific and Standardization Subcommittee on Neonatal Hemostasis. *Thromb Haemost* 1991; **65**: 323–5.

54 Buck ML. Anticoagulation with warfarin in infants and children. *Ann Pharmacother* 1996; **30**: 1316–22.

55 Michelson AD, Bovill E, Monagle P, Andrew M. Antithrombotic therapy in children. *Chest* 1998; **114**: 748S–69S.

8

Modalities for assessing deep vein thrombosis and pulmonary embolism

C GREGORY ELLIOTT

DIAGNOSIS OF VENOUS THROMBOEMBOLISM

The diagnoses of deep vein thrombosis and acute pulmonary embolism remain a challenge for the primary care physician. Often, these diagnoses are not made prior to death, in part because of the nonspecificity of the symptoms, signs, and laboratory abnormalities which accompany venous thromboembolism. Symptoms of pulmonary embolism such as dyspnea or pleuritic chest pain may be erroneously attributed to common diseases which mimic pulmonary embolism (e.g., pneumonia), or which coexist with pulmonary embolism (e.g., chronic obstructive pulmonary disease). Furthermore, a diagnosis of deep vein thrombosis or pulmonary embolism based upon the history, physical examination, and basic laboratory studies is often wrong. Objective tests, such as pulmonary angiography, confirm the diagnosis of acute pulmonary embolism for only one in three patients referred for angiography.[1] Similarly, venography confirms the diagnosis of acute deep vein thrombosis in approximately one in five patients who are believed to have this diagnosis on clinical grounds.[2]

The requirement for the objective confirmation of clinically suspected deep vein thrombosis and acute pulmonary embolism presents additional challenges for the primary care physician. Which tests should be performed? In what sequence? When is additional testing needed? Why? What is the role of newer technologies such as contrast-enhanced spiral computed tomography, magnetic resonance angiography, D-dimers? Is one diagnostic strategy more cost effective than another?

The purpose of this chapter is to describe the current diagnostic approach to pulmonary embolism and deep vein thrombosis.

DEEP VEIN THROMBOSIS

Deep vein thrombosis remains a common clinical problem for the primary care physician. The diagnosis requires clinical suspicion *and* objective confirmation.[3] Although a number of objective tests are available to confirm the clinician's suspicion of deep vein thrombosis, compression ultrasonography with venous imaging is the preferred initial diagnostic test.

Clinical suspicion

As with pulmonary embolism, historical information and findings on physical examination influence the physician's suspicion that deep vein thrombosis is present. The most common symptom is pain, but patients may also complain of swelling or discoloration. Physical findings include tenderness over the deep veins of the lower extremity, swelling, venous distention, or a cyanotic or reddish purple discoloration. Homan's sign (discomfort in the upper calf on forced dorsiflexion) is both insensitive and nonspecific; whereas phlegmasia cerulea dolens (marked swelling and cyanosis with obstructive iliofemoral vein thrombosis) is more specific. Risk factors for venous thrombosis (Table 8.1) also strengthen the clinician's suspicion, whereas evidence of competing diagnoses (Table 8.2) decrease clinical suspicion.

Table 8.1 *Common risk factors for venous thromboembolism*

Age > 40 years
Cancer
Recent surgery or major trauma
Previous venous thromboembolism
Immobility[a]
Oral contraceptives

[a]Includes major medical illness, e.g., stroke, congestive heart failure, and immobility associated with prolonged travel.

Table 8.2 *Differential diagnosis of deep vein thrombosis*

Muscle tear	Cellulitis
Muscle ache	Myositis
Muscle hematoma	Lymphangitis
Ruptured Baker's cyst	Postphlebitic syndrome

Although a diagnosis of deep vein thrombosis based upon clinical features is unreliable, physicians can provide accurate estimates of the likelihood of deep vein thrombosis. For example, a clinical model based upon signs and symptoms, risk factors, and potential alternative diagnoses permitted physicians to identify subgroups of patients for whom the likelihood of deep vein thrombosis was high (85% prevalence), intermediate (33% prevalence), or low (5% prevalence).[4] Major points that suggest that deep vein thrombi are present include cancer diagnosed or treated within the previous 6 months, immobility for more than 3 days, major surgery within 4 weeks, calf swelling, tenderness localized to deep veins, and/or a strong family history. Features such as pitting edema, erythema, or dilated superficial veins were less predictive of deep vein thrombosis.

Diagnostic testing (Fig. 8.1)

COMPRESSION ULTRASONOGRAPHY WITH VENOUS IMAGING

Compression ultrasonography with venous imaging involves visualizing the deep veins of the lower extremity and applying pressure with the transducer over the entire length of the deep venous system.[5] The examination may be limited to the common femoral and the popliteal veins in some centers. The diagnosis of deep vein thrombosis requires demonstration of a noncompressible deep venous segment.[6] For outpatients who present with symptoms and signs of deep vein thrombosis, compression ultrasonography is a sensitive and specific test to confirm proximal deep vein thrombosis (Table 8.3).

Table 8.3 *Compression ultrasonography in patients with clinically suspected deep vein thrombosis*[a]

	Sensitivity (%)	Specificity (%)
Proximal	96	98
Calf only	87	95

[a]Data for deep vein thrombosis confirmed by venography pooled from nine prospective studies.

Compression ultrasonography has limitations. It does not detect isolated iliac vein thrombosis, and it is less sensitive than venography for the detection of isolated calf vein thrombosis. Similarly, the sensitivity of compression ultrasonography is low for the detection of both calf and proximal deep vein thrombi in asymptomatic, high-risk patients, e.g., patients who have just undergone hip or knee replacement (Table 8.4).

Table 8.4 *Compression ultrasonography for the detection of proximal deep vein thrombi in asymptomatic, high-risk patients*[a]

Sensitivity (%)	Specificity (%)	Positive predictive value (%)
62	97	79

[a]Data pooled from eight prospective studies.

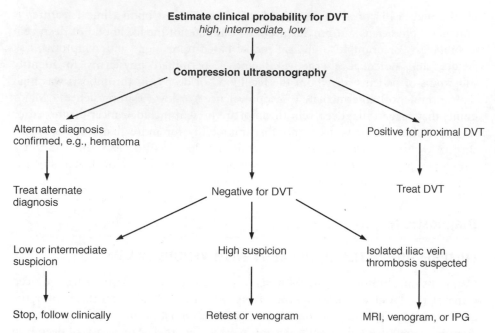

Figure 8.1 *A guide to the diagnosis of deep vein thrombosis. The exact approach may differ based upon clinical circumstances. For example, when the physician's suspicion is low and compression ultrasonography is positive, additional testing may be necessary, especially if risks for bleeding are present. (DVT = deep vein thrombosis; MRI = magnetic resonance imaging; IPG = impedance plethysmography.)*

Figure 8.1 outlines an approach to the outpatient suspected of having symptomatic, acute, proximal, deep vein thrombosis. Compression ultrasonography is the test of choice for the vast majority of patients in whom acute, proximal, deep vein thrombosis is suspected. When compression ultrasonography is negative, the physician must decide whether additional study is needed. Venography, impedance plethysmography, or magnetic resonance imaging is necessary when the physician suspects isolated iliac vein thrombosis. Because isolated iliac vein thrombosis may complicate pregnancy, magnetic resonance imaging or impedance plethysmography may be preferable to venography in pregnant patients.[7,8] Identification of an alternative diagnosis permits definitive treatment without additional study. Similarly, clinical follow-up without additional testing is appropriate for most patients, except those for whom the physician strongly suspects a falsely negative test. In this situation, either venography or repeat compression ultrasonography is appropriate. One clinical trial has shown a low rate (0.6% over 3 months) of venous thromboembolism when limited examinations of proximal deep veins were negative on two occasions (day 1, and a single repeated test done 5–7 days later) and anticoagulants were not given.[9]

MAGNETIC RESONANCE IMAGING

Magnetic resonance imaging appears to be a sensitive and specific method to confirm clinically suspected acute deep vein thrombi (Table 8.5). Limited data

Table 8.5 *Magnetic resonance imaging for acute deep vein thrombosis*[a]

	Sensitivity (%) (95% CI)	Specificity (%) (95% CI)
Pelvic veins	100	95
	(66–100)	(85–99)
Thigh veins	100	100
	(79–100)	(92–100)
Calf veins	87	97
	(60–98)	(85–100)

[a]Data from Evans et al. (1993).[10]

suggest that the sensitivity of this test is at least 80% for proximal deep vein thrombi.[10] Magnetic resonance imaging appears especially useful for the examination of pelvic veins, which are not easily evaluated by compression ultrasonography.

The utility of magnetic resonance imaging depends upon the active involvement of an experienced radiologist. Thus, the procedure is not widely available. Furthermore, patients with metallic devices, e.g., pacemakers, are not eligible.

CONTRAST VENOGRAPHY

Contrast venography is the reference standard for the diagnosis of deep vein thrombosis. Compression ultrasonography has become the preferred test for the evaluation of symptomatic deep vein thrombosis because it offers comparable diagnostic accuracy for proximal vein thrombi without the additional costs and risks of contrast venography. Idiosyncratic reactions (urticaria, angioedema, bronchospasm, or cardiovascular collapse), transient renal failure, or phlebitis may complicate venography (Table 8.6).

Table 8.6 *Complications of contrast venography*

Idiosyncratic
Urticaria
Angioedema
Bronchospasm
Cardiovascular collapse
Renal failure
Superficial or deep vein thrombophlebitis

Contrast venography remains useful for the occasional patient whose presentation suggests pelvic vein thrombosis or patients with negative compression ultrasonography in the face of very high clinical suspicion for proximal deep vein thrombosis. It is also the most useful test for the diagnosis of recurrent venous thrombosis. Although venography is more accurate than compression ultrasonography for the detection of isolated calf thrombosis, most physicians choose to follow up patients if compression ultrasonography is negative.

IMPEDANCE PLETHYSMOGRAPHY

Impedance plethysmography measures the impedance to electrical current passing between two electrodes on the calf. Impedance changes when blood pools in the leg following inflation of a tourniquet, and again as blood leaves the leg when the tourniquet deflates. Obstruction to the outflow of blood by proximal vein thrombosis *or* extrinsic compression of the vein alters the change in impedance. Thus, impedance plethysmography can only detect proximal deep vein thrombosis, and false-positive results are possible. Clinical observations suggest that false-positive results occur more frequently with impedance plethysmography than with compression ultrasonography,[2] and that compression ultrasonography is somewhat more sensitive and specific than impedance plethysmography for the evaluation of symptomatic outpatients.[11]

Impedance plethsymography can diagnose recurrent proximal deep vein thrombosis when impedance plethysmography has returned to normal following the previous episode of deep vein thrombosis. It is also less expensive than compression ultrasonography and it requires less technical expertise.

PULMONARY EMBOLISM

Clinical suspicion

Clinical suspicion remains a critical, but poorly defined, step in the diagnosis of acute pulmonary embolism. The decision to evaluate a patient for suspected pulmonary embolism reflects the physician's assessment of symptoms, signs, laboratory abnormalities, and the presence of risk factors (Tables 8.7, 8.8, and 8.9). The majority of patients with acute pulmonary embolism complain of dyspnea or pleuritic-type chest pain, and most patients with acute pulmonary embolism have tachypnea (respiratory rate $\geq$ 20/minute). The presence of risk factors, such as immobility, recent trauma or surgery, or underlying malignancy, should increase the level of clinical suspicion when symptoms or signs of pulmonary embolism are present.

The results of basic and more advanced laboratory studies may also suggest the diagnosis of pulmonary embolism. Chest radiographs, electrocardiograms, and arterial blood gases are often abnormal in patients with acute pulmonary embolism.

Table 8.7 *Symptoms which commonly suggest acute pulmonary embolism in patients without prior heart or lung disease*[a]

Symptom	%
Dyspnea	73
Pleuritic chest pain	66
Cough	37
Leg swelling	28
Leg pain	26
Hemoptysis	13
Palpitation	10
Wheezing	9
Ischemic chest pain	4

[a]Data from Stein et al. (1991).[34]

Cardiomegaly is the most common chest radiographic abnormality (Table 8.10), and abnormalities of T waves and ST segments are the most common electrocardiographic abnormalities (Table 8.11). More recently, investigators have added the

Table 8.8 *Signs which accompany acute pulmonary embolism in patients without prior heart or lung disease*[a]

Sign	%
Tachypnea (≥ 20/minute)	70
Rales	51
Tachycardia (> 100/minute)	30
Fourth heart sound	24
Increased P2	23
Diaphoresis	11
Temperature > 38.5°C	7
Wheezing	5
Right ventricular lift	4
Pleural friction rub	3

[a]Data from Stein et al. (1991).[34]

Table 8.9 *Basic laboratory abnormalities which accompany acute pulmonary embolism in patients without prior heart or lung disease*[a]

Laboratory abnormality	%
Alveolar–arterial oxygen tension gradient > 20 mmHg	86
Abnormal chest radiograph (see Table 8.10)	84
Abnormal electrocardiogram (see Table 8.11)	70

[a]Data from Stein et al. (1991).[34]

Table 8.10 *Chest radiographic abnormalities which may suggest acute pulmonary embolism*[a]

Cardiomegaly	27
Enlarged descending pulmonary artery	19
Elevated hemidiaphragm	20
Atelectasis	18
Lung density compatible with pulmonary infarction	
Truncated wedge-shaped area with indistinct borders ('Hampton hump')	5
Radiolucent area ('Westermark sign')	8
Pleural effusion (small)	23

[a]Data from Elliott et al. (2000).[35]

Table 8.11 *Electrocardiographic abnormalities accompanying acute pulmonary embolism in patients without prior heart or lung disease*[a]

Abnormality	%
ST segment and T wave abnormalities	49
P pulmonale *or* right bundle branch block, or right axis	6
Rhythm disturbances	
Atrial fibrillation	4
Atrial flutter	1

[a]Data from Stein et al. (1991).[34]

echocardiographic findings of abnormal right ventricular wall motion to the list of laboratory abnormalities which may indicate the presence of acute pulmonary embolism.[12] For some patients, transthoracic or transesophageal echocardiography may actually confirm the diagnosis of venous thromboembolism when thrombi are visualized in the right heart or central pulmonary arteries.

The exact threshold for ordering diagnostic tests remains uncertain, but, as a general rule, the physician should order diagnostic tests whenever clinical information does not allow confident exclusion of pulmonary embolism. Alternative diagnoses (e.g., status asthmaticus, pneumothorax) may eliminate clinical suspicion of acute pulmonary embolism for some patients. In contrast, additional tests to confirm or exclude the diagnosis of pulmonary embolism are usually required for some presentations, e.g., sudden dyspnea and arterial hypoxemia accompanied by a normal chest radiograph following major surgery.

Once a physician suspects pulmonary embolism, it is important to estimate the level of suspicion. The Prospective Investigation of Pulmonary Embolism Diagnosis (PIOPED) provided strong evidence that the strength of clinical suspicion before lung scanning influences the likelihood that pulmonary embolism is responsible for abnormalities detected by ventilation and perfusion lung scans (Table 8.12).[1] For example, 40% of patients had pulmonary emboli identified by pulmonary arteriography when a physician strongly suspected acute pulmonary embolism and the ventilation and perfusion lung scan pattern was consistent with a low probability for acute pulmonary embolism. Conversely, only 4% of patients had acute pulmonary embolism when a low-probability ventilation and perfusion lung scan pattern was accompanied by a low pretest clinical suspicion.

Table 8.12 *Influence of pretest clinical suspicion upon the likelihood that lung scan patterns are due to pulmonary embolism*[a]

| Scan pattern | Pretest clinical suspicion for pulmonary embolism | | |
	High (80–100)	Intermediate (20–79)	Low (0–19)
High	96	88	56
Intermediate	66	28	16
Low	40	16	4

[a]Data from the PIOPED Investigators.[1]

Exact definitions of the degree of clinical suspicion are not available. At present, the level of suspicion represents the physician's gestalt of available clinical information. One proposed scheme considers pulmonary embolism to be highly probable when patients with one or more risk factors have common symptoms, signs, or laboratory abnormalities of pulmonary embolism for which there is no alternative diagnosis.[13] Conversely, pulmonary embolism is much less likely (low a priori suspicion) when no risk factor is present and another condition can explain the symptoms, signs, or laboratory abnormalities which suggest acute pulmonary embolism. Clinical data which do not meet criteria for high or low a priori suspicion represent an intermediate clinical suspicion for acute pulmonary embolism.

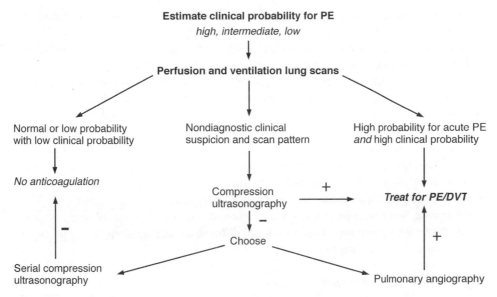

Figure 8.2 *A guide to the evaluation of clinically suspected acute pulmonary embolism (PE). The exact approach may differ based upon clinical circumstances. (DVT = deep vein thrombosis.)*

Diagnostic testing (Fig. 8.2)

VENTILATION AND PERFUSION LUNG SCANS

Perfusion lung scans remain the cornerstone for the evaluation of clinically suspected acute pulmonary embolism. A normal perfusion lung scan excludes clinically important pulmonary embolism, and provides sufficient evidence to withhold anticoagulant therapy.[14] Conversely, an abnormal perfusion lung scan often results from diseases other than pulmonary embolism. Combining abnormal perfusion lung scans with pulmonary ventilation scans permits an estimate of the likelihood that a patient has acute pulmonary embolism. Furthermore, when the physician combines pretest clinical suspicion with well-defined ventilation and perfusion lung scan patterns, precise estimates of the likelihood that acute pulmonary embolism will be found on pulmonary angiography are possible (Table 8.12).

APPROACH TO THE PATIENT WITH NONDIAGNOSTIC LUNG SCANS

Unfortunately, the combination of clinical suspicion and lung scan results often does not permit confident confirmation or exclusion of pulmonary embolism. Knowledgeable experts agree that all intermediate lung scan patterns, regardless of clinical suspicion, are nondiagnostic.[13,15,16] Similarly, lung scan patterns which conflict with the clinical estimate, e.g., low-probability scans and high clinical probability *or* high-probability scans and low clinical probability, are nondiagnostic. There is also general agreement that intermediate clinical suspicion and high-probability or low-probability lung scan patterns are nondiagnostic; and that low-probability lung scan patterns in combination with a low clinical suspicion permit the physician to withhold treatment without additional diagnostic tests for acute pulmonary embolism.

Additional diagnostic tests are essential when the clinical evaluation combined with lung scan results does not confirm or exclude acute pulmonary embolism.

The approach to the patient who requires additional diagnostic tests remains controversial. The primary care physician must consider regional expertise and resources. One approach is to perform pulmonary angiography. A negative pulmonary angiogram provides sufficient evidence to withhold anticoagulant therapy.[17,18] Another approach is to perform impedance plethysmography or compression ultrasonography examinations of the lower extremities. If these studies are positive, the physician treats the patient for venous thromboembolism. If the first study is negative, serial examinations of the lower extremities are necessary. The latter approach is not appropriate for patients with limited cardiopulmonary reserve (Table 8.13). These patients should undergo pulmonary angiography if compression ultrasonography is negative.

Table 8.13 *Limited cardiorespiratory reserve*[a]

Hypotension (systolic blood pressure < 90 mmHg)
Acute tachyarrhythmia
Abnormal spirometry (FEV$_1$ < 1.0 L, FVC < 1.5 L)
Abnormal ABG (PaO$_2$ < 50 mmHg or PaCO$_2$ > 45 mmHg)
Pulmonary edema
Right ventricular failure

[a]These patients require definitive diagnosis by pulmonary angiography (or other technique) when ventilation and perfusion lung scans are not diagnostic.[21]
(FEV$_1$ = forced expired volume in 1 second; FVC = forced vital capacity; PaO$_2$ = partial pressure of oxygen in the arterial blood; PaCO$_2$ = partial pressure of carbon dioxide in the arterial blood.)

PULMONARY ANGIOGRAPHY

Pulmonary angiography is invasive, expensive, and not always readily available. The technique involves venous catheterization, with passage of the catheter into the main pulmonary arteries. Current techniques call for selective injections of contrast into the right and left pulmonary artery. Reduction of the injection flow rate of contrast and the total contrast volume injected is appropriate when pulmonary hypertension is present. A history of life-threatening reaction to contrast dye is a strong contraindication to pulmonary angiography, whereas pulmonary hypertension is not. Although many complications are possible, major complications are rare (Table 8.14), occurring in approximately 1% of patients.[19] Major complications are more likely in critically ill patients and older patients. Pulmonary angiography costs approximately $2000 (hospital plus professional fees; 1999 figure).

Lower extremity studies to detect deep vein thrombosis

Because pulmonary angiography is expensive, invasive, and not always readily available, physicians have examined less expensive noninvasive tests. Impedance plethysmography and compression ultrasonography with venous imaging may detect deep vein thrombi in patients suspected of having pulmonary embolism, and permit the initiation of antithrombotic therapy. Conversely, serial negative studies of the legs

Table 8.14 *Complications of pulmonary angiography*[a]

Complication	%
Death[b]	0.5
Renal failure (dialysis)	0.3
Respiratory failure (CPR or intubation)	0.4
Hematoma (requiring transfusion)	0.2
Bronchospasm	0.2
Hypotension	0.2
Urticaria	1.4

[a]Data from Stein et al. (1992).[19]
[b]Not clearly attributable to the procedure, as the patients had severe cardiorespiratory impairment before pulmonary angiography.
(CPR = cardiopulmonary resuscitation.)

may permit anticoagulant therapy to be withheld safely because recurrent pulmonary embolism is unlikely when proximal deep vein thrombi are not present.

Impedance plethysmography can be used to diagnose proximal deep vein thrombosis. This technique is relatively inexpensive, although it requires technical expertise.[20] When serial studies are performed, impedance plethysmography provides a noninvasive alternative to pulmonary angiography for patients with nondiagnostic ventilation and perfusion lung scans and adequate cardiorespiratory reserve. A prospective study found that only 12 of 627 patients with clinically suspected pulmonary embolism, nondiagnostic lung scans, and repeatedly negative impedance plethysmography had symptomatic pulmonary embolism or deep vein thrombosis during a 3-month follow-up period, even though they did not receive anticoagulant therapy.[21] An additional 16 patients had proximal deep vein thrombosis detected when impedance plethysmography was repeated on four occasions during the 2 weeks immediately after the first presentation, underscoring the importance of *serial* studies for this noninvasive strategy. Using this strategy, the risk for symptomatic recurrence is less than 3%. Thus, serial impedance plethysmography represents a clinically validated, noninvasive strategy for the primary care physician to use when confronted with nondiagnostic combinations of clinical suspicion and lung scans and a negative initial study of the leg veins. The requirement for four tests over 2 weeks and the need for technical expertise are both practical barriers to this strategy. Furthermore, impedance plethysmography is neither as sensitive nor as specific for the diagnosis of proximal deep vein thrombosis as compression ultrasonography with B mode venous imaging.[2]

Compression ultrasonography is an alternative for the evaluation of patients with suspected pulmonary embolism and nondiagnostic ventilation and perfusion lung scans.[22] Compression ultrasonography with B mode venous imaging is useful when proximal deep vein thrombi are present.[22] Identification of proximal deep vein thrombi by compression ultrasonography is an indication for treatment, and avoids pulmonary angiography. Unfortunately, although bilateral contrast venography often identifies deep vein thrombi after a patient has had symptomatic pulmonary embolism,[23] bilateral compression ultrasonography limited to the common femoral and popliteal veins rarely identifies proximal deep vein thrombi in patients suspected of having pulmonary embolism.[24] Thus, if the practitioner chooses compression ultrasonography, and the test is negative, either compression ultrasonography should be repeated serially (days 2, 7, and 14)[22] to exclude subsequent extension of calf vein thrombi into popliteal or more proximal veins *or* pulmonary angiography should be performed, because negative bilateral compression ultrasonography cannot exclude the diagnosis of pulmonary embolism.

NEW TECHNOLOGIES

A number of new technologies may eliminate or greatly reduce the need for pulmonary angiography. Contrast-enhanced spiral computed tomography and magnetic resonance angiography are sensitive and specific for the diagnosis of large central pulmonary emboli,[25,26] and it is likely that technologic advances will occur rapidly to improve the accuracy of these techniques for the evaluation of more peripheral pulmonary vessels.[27] For the present, these techniques cannot be used routinely to evaluate suspected pulmonary embolism. In cases where they are used, the primary care physician should not forget that smaller, more peripheral thromboemboli may be missed with the current technology.

Magnetic resonance angiography

A few medical centers have combined fast magnetic resonance hardware with dynamic gadolinium enhancement in order to perform high-resolution pulmonary angiography. This approach avoids the risks of pulmonary angiography. Furthermore, when experienced physicians perform and interpret these studies, the sensitivity and specificity of magnetic resonance angiography for the evaluation of thromboemboli in main and segmental pulmonary arteries appear acceptable.[25]

Spiral computed tomography

Spiral computed tomography is more widely available than magnetic resonance angiography. The patient moves continuously through the scanner. The rotating gantry and detector system assemble images rapidly while the patient performs a breath-hold maneuver. Vascular imaging requires a bolus of contrast material. Thus, unlike magnetic resonance angiography, the risks associated with contrast materials are not avoided. Spiral computed tomography can detect thromboemboli in main, lobar, or segmental pulmonary arteries, with sensitivities reported between 73% and 97% and specificities of 86–98%.[28]

Contrast-enhanced electron-beam computer tomography

This technique does not require breath holding because scanning times are very short, and it reduces artifacts from respiratory and cardiac motion. Like spiral computed tomography, this technique requires a bolus of contrast and, like spiral computed tomography, it permits evaluation of other mediastinal structures, e.g., lymph nodes, pericardium, etc.

D-dimer

D-dimer is a unique degradation product released into the circulation by endogenous fibrinolysis of a cross-linked fibrin clot. Recently, investigators have evaluated serum assays for D-dimer as screeing tests for venous thromboembolism.[29,30] Two assays, a latex and an enzyme-linked immunosorbent assay (ELISA), are available.

The ELISA assay takes time and is labor intensive, whereas the latex assay is not sensitive enough to exclude venous thromboembolism. For these reasons, D-dimer assays are not widely employed for the evaluation of clinically suspected acute pulmonary embolism. However, available evidence suggests that the ELISA assay, because of its high sensitivity and high negative predictive value for acute venous thromboembolism, may permit thromboembolism to be excluded.[29] Whole-blood assays (Simpli RED) show promise as rapidly available screening tests.[30] At present, D-dimer assays require further validation and standardization before they can be considered appropriate screening tests for venous thromboembolism.

Cost effectiveness

The most cost effective approach to the diagnosis of pulmonary embolism remains controversial.[31-3] Strategies which use perfusion lung scans, D-dimer ELISA assays, impedance plethysmography, or compression ultrasonography to minimize the number of pulmonary arteriograms while maintaining diagnostic accuracy are most cost effective. For example, a strategy which performs pulmonary angiography on all patients with an abnormal non-high-probability lung scan maintains diagnostic accuracy, but requires pulmonary angiography for more than 50% of patients with clinically suspected pulmonary embolism. In contrast, a strategy which only performs pulmonary angiography after a negative compression ultrasonography examination of the legs, and does not do so with low clinical suspicion and a low-probability pattern on ventilation and perfusion lung scanning, is less expensive and requires that few patients undergo pulmonary angiography. One study has compared the costs that would have been incurred to evaluate a large cohort of patients, emphasizing correct diagnosis and management for each patient.[33] A strategy based upon the use of ventilation–perfusion lung scans, serial impedance plethysmography, and pulmonary angiography was most cost effective (Table 8.15).

Table 8.15 *Costs of alternative strategies for evaluating suspected pulmonary embolism*[a]

Strategy[b]	Cost per patient who required treatment – 1992 US dollars	Cost per patient correctly not treated – 1992 US dollars
1	14 421	5978
2	14 047	5865
3	14 407	6016
4	12 639	4333
5	13 842	4745

[a]Adapted from Hull et al. (1996).[33]
[b]Strategy 1: ventilation–perfusion lung scans and pulmonary angiography. Strategy 2: ventilation–perfusion lung scans, single bilateral impedance plethysmography, and pulmonary angiography. Strategy 3: ventilation–perfusion lung scans, single bilateral compression ultrasonography, and pulmonary angiography. Strategy 4: ventilation–perfusion lung scans, serial bilateral impedance plethysmography, and pulmonary angiography. Strategy 5: ventilation–perfusion lung scans, serial bilateral compression ultrasonography, and pulmonary angiography.

SUMMARY

Deep vein thrombosis

The clinical diagnosis of deep vein thrombosis is unreliable, and objective testing is necessary to confirm or exclude the diagnosis. Although contrast venography is the reference standard, compression ultrasonography with venous imaging is the preferred test, because it is noninvasive and comparably accurate for the detection of symptomatic proximal deep vein thrombi.

Recurrent deep vein thrombosis

This diagnosis remains difficult. Contrast venography is the reference standard against which impedance plethysmography has been validated.

Isolated pelvic vein thrombosis

Contrast venography and magnetic resonance imaging are the most sensitive and specific tests. Compression ultrasonography is less reliable.

Pulmonary embolism

The first step in the evaluation of pulmonary embolism is an estimate of clinical suspicion followed by perfusion and ventilation lung scans. A normal lung scan excludes pulmonary embolism, whereas high-probability scan patterns accompanied by high clinical suspicion usually provide sufficient evidence to treat the patient for pulmonary embolism. Additional diagnostic testing is necessary when ventilation and perfusion lung scan patterns are nondiagnostic. Pulmonary angiography, although expensive and invasive, is the definitive test. Serial, noninvasive, lower extremity tests (impedance plethysmography or compression ultrasonograpy) may subsititute for pulmonary angiography for patients who have adequate cardiopulmonary reserve.

REFERENCES

1 PIOPED Investigators. Value of the ventilation/perfusion scan in acute pulmonary embolism. *J Am Med Assoc* 1990; **263**: 2753–9.
2 Heijboer H, Buller HR, Lensing AWA. A comparison of real-time compression ultrasonography with impedance plethysmography for the diagnosis of deep-vein thrombosis in symptomatic outpatients. *N Engl J Med* 1993; **329**: 1365–9.
3 Wheeler HB, Hirsh J, Wells P, Anderson FA. Diagnostic tests for deep vein thrombosis. *Arch Intern Med* 1994; **154**: 1921–8.
4 Wells PS, Hirsh J, Anderson DR, et al. Accuracy of clinical assessment of deep-vein thrombosis. *Lancet* 1995; **345**: 1326–30.

5 Talbot SR. B-mode evaluation of peripheral veins. *Semin Ultrasound CTMR* 1988; **9**: 295–319.

6 Lensing AW, Prandoni P, Brandjes D. Detection of deep-vein thrombosis by real-time B-mode ultrasonography. *N Engl J Med* 1989; **320**: 342–5.

7 Hull RD, Raskob GE, Carter CJ. Serial impedance plethysmographhy in pregnant patients with clinically suspected deep-vein thrombosis. Clinical validity of negative findings. *Ann Intern Med* 1990; **112**: 663–7.

8 Spritzer CE, Evans AC, Kay HH. Magnetic resonance imaging of deep venous thrombosis in pregnant women in lower extremity edema. *Obstet Gynecol* 1995; **85**: 603–7.

9 Birdwell GB, Raskob GE, Whitsett TL, et al. The clinical validity of normal compression ultrasonography in outpatients suspected of having deep vein thrombosis. *Ann Intern Med* 1998; **128**: 1–7.

10 Evans AJ, Sostman HD, Knelson MH,et al. Detection of deep vein thrombosis: prospective comparison of MRI with contrast venography. *Am J Roentgenol* 1993; **161**: 131–9.

11 Wells PS, Hirsh J, Anderson DR, et al. Comparison of the accuracy of impedance plethysmography and real-time compression ultrasonography in outpatients with clinically suspected deep vein thrombosis. *Thromb Haemost* 1995; **74**: 1423–7.

12 Wolfe MW, Lee RT, Feldstein ML, Parker JA, Come PC, Goldhaber SZ. Prognostic significance of right ventricular hypokinesis and perfusion lung scan defects in pulmonary embolism. *Am Heart J* 1994; **127**: 1371–5.

13 Hyers TM. Diagnosis of pulmonary embolism. *Thorax* 1995; **50**: 930–2.

14 Hull RD, Raskob GE, Coates G, et al. Clinical validity of a normal perfusion lung scan in patients with suspected pulmonary embolism. *Chest* 1990; **97**: 23–6.

15 Elliott CG. Pulmonary embolism. In: Donald F, Tierney MD, eds *Current pulmonology*. Chicago: Mosby-Year Book, Inc., 1995: 51–85.

16 Kelley MA, Carson JL, Palevsky HI, et al. Diagnosing pulmonary embolism: new facts and strategies. *Ann Intern Med* 1991; **114**: 300–6.

17 Noveline RA. The clinical course of patients with suspected pulmonary embolism and a negative pulmonary angiogram. *Radiology* 1978; **126**: 561–7.

18 Henry JW, Relya B, Stein PD. Continuing risk of thromboemboli among patients with normal pulmonary angiograms. *Chest* 1995; **107**: 1375–8.

19 Stein PD, Athanasoulis C, Alavi A, et al. Complications and validity of pulmonary angiography in acute pulmonary embolism. *Circulation* 1992; **85**: 462–8.

20 Anderson FA, Cardullo PA, Wheeler HB. Problems commonly encountered in IPG testing and their solution. *Bruit* 1980; **IV**: 21–4.

21 Hull RD, Raskob GE, Ginsberg JS, et al. A noninvasive strategy for the treatment of patients with suspected pulmonary embolism. *Arch Intern Med* 1994; **154**: 289–97.

22 Wells PS, Ginsberg JS, Anderson DR, et al. Use of a clinical model for safe management of patients with suspected pulmonary embolism. *Ann Intern Med* 1998; **129**: 997–1005.

23 Hull RD, Hirsh J, Carter CJ, et al. Pulmonary angiography, ventilation lung scanning, and venography for clinically suspected pulmonary embolism with abnormal perfusion lung scan. *Ann Intern Med* 1983; **98**: 891–9.

24 Turkstra F, Kuiker PMM, van Beek EJR, Brandjes DPM, ten Cate JW, Buller HR. Diagnostic utility of ultrasonography of leg veins in patients suspected of having pulmonary embolism. *Ann Intern Med* 1997; **126**: 775–81.

25 Meany JFM, Weg JG, Chenevert TL, Stafford-Johnson D, Hamilton BH, Prince MR.

Diagnosis of pulmonary embolism with magnetic resonance angiography. *N Engl J Med* 1997; **336**: 1422–7.

26 Remy-Jardin M, Remy J, Deschildre F, et al. Diagnosis of pulmonary embolism with spiral CT: comparison with pulmonary angiography and scintigraphy. *Radiology* 1996; **200**: 699–706.

27 Woodard PK. Pulmonary arteries must be seen before they can be assessed. *Radiology* 1997; **204**: 11–12.

28 Tapson VF. Pulmonary embolism – new diagnostic approaches. *N Engl J Med* 1997; **336**: 1449–51.

29 Perrier A, Desmarais S, Goehring C, et al. D-dimer testing for suspected pulmonary embolism in outpatients. *Am J Respir Crit Care Med* 1997; **156**: 492–6.

30 Ginsberg JS, Kearon C, Douketis J, et al. Bedside blood test can help diagnose deep vein thrombosis. *Arch Intern Med* 1997; **157**: 1077–81.

31 Oudkerk M, van Beek EJR, van Putten WLJ, Buller HR. Cost-effectiveness analysis of various strategies in the diagnostic management of pulmonary embolism. *Arch Intern Med* 1993; **153**: 947–54.

32 Perrier A, Buswell L, Bounameaux H, et al. Cost-effectiveness of noninvasive diagnostic aids in suspected pulmonary embolism. *Arch Intern Med* 1997; **157**: 2309–16.

33 Hull RD, Feldstein W, Stein PD, Pineo GF. Cost-effectiveness of pulmonary embolism diagnosis. *Arch Intern Med* 1996; **156**: 68–72.

34 Stein PD, Terrin ML, Hales CA, et al. Clinical, laboratory, roentgenographic, and electrocardiographic findings in patients with acute pulmonary embolism and no pre-existing cardiac or pulmonary disease. *Chest* 1991; **100**: 598–603.

35 Elliott CG, Goldhaber SZ, Visani L, DeRosa M. Chest radiographs in acute pulmonary embolism. *Chest* 2000; **118**: 33–8.

9

Prophylaxis for deep vein thrombosis and pulmonary embolism in the surgical and medical patient

GENO J MERLI

INTRODUCTION

The Fifth Consensus Conference on Antithrombotic Therapy provides the most up-to-date guidelines for the prevention of deep vein thrombosis and pulmonary embolism in surgical and nonsurgical patients.[1] These recommendations have become a major guideline for clinicians managing patients in the perioperative period. Despite these recommendations, there continues to remain a concern for balancing the risk of major postoperative bleeding versus the benefit of preventing thrombosis. In an attempt to resolve this issue, clinicians have requested evidence-based guidelines for identification of high-risk groups for whom prophylaxis must be utilized as well as mechanical and pharmacologic options for preventing deep vein thrombosis/pulmonary embolism. In addition, the perioperative management of patients on long-term anticoagulation for prosthetic valves, atrial fibrillation, or recurrent deep vein thrombosis/pulmonary embolism will require guidelines. The focus of this chapter is to review the etiology, risk factor stratification, deep vein thrombosis/pulmonary embolism regimens of prophylaxis, and recommendations for managing patients on long-term anticoagulation.

ETIOLOGY OF DEEP VEIN THROMBOSIS

Stasis, intimal injury, and hypercoagulability are the three risk factors that contribute to the development of thrombosis in the postopertive period.[2]

Stasis results from the supine position and the effects of anesthesia. Venographic studies in supine patients demonstrated that there was delayed clearing of venographic contrast media from the soleal sinuses of the calf muscles.[3,4] Concomitant with this pooling is the vasodilatory effect of anesthesia, which increases venous capacitance and decreases venous return from the lower extremities.[5,6] Venous thrombi composed of platelets, fibrin, and red blood cells develop behind the venous valve cusps or the intramuscular sinuses of the calf secondary to decreased blood flow and stasis.[7]

Intimal injury from excessive vasodilatation caused by vasoactive amines, anesthesia, and surgical manipulation, such as positioning, tourniquets, and vessel traction, all contribute to endothelial damage and the establishment of sites for clot formation.[8,9]

Stasis and surgery set up the appropriate conditions for the development of hypercoagulability. The impaired venous blood flow results in a decreased clearance of activated clotting factors, which subsequently set up clot formation on areas of intimal injury and low flow areas such as the posterior valve cusps.[10] Other factors have been assessed, such as fibrinopeptide A, platelet factor 4, beta thromboglobulin, antithrombin III, alpha-2-antiplasmin, factor VIII activity, von Willebrand factor antigen, tissue plasminogen activator inhibitor, D-dimers, thrombin antithrombin III complexes, fragment F 1+2, and decreased plasmin activity.[11] Recently, Confrencesco et al. evaluated D-dimers, thrombin antithrombin III, and fragment F 1+2 in patients undergoing total hip replacement.[12] These three tests did not demonstrate significant sensitivity and specificity when compared to venography as the thrombosis endpoint. None of these factors has been demonstrated to be sensitive and specific in predicting those patients at risk for developing deep vein thrombosis in the postoperative period.

Stasis, intimal injury, and hypercoagulability are the three major factors that contribute to the development of deep vein thrombosis/pulmonary embolism in the postoperative period. The use of pharmacologic and mechanical modalities serves to reverse or prevent thromboembolic complications.

RISK FACTOR ASSESSMENT

When assessing the patient's risk for deep vein thrombosis/pulmonary embolism prior to surgery, age, length and type of surgery, previous deep vein thrombosis/pulmonary embolism, and secondary risk factors must be considered. The secondary

Table 9.1 *Clinical risk factors for developing deep vein thrombosis/pulmonary embolism*

1   Age > 40 years
2   Prolonged immobilization
3   Previous deep vein thrombosis/pulmonary embolism
4   Cancer
5   Obesity
6   Varicose veins
7   Congestive heart failure
8   Stroke
9   Inflammatory bowel disease
10 Nephrotic syndrome
11 Estrogen use
12 Hereditary or acquired thrombotic disorders
13 Major surgery: abdomen, pelvis, lower extremities
14 Fractures: pelvis, hip, leg
15 Indwelling catheters

risk factors are numerous (Table 9.1) but the following are most significant: obesity, varicose veins, estrogen use, malignancy, paralysis, and prolonged immobilization.[1] Patients are classified as low, moderate, high, or very high risk for developing postoperative deep vein thrombosis/pulmonary embolism, and appropriate prophylaxis should be applied for each of the categories (Table 9.2).[1]

Table 9.2 *Deep vein thrombosis/pulmonary embolism risk classification*

Risk categories	Calf deep vein thrombosis (%)	Proximal deep vein thrombosis (%)	Fatal pulmonary embolism (%)
Low risk	2	< 0.4	< 0.002
a. Age < 40 years			
b. Minor surgery			
c. No secondary risk factors			
Moderate risk	10–20	4–8	0.1–0.4
a. Age > 40 years			
b. Major surgery			
c. No secondary risk factors			
High risk	20–40	4–8	0.4–1
a. Age > 40 years			
b. Major surgery			
c. Secondary risk factors			
d. Age > 60, years major surgery, no risk factors			
Very high risk	40–80	10–20	1–5
a. Age > 40 years			
b. Major surgery			
c. Previous deep vein thrombosis/pulmonary embolism, cancer, hypercoagulable state			
d. Orthopedic surgery, multiple trauma, acute spinal cord injury			

(DVT = deep vein thrombosis; PE = pulmonary embolism.)
Secondary risk factors: obesity, varicose veins, estrogen use, malignancy, immobilization, and paralysis.
Adapted from Clagett et al. (1998).[1]

Low-risk patients are aged over 40, without secondary risk factors, and undergoing uncomplicated minor surgery. This group of patients has a 2% risk of calf deep vein thrombosis, a 0.4% risk of proximal vein deep vein thrombosis, and a 0.002% risk of fatal pulmonary embolism if prophylaxis is not used.

Moderate-risk patients are over the age of 40, having major surgery, and with no secondary risk factors (obesity, varicose veins, estrogen use, malignancy, paralysis, and prolonged immobilization). Without prophylaxis, this group has a 10–20% risk of developing calf vein thrombosis, a 2–4% risk of proximal vein clot, and a 0.1–0.4% risk of fatal pulmonary embolism.

The high-risk group comprises those patients over the age of 40, having major surgery, and with the presence of one or more of the secondary risk factors (obesity, varicose veins, estrogen use, malignancy, paralysis, and prolonged immobilization). This group has a 20–40% risk of calf vein thrombosis, a 4–8% risk of proximal vein thrombosis, and a 0.4–1% risk of fatal pulmonary embolism if prophylaxis is not utilized.

The very high-risk group comprises patients over the age of 40, having major surgery for malignancy or an orthopedic procedure of the lower extremities, a previous history of deep vein thrombosis/pulmonary embolism, hip fracture, stroke, or spinal cord injury. This group has a 40–80% risk of calf vein thrombosis, a 10–20% risk of proximal vein thrombosis, and a 1–5% risk of fatal pulmonary embolism without the use of prophylactic regimens.

All patients should be risk stratified for deep vein thrombosis/pulmonary embolism prior to surgery in order to provide the most effective and safe prophylaxis for the prevention of this complication.

MODALITIES OF PROPHYLAXIS

At the present time, there are a number of recommended modalities of prophylaxis for deep vein thrombosis/pulmonary embolism. Each modality should be administered in its own specific regimen. In this section, each modality is reviewed with respect to dose, administration, and duration of therapy (Table 9.3).[11]

Fixed-dose heparin

Heparin is administered subcutaneously with 5000 units 2 hours prior to surgery. This is followed postoperatively with 5000 units subcutaneously every 8 or 12 hours until the patient is fully ambulatory or discharged. In double-blind trials, the incidence of major hemorrhagic events was 1.8% versus 0.8% in the controls.[13] This difference is not statistically significant. The incidence of minor bleeding such as injection site and wound hematomas has been reported to be significant, with 6.3% in the low-dose heparin and 4.1% in the controls.

Adjusted low-dose heparin

Adjusted low-dose heparin was developed for use in total hip replacement patients. In the original study of its use, prophylaxis with heparin was begun at 3500 units

Table 9.3 *Regimens of pharmacologic prophylaxis for deep vein thrombosis/pulmonary embolism*

I. Heparin
    A. 5000 U, subcutaneously, 2 hours prior to surgery then every 8 hours or 12 hours
    B. Maintain prophylaxis until discharge

II. Adjusted-dose heparin
    A. 3500 U, subcutaneously, 2 hours prior to surgery
    B. 3500 U, subcutaneously, every 8 hours postoperative (0800, 1600, 2400 hours)
    C. Begin adjusting the dose 6 hours following the 1600 hours' dose on the day of surgery, using the dosing schedule below. The first adjusted dose will be at 2400 hours
    D. If the patient returns from the procedure after 1600 hours, begin dosing adjustment as in E below
    E. Postoperative day 1: adjust the day's remaining heparin doses by an aPTT obtained 6 hours following the 0800 hours' heparin dose. Use the heparin-dosing schedule below
    F. Thereafter, adjust the dose every second day, 6 hours after the 0800 hours' dose
    G. After two to three adjustments, either begin warfarin (INR 2–3) or maintain the patient on the last total daily-adjusted dose of heparin, subcutaneously, every 12 hours for 7–10 days.
        < 36 s = + 1000 U
        36–40 s = + 500 U
        41–45 s = no additional heparin
        46–50 s = –500 U
        50 s = –1000 U

(To establish the above dosing scale, take the top normal aPTT of the laboratory and add or subtract by 4 s.)

III. Low molecular weight heparins (FDA-approved indications)
    A. Enoxaparin
        1. General surgery:
            a. 40 mg, subcutaneouslty daily beginning 12 hours postsurgery
        2. Orthopedic surgery (THR and TKR)
            a. 30 mg, subcutaneously, every 12 hours beginning 12–24 hours postsurgery
            b. 40 mg, subcutaneously daily beginning 12–24 hours postsurgery (European Dosing Schedule)
    B. Dalteparin
        1. General surgery
            a. 5000 U, subcutaneously, 10–12 hours prior to surgery, then once daily postsurgery
        2. Orthopedic surgery (THR)
            a. 5000 U, subcutaneouslty, 8–12 hours prior to surgery, then once daily 12 hours postsurgery
    C. Ardeparin
        1. Orthopedic surgery (TKR)
            a. 50 U/kg twice daily starting 12–24 hours postsurgery

IV. Warfarin
    A. Method 1
        1. 10 mg, by mouth, the evening prior to surgery
        2. 5 mg, by mouth, the evening of surgery   *continued*

Table 9.3 *continued*

3. Adjust warfarin dose daily to an INR of 2–3
4. Maintain warfarin for 7–10 days or 4–6 weeks for extended prophylaxis with a target INR of 2–3
  B. Method 2
1. Begin warfarin at home 12–14 days prior to admission
2. Maintain the prothrombin time at 1.5–3 s beyond control
3. Postoperative day 1: begin adjusting dose to maintain an INR of 2–3
4. Maintain warfarin for 7–10 days or 4–6 weeks for extended prophylaxis with a target INR of 2–3
  C. Method 3
1. 10 mg, by mouth, the evening of surgery
2. No warfarin on postoperative day 1
3. Postoperative day 2: begin warfarin and adjust dose to achieve an INR 2–3
4. Maintain warfarin for 7–10 days or 4–6 weeks for extended prophylaxis with a target INR of 2–3

V. External pneumatic compression devices
  A. Extremity sleeves or foot pumps must be applied prior to or at the time of surgery
  B. These devices should be worn continuously except for during therapy, ambulating, testing, or bathroom visits
  C. If the patient has been at bed rest or immobilized for over 72 hours without prophylaxis, the extremity should be screened for deep vein thrombosis prior to placing the compression devices

(aPTT = activated partial thromboplastin time; INR = International Normalized Ratio; THR = total hip replacement; TKR = total knee replacement.)

delivered subcutaneously every 8 hours, 2 days prior to surgery.[14] Adjustments were made on a sliding scale in order to maintain the activated partial thromboplastin time (aPTT) at the top-normal level of the laboratory. The current practice of same-day admission does not practically allow for compliance with the above regimen.

We begin heparin at 3500 units delivered subcutaneously 2 hours prior to surgery, followed postoperatively by 3500 units delivered subcutaneously every 8 hours, beginning with the evening of the procedure.[11] The first heparin dose is adjusted according to the aPTT 6 hours after the postoperative afternoon dose. If surgery goes beyond the 1600-hour time, then the first adjustment should begin after the following morning dose, as noted in Table 9.3. The second adjustment is completed 6 hours after the morning dose on postoperative day 1, then every 2 days for two to three adjustments. The heparin dose is derived from a sliding scale schedule of 4 seconds plus or minus the top-normal of the laboratory. The object is to maintain the aPTT at a range within 4 seconds of the top-normal level. The dose of heparin is adjusted for 7–10 days postoperatively, after which time warfarin – International Normalized Ratio (INR) of 2–3 – or the last total daily adjusted dose of heparin is given every 12 hours until the patient is discharged. Two studies have reported no increase in the risk of major bleeding with this regimen.[14]

Low molecular weight heparin

Low molecular weight heparins (LMWHs) are better absorbed, have a longer duration of action, and are more effective anticoagulants than unfractionated heparin (UFH). This group of heparins was observed to have a more significant inhibitory effect on factor Xa than IIa, as well as a lower bleeding risk than standard heparin.[15] Currently, six LMWH preparations are approved for use in Europe, and in the USA enoxaparin, dalteparin, and ardeparin are available for deep vein thrombosis/pulmonary embolism prophylaxis (Table 9.3). Each of these LMWHs has a different molecular weight, anti-Xa to anti-IIa activity, rates of plasma clearance, and recommended dosage regimens.[15] LMWHs are not bound to plasma proteins, endothelial cells, or macrophages like UFH.[14] This lower affinity contributes to a longer plasma half-life, more complete plasma recovery at all concentrations, and a clearance independent of dose and plasma concentration. Enoxaparin is initiated following orthopedic surgery (total hip replacement and total knee replacement) at 30 mg subcutaneously, every 12 hours, and in general surgery at 40 mg subcutaneously once daily. Dalteparin is administered at 5000 units subcutaneously once daily for general surgery and orthopedic surgery (total hip replacement). Ardeparin is administered at 50 IU/kg subcutaneously every 12 hours for orthopedic surgery (total knee replacement).

Warfarin

Warfarin prophylaxis can be administered by three methods (Table 9.3). The first regimen is to give warfarin 10 mg on the evening before surgery.[16] This dose is followed by 5 mg on the evening of surgery. The daily dose is determined by the INR. The INR sought is 2–3. The second regimen initiates warfarin therapy 10–14 days prior to surgery.[17] The warfarin is adjusted to maintain a prothrombin time at 1.5–3 seconds longer than the laboratory control value prior to surgery. Postoperatively, on day 1 the dose of warfarin is regulated to maintain an INR of 2–3. The third regimen begins with 10 mg of warfarin on the evening of surgery.[18] No warfarin is given on postoperative day 1. On the second postoperative day, warfarin dosing is begun to maintain an INR of 2–3. If the patient is unable to take anything by mouth, warfarin can be administered intravenously at the same dose as the oral preparation. This approach is reserved for special circumstances, because other forms of pharmacological prophylaxis could be used. Any of the three prophylaxis methods with warfarin should be maintained for 7–10 days. Out-of-hospital prophylaxis is discussed in the section on extended prophylaxis. The incidence of major postoperative bleeding with warfarin therapy has varied from 5% to 10%. The rare complication of warfarin skin necrosis has never been reported in studies using this drug as prophylaxis for deep vein thrombosis/pulmonary embolism.

External pneumatic compression devices

External pneumatic compression devices are mechanical methods of improving venous return from the lower extremities by compression of either the gastrocnemius–soleus muscle group or plantar surface of the foot.[19] Either type of device is placed on the patient on the morning of surgery and worn throughout the surgical procedure. The sleeves are worn continuously for 48 hours postoperatively. If the patient is ambulatory, the sleeves can be discontinued and/or replaced by subcutaneous UFH or LMWH until discharge. If the patient is not ambulatory, the sleeves should be maintained until the patient is more active. In this latter group, the patient may not tolerate the sleeves due to increased warmth, sweating, or disturbance of sleep. Subcutaneous UFH or LMWH can be substituted until discharge or the patient is ambulatory. Bedbound patients wearing the sleeves may have them temporarily removed for skin care, bathing, physical therapy, or bedside commode use. Each manufacturer has specifications on the operation and cycle time of their respective device, but there has not been shown to be a statistically significant difference in the incidence of deep vein thrombosis with the brand employed. If the patient has been at bed rest or immobilized for over 72 hours without any form of prophylaxis, the placement of external pneumatic compression devices is not recommended because of the possibility of disturbing newly formed clot.[11] Assessment of the lower extremity with venous imaging is recommended.

Inferior vena cava filters

The use of inferior vena cava filters as prophylaxis for pulmonary embolism for patients at extremely high risk for postoperative deep vein thrombosis and bleeding has been advocated in a number of studies.[1] Decousus et al. randomized patients with acute deep vein thrombosis on constant infusion heparin or LMWH to either inferior vena cava filters or no filter placement.[20] The 2-week incidence of subsequent pulmonary embolism was significantly reduced in the patients receiving the filters; however, the 2-year cumulative rate of recurrent deep vein thrombosis was subsequently increased in the patients with inferior vena cava filters. During each of the time periods studied, there was no difference in mortality in either of the two groups. Clagett et al. recommend the placement of an inferior vena cava filter as prophylaxis for major surgery when the patient has significant cardiopulmonary disease that would be exacerbated by a postoperative pulmonary embolism or cannot receive any form of prophylaxis following a high-risk surgical procedure.[1]

PROPHYLAXIS FOR SURGERY

General surgery

The incidence of deep vein thrombosis in general surgery has been documented to be 20–30%.[1] These studies evaluated a wide range of patients undergoing a variety of surgical procedures. The recommended prophylaxis has been tailored to the risk classification listed in Table 9.2. In high-risk general surgery, low-dose heparin or LMWH should be used. In very high-risk general surgery, external pneumatic compression devices plus low-dose heparin or LMWH are recommended. Prophylaxis should be maintained until the time of discharge.

Orthopedic surgery

Prophylaxis for deep vein thrombosis/pulmonary embolism in this surgical group has been strongly advocated by the American College of Chest Physicians Consensus Conference on Antithrombotic Therapy and in many subsequent articles.[1] Total hip replacement and fractured hips comprise the predominant procedures performed in the geriatric patient. In these types of surgery deep vein thrombosis may occur as isolated proximal, proximal and distal, or isolated distal thrombosis. This incidence of fatal pulmonary embolism in total joint replacement patients not receiving prophylaxis has been reported to be 1–5%.[1] This high incidence of fatal pulmonary embolism is unacceptable for patients undergoing these procedures. In order to understand the approach to prophylaxis, the predominant orthopedic procedures are reviewed below.

The incidence of deep vein thrombosis without prophylaxis in total hip replacement is approximately 45–50%.[11] Enoxaparin, danaparoid, dalteparin, and warfarin are currently the pharmacologic agents of choice for deep vein thrombosis prophylaxis. Warfarin may be administered by any of the methods listed in Table 9.3. Enoxaparin, danaparoid, and dalteparin are also Food and Drug Administration (FDA) approved agents and dosed as listed in Table 9.3. Leyvraz et al. adapted an adjusted low-dose heparin regimen that was effective in reducing the incidence of deep vein thrombosis in total hip replacement.[13] Although effective, this regimen is labor intense and not often used. External pneumatic compression sleeves have been effective in total hip replacement but these devices must be worn at least 23 hours per day for 5–7 days. This is no longer practical with a stay in hospital of 3–4 days and early mobilization of patients. This mechanical prophylaxis does not increase the risk of perioperative bleeding and has been shown to be effective in reducing deep vein thrombosis, but is recommended as an adjuvant therapy for prophylaxis.

Hip fractures have been shown to have a deep vein thrombosis incidence without prophylaxis of 40–45%.[11] By extrapolation of the data from total hip replacement, enoxaparin, dalteparin, adjusted low-dose heparin, and warfarin should be routinely used as deep vein thrombosis prophylaxis. External pneumatic compression sleeves may be used alone or combined with pharmacological prophylaxis in this patient group.

The incidence of deep vein thrombosis without prophylaxis in total knee replacement has been reported to be 72%.[11] This high rate is attributed to the procedure and tourniquet application. Enoxaparin and ardeparin have been recommended as the most effective prophylaxis for deep vein thrombosis/pulmonary embolism prevention. In addition, warfarin (INR 2–3) has also been included as a regimen for prophylaxis.

Extended prophylaxis

The duration of risk for the development of deep vein thrombosis following orthopedic surgery has become an important issue due to the dramatic reduction in the length of stay in hospital following procedures. All of the above information has focused on a defined time period of prophylaxis during hospitalization and has not assessed the risk of thrombosis after discharge. All the patients involved in the deep vein thrombosis/pulmonary embolism prophylaxis trials received a venogram at the time of discharge in order to assess the incidence of deep vein thrombosis. Despite a variety of effective prophylactic regimens, the incidence of deep vein thrombosis at the time of discharge in total hip or knee surgery is not zero. The question is whether these asymptomatic thrombi are clinically significant or will progress to clinical significance.

Three recent studies have addressed the issue of extended prophylaxis. Planes et al. randomized patients to either LMWH (enoxaparin 40 mg subcutaneously, once daily) or placebo for 21 days following total hip replacement surgery.[21] Patients were screened with bilateral leg venography followed by randomization to either enoxaparin or placebo. After 21 days, bilateral leg venography was repeated. Deep vein thrombosis was documented in 7.1% of the enoxaparin group and in 19.3% of those receiving placebo ($p = 0.18$).

Bergqvist et al. treated patients with enoxaparin 40 mg subcutaneously every day for 10 days following total hip replacement and then randomized the patients to enoxaparin or placebo without objective predischarge studies.[22] Bilateral leg venography was performed between days 19 and 21, which revealed a 34.7% incidence of deep vein thrombosis in the placebo group and 16.7% in those on enoxaparin. In this trial, 10 patients (8%) in the placebo group had symptomatic deep vein thrombosis and nonfatal pulmonary embolism compared with two patients (1.7%) in the enoxaparin arm.

The third study by Dahl et al. treated patients following total hip replacement with subcutaneous dalteparin 5000 U, preoperatively for a mean of 7 days, and dextran 70 on the day of surgery and on the first postoperative day.[23] All patients had bilateral leg venography and a ventilation perfusion scan at discharge from the hospital. Patients with negative or isolated calf or popliteal deep vein thrombosis were randomly assigned to dalteparin 5000 U subcutaneously every day or placebo for an additional 28 days. At 28 days, bilateral leg venography demonstrated a 31.7% incidence of deep vein thrombosis in the placebo group and 19.3% in the dalteparin arm. The 35-day incidence of symptomatic deep vein thrombosis in the LMWH group was 3.5% and in the placebo group it was 2.8%. The combined prevalence of symptomatic pulmonary embolism and new high-probability lung scans was 6.6% in the placebo arm compared with 3.6% in the LMWH arm. All three studies had no major bleeding.

Extended prophylaxis based on the preceding studies raises the issue of the clinical meaning of asymptomatic deep vein thrombosis discovered by an objective test. The American College of Chest Physicians Consensus Conference recommends a minimum of 7–10 days' duration of prophylaxis with LMWH or warfarin for patients undergoing total hip or total knee replacement procedures.[1] Extended prophylaxis with LMWH (enoxaparin 40 mg subcutaneously, once daily) for 29–35 days following discharge offers additional protection.[1] Adjusted-dose warfarin (INR 2–3) has been advocated by nonrandomized trial as an alternative prophylaxis for deep vein thrombosis/pulmonary embolism.

Neurosurgery

Craniotomies and spinal surgeries have been the predominant neurosurgical procedures evaluated for prophylaxis. There are six major neurosurgical prophylaxis studies in the literature.[11] Three of the six trials evaluated both craniotomy and spinal surgery; two studies assessed only craniotomy and aneurysm resection. In these studies, the incidence of deep vein thrombosis ranged between 19% and 43%. Intracranial (versus spinal) surgery, malignant (versus benign) tumors, duration of surgery (> 4 hours), and leg weakness were documented as risk factors that increased the incidence of postoperative deep vein thrombosis.[1] External pneumatic compression devices have been the primary prophylaxis measures studied in this population. A reduction in the incidence of deep vein thrombosis from 19% to 1.5% has been demonstrated in a number of trials. Recently, two large randomized trials compared elastic stockings alone with elastic stockings and LMWH (e.g., enoxaparin 40 mg subcutaneously, once daily; nadroparin 7500 U subcutaneously, once daily).[24,25] Both studies demonstrated a significant reduction in proximal deep vein thrombosis and in the overall incidence of deep vein thrombosis in the patients treated with either enoxaparin or nadroparin plus elastic stockings versus stockings alone. In addition, these trials did not demonstrate an increased risk of intracranial hemorrhage.

Because neurosurgeons would be concerned about any bleeding, it is recommended that external pneumatic compression devices with or without elastic stockings be used in patients undergoing intracranial surgery.[1] LMWH or low-dose UFH may be an acceptable alternative.[1]

Anesthesia considerations

Recently, the FDA Public Health Advisory reported cases of epidural or spinal hematoma following the use of prophylactic LMWH.[26] Approximately 75% of the cases occurred with orthopedic surgery. In a recent review of neuraxial complications of anticoagulants in patients receiving anesthesia, the following recommendations were made: regional anesthesia should be avoided in patients with an abnormal clinical bleeding history or in patients receiving other drugs that affect hemostasis; the insertion of the spinal needle should be delayed for 10–12 hours after the initial LMWH prophylaxis dose; regional anesthesia should be avoided in patients with a hemorrhagic aspirate during the initial spinal needle placement; and subsequent LMWH prophylaxis doses should be delayed for at least 12 hours after spinal needle placement or epidural catheter.[26–8] All patients should be monitored carefully for early signs of cord compression, such as progressive numbness, weakness, or bowel and bladder dysfunction.

MEDICAL PATIENTS

The above data support the clinical effectiveness of routine deep vein thrombosis/pulmonary embolism prophylaxis in surgical patients, but the application of these approaches in general medical patients remains controversial. The American College of Physicians has made prophylaxis recommendations for stroke and myocardial infarction patients with unfractionated heparin or LMWH.[1] This section focuses on the hospitalized general medical patient with respect to deep vein thrombosis/pulmonary embolism prophylaxis (Table 9.4).

Table 9.4 *Deep vein thrombosis/pulmonary embolism prophylaxis in hospitalized medical patients*

Study	Number of patients	Regimen	Deep vein thrombosis	Major bleeding
Harenberg et al.[29,a]	710	UFH	4 (1%)	4 (1%)
	726	Nadroparin[a]	6 (1%)	5 (1%)
Bergmann et al.[30,b]	216	UFH	10 (5%)	4 (2%)[d]
	207	Enoxaparin	10 (5%)	2 (1%)[d]
Samama et al.[31,c]	288	Placebo	43 (15%)	7 (2%)
	291	Enoxaparin	16 (5%)	12 (4%)
	287	Enoxaparin	43 (15%)	4 (1%)

[a]Nadroparin = 3600 U, subcutaneously daily; UFH = 5000 U, subcutaneously, every 8 hours
[b]Enoxaparin = 20 mg, subcutaneously daily; UFH = 5000 U, subcutaneously, every 12 hours
[c]Enoxaparin = 40 mg, subcutaneously daily; Enoxaparin 20 mg, subcutaneously daily
[d]4/223 evaluable patients; 2/216 evaluable patients
(UFH = unfractionated heparin.)

Three large randomized trials evaluated LMWHs with unfractionated heparin in hospitalized patients with acute medical illnesses. Harenberg et al. completed a multicenter, randomized, double-blind study comparing nadroparin (3600 U, subcutaneously once daily) with unfractionated heparin (5000 U, subcutaneously every 8 hours) in hospitalized, bedridden patients.[29] The endpoints of this study were symptomatic thromboembolic disease or asymptomatic proximal clot detected on compression ultrasound on days 1 and 10. Six out of 710 patients (1%) had deep vein thrombosis in the nadroparin group, and 4 of 726 patients (1%) developed deep vein thrombosis in the UFH arm. The incidence of major bleeding was 1% in the nadroparin patients and 1% with UFH.

The second study, by Bergmann et al. was a multicenter, randomized, and double-blinded trial comparing enoxaparin (20 mg, subcutaneously once daily) with UFH (5000 U, subcutaneously every 12 hours) in hospitalized patients with acute medical illnesses.[30] Radiolabeled fibrinogen scanning and clinical pulmonary embolism were the efficacy endpoints of this trial. The incidence of thomboembolic events was 4.8% (10/207 patients) in the enoxaparin group and 4.6% (10/216 patients) in the UFH patients. The incidence of major bleeding was 1% (2/216 patients) with enoxaparin and 2% (4/223 patients) in the UFH group.

The third study, by Samama et al. was a randomized, double-blind; trial involving 1102 hospitalized patients older than age 40 years.[31] Patients received prophylaxis with enoxaparin 40 mg, subcutaneously once daily; enoxaparin 20 mg, subcutaneously once daily, or placebo. Bilateral leg venography or compression ultrasound (only if venography could not be performed) was the study endpoint between days 6 and 14. In addition, patients were followed for 3 months after completing the initial prophylaxis phase. The incidence of deep vein thrombosis was 5.5% (16/291) in the 40-mg enoxaparin cohort, whereas the 20-mg enoxaparin group had a 15% (43/287) incidence of thrombotic events. The placebo group had a 14.9% (43/288) incidence of deep vein thrombosis. Major bleeding was reported in 2% of the placebo group, in 1% in the enoxaparin 20 mg arm, and in 3.4% in the enoxaparin 40 mg arm. This difference was not statistically significant.

The recommendations for hospitalized medical patients are UFH 5000 U, subcutaneously every 8–12 hours or LMWH (enoxaparin 40 mg, subcutaneously once daily). None of the LMWHs is approved for this indication, but, because of enoxaparin's availability for other FDA-approved indications, this agent could be used for prophylaxis of deep vein thrombosis/pulmonary embolism in hospitalized medical patients.

CONCLUSION

All the above recommendations are evidence based as well as being supported by expert panel review. These recommendations serve to provide clinicians with a variety of management strategies for the prevention of deep vein thrombosis/pulmonary embolism in the postoperative period and in hospitalized medical patients.

REFERENCES

1 Clagett P, Anderson F, Geerts W, et al. Prevention of venous thromboembolism. *Chest* 1998; **114**: 531S–60S.

2 Virchow R. Neuer fall von todlichen. Emboli der lungenarterie. *Arch Pathol Anat* 1856; **10**: 225–8.

3 Nicolaides A, Kakkar V, Field E, et al. Venous stasis and deep vein thrombosis. *Br J Surg* 1972; **59**: 713–16.

4 Nicolaides A, Kakkar V, Renney J. Soleal sinuses and stasis. *Br J Surg* 1970; **57**: 307.

5 Lindstrom B, Ahlman H, Jonsson O, et al. Influence of anesthesia on blood flow to the calves during surgery. *Acta Anesth Scand* 1984; **28**: 201–3.

6 Lindstrom B, Ahlman H, Jonsson O, et al. Blood flow in the calves during surgery. *Acta Chir Scand* 1977; **143**: 335–9.

7 Sevitt S. Pathology and pathogenesis of deep vein thrombi. In: Bergan J, Yao J eds *Venous problems*. Chicago: Year Book Medical Publishing, 1976: 257–69.

8 Comerota A, Stewart G, Alburger P, et al. Operative venodilation: a previously unsuspected factor in the cause of postoperative deep vein thrombosis. *Surgery* 1989; **106**: 301–9.

9 Stewart G, Alburger P, Stone E, et al. Total hip replacement induces injury to remote veins in a canine model. *J Bone Joint Surg* 1983; **65A**: 97–102.

10 Hamer J, Malone P, Silver I. The PO_2 in venous valve pockets: its possible bearing on thrombogenesis. *Br J Surg* 1981; **68**: 166–70.

11 Merli G. Deep vein thrombosis and pulmonary embolism prophylaxis in the surgical patient. In: Merli G, Weitz H eds *Medical care of the surgical patient*, 2nd edn. Philadelphia, PA: WB Saunders, 1998: 70–87.

12 Confrancesco E, Cortellaro M, Leonardi P, et al. Markers of hemostatic system activation during thromboprophylaxis with recombinant hirudin in total hip replacement. *Thromb Haemost* 1996; **75**: 407–11.

13 Clagett G, Reisch J. Prevention of venous thromboembolism in general surgical patients: results of meta-analysis. *Ann Surg* 1988; **208**: 227–39.

14 Leyvraz P, Richard J, Bachmann F, et al. Adjusted versus fixed dose subcutaneous heparin in the prevention of deep vein thrombosis after total hip replacement. *N Engl J Med* 1983; **309**: 954–8.

15 Hirsh J, Levine M. Low molecular weight heparin. *Blood* 1992; **79**: 1–17.

16 Harris W, Salzman E, Athanasoulis C. Comparison of warfarin, low molecular weight dextran, aspirin, and subcutaneous heparin in prevention of venous thromboembolism following total hip replacement. *J Bone Joint Surg* 1974; **56**: 1555–62.

17 Francis C, Marder V, Evart C, et al. Two-step warfarin therapy: prevention of postoperative venous thrombosis without excessive bleeding. *JAMA* 1983; **249**: 374–8.

18 Amstutz H, Friscia D, Dorey F, et al. Warfarin prophylaxis to prevent mortality from pulmonary embolism after total hip replacement. *J Bone Joint Surg* 1989; **71A**: 321–6.

19 Caprini J, Scurr J, Hasty J. Role of compression modalities in a prophylactic program for deep vein thrombosis. *Semin Thromb Hemost* 1988; **14**: 77–87.

20 Decousus H, Leizorovicz A, Parent F, et al. A clinical trial of vena caval filters in the prevention of pulmonary embolism in patients with proximal deep vein thrombosis. *N Engl J Med* 1998; **338**: 409–15.

21 Planes A, Vochelle N, Darmon J, et al. Risk of deep venous thrombosis after hospital discharge in patients having undergone total hip replacement: double-blind randomized comparison of enoxaparin versus placebo. *Lancet* 1996; **348**: 224–8.

22 Bergqvist D, Benoni G, Bjurgell O, et al. Low molecular weight heparin (enoxaparin) as prophylaxis against venous thromboembolism after total hip replacement. *N Engl J Med* 1996; **335**: 696–700.

23 Dahl O, Andreassen G, Aspelin T, et al. Prolonged thromboprophylaxis following hip replacement surgery: results of a double blind, prospective, randomized, placebo controlled study with dalteparin (Fragmin). *Thromb Haemost* 1997; **77**: 26–31.

24 Nurmohamed M, van Riel A, Henkens C, et al. Low molecular weight heparin and compression stockings in the prevention of venous thromboembolism in neurosurgery. *Thromb Haemost* 1996; **75**: 233–8.

25 Agnelli G, Piovella F, Buoncristiani P, et al. Enoxaparin plus compression stockings compared with compression stockings alone in the prevention of venous thromboembolism after elective neurosurgery. *N Engl J Med* 1998; **339**: 80–5.

26 Lumpkin M. FDA alert: FDA Public Advisory. *Anesthesiology* 1998; **88**: 27A–28A.

27 Horlocker T, Heit J. Low molecular weight heparin: biochemistry, pharmacology, perioperative prophylaxis regimens, and guidelines for regional anesthetic management. *Anesth Analg* 1997; **85**: 874–85.

28 American Society of Regional Anesthesia Consensus Statements on Neuraxial Anesthesia and Anticoagulation. Developed from the American Society of Regional Anesthesia Consensus Conference, Chicago Illinois, May 2–3, 1998.

29 Harenberg J, Roebruck P, Heene D, et al. Subcutaneous low molecular weight heparin versus standard heparin and the prevention of thromboembolism in medical inpatients. *Haemostasis* 1996; **26**: 127–39.

30 Bergmann J, Neuhart E. A multi-center randomized double blind study of enoxaparin compared with unfractionated heparin in the prevention of venous thromboembolic disease in elderly inpatients bedridden for an acute medical illness. *Thromb Haemost* 1996; **76**: 529–34.

31 Samama M, Cohen A, Darmon J, et al. A comparison of enoxaparin with placebo for the prevention of venous thromboembolism in acutely ill medical patients. *N Engl J Med* 1999; **341**: 793–800.

10

Treatment of venous thromboembolic disease

JAMIE C HEY, JOHN SPANDORFER

INTRODUCTION

Deep venous thrombosis and pulmonary embolism are relatively common medical conditions that have potentially serious sequelae. Deep vein thrombosis of the lower extremity treated with anticoagulation is associated with up to a 40% incidence of pulmonary embolism, although many are asymptomatic.[1] Deep vein thrombosis is also associated with a postthrombotic syndrome in approximately 30–60% of treated cases.[2,3] This syndrome can be a source of serious morbidity for those afflicted. Untreated pulmonary embolism has a mortality rate that has been reported to be as high as 30%; however, there is evidence that asymptomatic pulmonary embolism occurs in many patients, with uncertain significance.[4,5] In addition to the mortality associated with acute pulmonary embolism, recurrent events are a known cause of secondary pulmonary hypertension. Deep vein thrombosis and pulmonary embolism exist as a spectrum referred to as venous thromboembolic disease, and are linked by our diagnostic and therapeutic approaches to them. The diagnosis of venous thromboembolism is discussed elsewhere; this chapter deals with therapy.

The goal of therapy for venous thromboembolic disease is to prevent the acute mortality and long-term complications discussed above. This goal is primarily achieved by decreasing the recurrence of thrombus formation, which can lead to vascular damage and embolization. The standard treatment for both disorders is anticoagulation beginning with heparin and continuing with warfarin. It should be stressed that, as in all areas of medicine, treatment must be individualized and that there are appropriate alternatives to the standard regimen. This chapter addresses the use of heparin and warfarin and briefly describes alternative forms of treatment.

HEPARIN

Unfractionated heparin (UFH) has been used for many years in the treatment of thromboembolic disease. The first controlled trial providing evidence of its efficacy appeared in 1960.[4] Since that time, there has been a wealth of literature confirming the usefulness of heparin as well as refining the methods of administration. UFH has for years been used as the standard treatment for acute deep vein thrombosis. With the recent approval of low molecular weight heparins (LMWHs) for deep vein thrombosis treatment, it is expected that the use of LMWHs for this indication will increase.

Mechanism of action and monitoring

UFH consists of a mixture of sulfated polysaccharides. Heparin binds to serum proteins, including antithrombin III and the proteases of the coagulation cascade. The mechanism of action appears to lie chiefly in its interaction with antithrombin III.[5] The strength of this inhibition of thrombin varies with the molecular weight of the individual heparin molecules.[6] The binding of heparin to antithrombin III increases its capacity to inhibit the coagulation proteases, most importantly Xa and thrombin, thus inhibiting clot formation.

Monitoring of UFH administration is done routinely using the activated partial thromboplastin time (aPTT). Most studies evaluating the efficacy of heparin dosing use this test as a measure of activity. However, the aPTT response to heparin is dependent on the reagent used.[7] This presents a problem with standardization, much the way the prothrombin time (PT) did in monitoring warfarin therapy before the development of the International Normalized Ratio (INR). Other methods of monitoring heparin activity include measuring heparin levels using a protamine titration assay and measuring antifactor Xa activity. However, the aPTT remains the most used and studied test, and the others are reserved for patients in whom the aPTT reponse to heparin is inaccurate or for establishing a therapeutic range for heparin therapy in the laboratory.

As mentioned earlier, the action of heparin on antithrombin III-mediated thrombin inhibition varies with the molecular weight of the individual heparin molecules. LMWH contains smaller fractions of polysaccharides than the unfractionated form. These smaller molecules retain the ability to inhibit factor Xa, but have different pharmacokinetics and bioavailability profiles from UFH. The half-life of LMWH is longer than that of UFH and it has a greater bioavailability. The potential clinical advantages of LMWH relate, in part, to these differences. Of note, the aPTT is not sensitive to the effects of LMWH; thus, antifactor Xa activity is used if monitoring of anticoagulation is needed.[8] The anticoagulant response to a given subcutaneous dose of LMWH is proportional to patient weight and is more predictable than with UFH.[9,10] Fixed-dose LMWH, based on weight, is as effective as adjusted-dose LMWH guided by antifactor Xa activity in preventing the recurrence of deep vein thrombosis after an initial episode.[11] Thus, most of the clinical studies comparing intravenous UFH to subcutaneous LMWH have done so without adjusting the dose. This translates to much simpler drug administration and patient care.

Administration

UFH is routinely administered as subcutaneous boluses or continuous intravenous infusion. Intermittent intravenous bolus therapy is no longer used because of reports of a higher rate of bleeding.[12] Both subcutaneous and intravenous UFH have been shown to be effective in preventing recurrent events of venous thromboembolic disease as long as therapeutic levels of anticoagulation are achieved.[13–15] Intravenous UFH beginning with a large bolus followed by the continuous infusion is the more commonly used and most studied method. Because patients vary in their response to UFH, and because reaching the target level of anticoagulation early is crucial in the prevention of recurrence, several different approaches of initiating and adjusting

Table 10.1 *Nomograms of unfractionated heparin dosing for deep vein thrombosis*

Weight-based nomogram[18]
Initial: bolus of 80 U/kg, then infusion of 18 U/kg, measure aPTT 6 hours later
Heparin adjustments (aPTT should be rechecked 6 hours after change):

aPTT (s)	Adjustment
<35	80 U/kg bolus, increase rate by 4 U/kg per hour
35–45	40 U/kg bolus, increase rate by 2 U/kg per hour
46–70	No change
71–90	Decrease infusion by 2 U/kg per hour
>90	Stop infusion 1 hour, decrease rate by 3 U/kg per hour

Hull nomogram[19]
Initial: bolus of 5000 U, then infusion of 40 000 U/24 hours if low risk of bleeding or 30 000 U/24 hours if high risk of bleeding
Heparin adjustments (aPTT should be rechecked 6 hours after change):

aPTT (s)	Adjustment
≤45	Increase rate by 240 U/hour
46–54	Increase rate by 120 U/hour
55–85	No change
86–110	Stop heparin for 1 hour, decrease rate by 120 U/hour
>110	Stop heparin for 1 hour, decrease rate by 240 U/hour

Cruickshank method[17]
Initial: bolus of 5000 U, followed by 1280 U/hour
Heparin adjustments (aPTT should be rechecked 6 hours after change):

aPTT (s)	Adjustment
<50	Bolus 5000 U, increase rate by 120 U/hour
50–59	Increase rate by 120 U/hour
60–85	No change
86–95	Decrease rate by 80 U/hour
96–120	Stop heparin for 30 minutes, decrease rate by 80 U/hour
>120	Stop heparin for 60 minutes, decrease rate by 160 U/hour

(aPTT = activated partial thromboplastin time.)

heparin have been evaluated. Nomograms that provide guidelines for the dosing of heparin have been shown to decrease the time needed to achieve the therapeutic range of anticoagulation, thereby decreasing the incidence of recurrent venous thromboembolic disease (Table 10.1).[16–19] Of these nomograms, the weight-based method is the most attractive as it was able to provide an early therapeutic aPTT in 97% of patients with a low incidence of bleeding.[18] This method is also simpler than others as it does not require any adjustments for individual patient bleeding risk. The traditional method of beginning each patient with the same bolus and infusion rate is associated with an unnecessarily high rate of recurrence due to failure to reach the therapeutic range early in the course of the thrombotic episode. Furthermore, even though many patients are 'over-anticoagulated' based on the aPTT using the more aggressive dosing nomograms, there is no clear increased risk of hemorrhage.[19] The aPTT should be monitored every 6 hours after beginning therapy until it is within the therapeutic range of 1.5–2.5 times control (or what has been established as a therapeutic range in the laboratory) and then daily afterward. The 6-hour point is used to allow for a steady state to be achieved.

When administering UFH subcutaneously, the regimen that has been used in the literature begins with a dose of 15 000 units every 12 hours. The aPTT should be measured 6 hours after a dose, and the next dose adjusted accordingly. It has been shown that this method of administering heparin long term following initial treatment with intravenous heparin was as effective as warfarin.[20] In this study, the aPTT was not followed after an appropriate dose was reached. Therefore 'adjusted-dose' subcutaneous heparin may avoid the need for long-term aPTT monitoring and increase patient convenience.

LMWHs are administered subcutaneously. Dosages of several LMWHs that have been evaluated in deep vein thrombosis treatment trials are listed in Table 10.2. Enoxaparin, the only LMWH that is Food and Drug Administration (FDA) approved for the treatment of deep vein thrombosis as of 1999, may be given at 1 mg/kg every 12 hours in the inpatient or outpatient setting. The FDA has also approved enoxaparin at 1.5 mg/kg every 24 hours for inpatients with deep vein thrombosis (for more information on treatment with LMWH see Chapter 5).[21]

Table 10.2 *Low molecular weight heparins and dosages used in the treatment of venous thromboembolic disease*

Drug	Mean molecular weight	Anti-XA : anti-IIA ratio	Dose	Frequency
Dalteparin (Fragmin)	6000	2.7	200 IU/kg	q 24
Enoxaparin (Lovenox)	4200	3.8	1 mg (100 IU)/kg	q 12
			or 1.5 mg/kg	q 24
Nadroparin (Fraxiparin)	4500	3.6	≤50 kg: 8200 IU	q 12
			50–70 kg: 12 300 IU	q 12
			>70 kg: 18 400 IU	q 12
Reviparin (Clivarin)	4000	3.5	35–45 kg: 3500 IU	q 12
			46–60 kg: 4200 IU	q 12
			>60 kg: 6300 IU	q 12
Tinzaparin (Innohep)	4500	1.9	175 IU/kg	q 24

Duration of heparin therapy

As noted above, subcutaneous heparin has been evaluated as long-term treatment of deep vein thrombosis in place of standard warfarin and is routinely used in this manner in venous thromboembolic disease complicating pregnancy. However, in most patients heparin is only used as the initial form of anticoagulation. Its role here is crucial as there is a high rate of recurrent episodes of venous thromboembolic disease if warfarin is used alone.[13] In the past, heparin was used for a prolonged period of time while waiting for the onset of action of warfarin, which was often started 4–5 days into the hospitalization. Studies documenting the safety of early administration of warfarin as well as a short course of heparin have helped to decrease the duration of the initial inpatient treatment.[15,19,22] Currently, the usual duration of therapy for heparin in acute venous thromboembolic disease should be 5 days, at which time it is discontinued if the INR has reached a therapeutic level.

Complications

The most common complication of heparin therapy is hemorrhage. In the treatment of thromboembolic disease, the incidence has been variously reported to be 0–30%, depending partly on the definition of bleeding and the method of UFH administration.[12,14,18,19,23] As mentioned earlier, intermittent intravenous bolus administration appears to have a higher complication rate than other forms of therapy. The risk of bleeding correlates more with the clinical risk factors for hemorrhage than with the level of anticoagulation determined by the aPTT.[19,23] The risk of bleeding on heparin increases with age, possibly because of increased sensitivity to its anticoagulant effects.[24,25] The presence of comorbid conditions, including heart, liver or kidney dysfunction, also increases the risk of bleeding during anticoagulation.[25]

The second most common complication of heparin therapy is thrombocytopenia, which may be associated with bleeding or thrombosis. Heparin-associated thrombocytopenia occurs in two forms: type I, a nonimmunologic, transient, mild thrombocytopenia related to direct heparin–platelet interactions; and type II, an antibody-mediated thrombocytopenia that is more likely to be severe and associated with thrombosis.[26] The incidence of UFH-associated thrombocytopenia is between 1% and 10%.[26] Long-term UFH has been associated with early development of osteoporotic fractures. In women receiving UFH for venous thromboembolic disease complicating pregnancy, the incidence is approximately 2%.[27] Therefore, heparin is not used for long term therapy unless there is a clear contraindication to warfarin.

Heparin also has metabolic effects. Hyperkalemia, metabolic acidosis, and hyponatremia, possibly related to aldosterone suppression, have been reported but are rare.[28] For further information on heparin-related complications, see Chapter 12.

Experience with LMWH in deep vein thrombosis treatment

The clinical evaluation of LMWH in the treatment of deep vein thrombosis has been extensive and includes meta-analyses and studies evaluating the treatment of outpatients.[29–39] This research has shown that LMWH is as safe and effective as unfractionated heparin in the treatment of deep vein thrombosis for both inpatients and outpatients (Tables 10.3 and 10.4). LMWH also appears to be as effective as UFH in patients with pulmonary embolism (for more information on LMWH and venous thromboembolic disease, see Chapter 5).[34]

Table 10.3 *Trials of low molecular weight heparin (LMWH) versus unfractionated heparin (UFH) for venous thromboembolic disease*

	Treatment	Recurrence (%)	Major bleeding (%)	Mortality (%)
Simonneau[33]	Enoxaparin n=67	0	0	4.5
	UFH n=67	0	0	3.0
Hull[29]	Tinzaparin n=213	2.8	0.5	4.7
	UFH n=219	6.8	5.0	9.6
Lindmarker[36]	Dalteparin n=101	5.0	1.0	2.0
	UFH n=103	2.9	0	2.9
Prandoni[32]	Nadroparin n=85	7.1	1.2	7.1
	UFH n=85	14.1	3.8	14.1
Columbus[34]	Reviparin n=510	5.3	3.1	7.1
	UFH n=511	4.9	2.3	7.6
Simonneau[35,a]	Tinzaparin n=304	1.6	2.0	3.9
	UFH n=308	1.9	2.6	4.5

[a]All patients had pulmonary embolism.

Table 10.4 *Outpatient trials of low molecular weight heparin (LMWH) versus unfractionated heparin (UFH) for deep vein thrombosis*

	Koopman et al.[37]		Levine et al.[30]	
	UFH (n=198)	LMWH[a] (n=202)	UFH (n=253)	LMWH[b] (n=247)
Recurrence (%)	8.6	6.9	6.7	5.3
Major bleeding (%)	2.0	0.5	1.1	2.0
Death (%)	6.3	4.0	6.7	4.5

[a]Nadroparin.
[b]Enoxaparin.

One advantage of LMWH over UFH is that it may be given easily in an outpatient setting. Studies by Levine et al. and Koopman et al. demonstrate that LMWH is as safe and effective as UFH among outpatients with deep vein thrombosis[23,27] (Table 10.4). Outpatient treatment of deep vein thrombosis clearly can save costs. An economic analysis found the costs to be 64% less when patients were treated with LMWH as outpatients compared to UFH as inpatients.[40] As stated earlier, and covered in Chapter 12, another advantage of LMWH is that it results in less heparin-induced thrombocytopenia and thrombosis than UFH.[26]

WARFARIN

Warfarin is routinely used in the treatment of venous thromboembolic disease. As with heparin, there has been extensive clinical research aimed at refining the method of warfarin administration in the treatment of deep vein thrombosis and pulmonary embolism.

Mechanism of action and monitoring

Warfarin is a vitamin K antagonist that produces its anticoagulant effect by preventing the formation of active coagulation factors, specifically factors VII, IX, X, and prothrombin.[41] Anticoagulation is achieved when the circulating activated factors are cleared and warfarin has successfully blocked their further production. Proteins C and S, two antithrombotic enzymes produced by the liver, are also dependent on vitamin K for activation. Thus, warfarin is theoretically capable of inducing an anticoagulant or procoagulant state depending on the relative decrease in levels of activated coagulation factors and proteins C and S. Traditionally, heparin and warfarin therapies have been overlapped for several days before heparin was discontinued, because heparin would protect against the temporary hypercoagulable state. In the treatment of venous thromboembolic disease, this dual therapy is, indeed, necessary. Initial therapy with warfarin alone has been associated with a high incidence of recurrence or extension of venous thromboembolic disease.[13]

Warfarin activity is measured using the PT. Because variations in the sensitivity of reagents used in different laboratories were creating confusion and making standardization of treatment difficult, the World Health Organization developed a reference thromboplastin. The PT ratio obtained using this reagent is reported as the INR. The recommended INR for the treatment of venous thromboembolic disease is 2–3.[41]

Administration

Early administration of warfarin in the treatment of venous thromboembolic disease has been shown to be safe.[15,22] Warfarin can be started on the first day of therapy, but its effect on the PT takes 36–72 hours after dosing because of the relatively long half-life of some of the activated coagulation factors. The initial response of the PT to warfarin is related to depletion of activated factor VII, which has the shortest half-life of the vitamin K-dependent factors. Full anticoagulation occurs when the active factors II, IX, and X are depleted. This takes several days of warfarin therapy and occurs no more quickly when therapy is begun with a large loading dose.[42] Warfarin is now routinely begun with smaller doses, i.e., 5–10 mg for 2–3 days and then adjusted to achieve the target INR. The PT should be followed daily or every other day while waiting to achieve the therapeutic range, and less frequently afterwards.

Duration of warfarin therapy

The duration of warfarin therapy has been the subject of numerous investigations.[43–8] The following conclusions from these studies have been made.[46–9]

1. Patients who have developed a deep vein thrombosis from transient causes, such as temporary immobilization or estrogen use, may be anticoagulated for 1–3 months.

2. Patients who have permanent risk factors such as severe obesity, are heterozygous for factor V Leiden mutation, or an idiopathic cause of the deep vein thrombosis, should be treated for at least 6 months.
3. Patients who have had recurrent deep vein thrombosis should be treated indefinitely.

Some authorities believe that patients who have protein C or S deficiency, antithrombin deficiency, or are homozygous for activated protein C should also be treated indefinitely, although the recommendations regarding anticoagulation in patients with hypercoagulable states are limited because these patients were excluded from the above studies.[49] When deciding how long to anticoagulate, the risk that the patient has for major bleeding complications also needs to be considered. For example, the patient who developed a postoperative deep vein thrombosis and is at high risk of bleeding because he is 85 years old may be treated with warfarin for 1 month rather than 3 months (see Chapter 3 for more information).

Complications

As with heparin, the major complication of warfarin therapy is bleeding. However, the risk of bleeding on warfarin is directly related to the level of anticoagulation as measured by the PT, whereas there is not as clear a correlation between the aPTT and the risk of bleeding on UFH.[19] This difference relates directly to clinical practice. UFH administration is aggressively aimed at early therapeutic anticoagulation, accepting 'overshooting' in some patients to prevent the recurrence of venous thromboembolic disease. Warfarin administration needs to be more precise to achieve the target range while limiting supratherapeutic anticoagulation. Because warfarin is always initiated with heparin therapy in place, delays in reaching the target INR may prolong hospitalizations, but should not affect outcome.

Studies distinguish minor from major bleeding. Major bleeding typically is defined by hemorrhage that involves the central nervous system or requires hospitalization, blood transfusion, surgical intervention, or results in death. Reports have demonstrated that the prevalence of major bleeding may vary from 0% to 19% of anticoagulated patients.[23] The wide variation in rates may be secondary to the different patient populations, definitions of bleeding, methods of monitoring bleeding, and intensity of anticoagulation. The risks of bleeding in prospective controlled clinical trials are significantly less than those reported in retrospective studies. Controlled trials may exclude patients who are at a higher risk for bleeding, such as patients who have comorbid diseases or are noncompliant. Rates of bleeding may vary in controlled trials because of the indication for anticoagulation or intensity of anticoagulation required (higher in patients with prosthetic valves). Retrospective studies may reflect more accurately the risk of bleeding in a general outpatient practice. For more detailed information on warfarin-related bleeding, see Chapter 13.

Thrombolysis

Thrombolytic therapy has been used in the treatment of deep vein thrombosis and pulmonary embolism. A listing of approved agents and their dosages is in Table 10.5.

Table 10.5 *Thrombolytic agents for the treatment of venous thromboembolic disease*

Drug	Dosage (continuous infusion)
Streptokinase	250 000-IU loading dose, followed by 100 000 IU/hour for 24 hours
Urokinase	4400 IU/kg body weight loading dose, followed by 2200 IU/kg for 12–24 hours
Tissue plasminogen activator	100 mg over 2 hours

In both deep vein thrombosis and pulmonary embolism, earlier resolution of thrombus has been observed when compared to anticoagulation alone, but there has not been a clear effect on morbidity or mortality.[50,51] In deep vein thrombosis, the theoretical benefits of clot lysis would include less embolization as well as less vascular damage, possibly limiting postthrombotic symptoms. However, the incidence of recurrent venous thromboembolic disease with appropriate standard treatment is quite low, and the development of the postthrombotic syndrome may be related more to the number of thrombotic episodes than to time to resolution of the initial thrombus, regardless of size.[3] Therefore, the use of thrombolytics may be of less benefit than anticipated in most patients, and their use has been associated with an increased risk of bleeding.[51] Because the risk–benefit ratio may not be better than anticoagulation, the use of thrombolytic therapy in most cases is limited. Future studies may be helpful in demonstrating which patients may most benefit from thrombolytic therapy for deep vein thrombosis.

Pulmonary embolism, compared to deep vein thrombosis, is associated with higher mortality rates and more significant morbidity, including pulmonary hypertension. Thrombolysis in routine clinical practice is reserved for unstable patients as a life-saving measure. However, it has been shown to be more effective than heparin at improving pulmonary perfusion, hemodynamics, and right ventricular function in stable ptients with acute pulmonary embolism.[52] Thrombolytics may also be associated with a decrease in the recurrence of pulmonary embolism.[52] Despite these benefits, their use in stable patients continues to be uncommon because of the increased risk of hemorrhage and the success of standard heparin and warfarin in preventing recurrence. Thrombolytics remain the preferred agent in unstable patients in the hope to decreasing pulmonary artery pressures and improving right ventricular function.

Inferior vena cava filter

In patients in whom therapeutic anticoagulation is contraindicated or has failed to prevent recurrence of venous thromboembolic disease, mechanical protection from pulmonary embolism using an inferior vena cava filter is needed. These devices have been in use for many years. There are several different types, which vary in the type of metal used and in structure. The filter is routinely placed via central venous catheterization below the level of the renal veins. In a review of 24 studies of inferior vena cava filters, it was found that pulmonary embolism after placement is rare.[53] Placement of these devices is associated with some risks, including filter misplacement or migration, inferior vena cava penetration, inferior vena cava obstruction, and insertion site bleeding, or deep vein thrombosis.[54] A recent, randomized trial of filter placement plus anticoagulation versus anticoagulation alone confirmed the early effectiveness of these filters for preventing pulmonary embolism in patients with deep vein thrombosis, but also pointed out their association with an increased risk of recurrent deep vein thrombosis.[55] Although complications are not common, it is prudent to reserve the use of filters for the above indications and not for routine pulmonary embolism prophylaxis. Appropriate anticoagulation is very successful at preventing the recurrence of pulmonary embolism, and additional intervention is usually not needed. For additional information on inferior vena cava filters, see Chapter 11.

SUMMARY

The management of venous thromboembolism is guided by extensive, high-quality clinical research. This work has refined the use of anticoagulation and continues to provide us with alternatives to traditional treatment. The appropriate use of heparin and warfarin has been shown to be very effective at achieving the goals of therapy, and failure to use these medications in the proper manner has been shown to increase the incidences of recurrence of disease and complications. As stated earlier, the approach to the patient with a deep vein thrombosis or pulmonary embolism must be individualized to reach a satisfactory outcome, and the internist must be well versed in this area to provide optimal care to his or her patients.

REFERENCES

1 Moser KM, Fedullo PF, Littejohn JK, Crawford R. Frequent asymptomatic pulmonary embolism in patients with deep venous thrombosis. *JAMA* 1994; **271**: 223–5.
2 Prandoni P, Lensing WA, Cogo A, Cuppini S, Villalta S, Carta M. The long-term clinical course of acute deep venous thrombosis. *Ann Intern Med* 1996; **125**: 1–7.
3 Prandoni P, Villalta S, Polistena P, Bernardi E, Cogo A, Gipolami A. Symptomatic deep-vein thrombosis and the post-thrombotic syndrome. *Haematologica* 1995; **80** (Suppl. 2): 42–8.
4 Barritt DW, Jordan SC. Anticoagulant drugs in the treatment of pulmonary embolism, a controlled trial. *Lancet* 1960; **1**: 1309–12.
5 Bjork I, Lindahl U. Mechanism of the anticoagulant action of heparin. *Mol Cell Biochem* 1982; **48**: 161–82.
6 Agnelli G. Pharmacological activities of heparin chains: should our past knowledge be revised? *Haemostasis* 1966; **26**: 2–9.
7 van den Besselar AM, Meeuwisse-Braun J, Bertina RM. Monitoring heparin therapy: relationships between the activated partial thromboplastin time and heparin assays based on ex-vivo heparin samples. *Thromb Haemost* 1990; **63**: 16–23.
8 Goran B, Aberg W, Johansson M, Tornebohm E, Granqvist S, Lockner D. Two daily subcutaneous injections of fragmin compared with intravenous standard heparin in the treatment of deep venous thrombosis. *Thromb Haemost* 1990; **64**: 506–10.

9   Handeland GF, Abildgaard U, Holm HA, Arnesen KE. Dose adjusted heparin treatment of deep venous thrombosis: a comparison of unfractionated and low molecular weight heparin. *Eur J Clin Pharmacol* 1990; **39**: 107–12.

10 Hirsh J, Arkentin TE, Raschke R, et al. Heparin and low-molecular-weight heparin: mechanisms of action, pharmacokinetics, dosing considerations, monitoring, efficacy, and safety. *Chest* 1998; **114**: 489S–510S.

11. Alhenc-Gelas M, Jestin-Le Guernic C, Vitoux JF, Khr A, Aiach M, Fiessinger JN. Adjusted versus fixed doses of the low-molecular-weight heparin fragmin in the treatment of deep vein thrombosis. *Thromb Haemost* 1994; **71**: 698–702.

12 Glazier RL, Crowell EB. Randomized prospective trial of continuous vs intermittent heparin therapy. *JAMA* 1976; **236**: 1365–7.

13 Brandjes DP, Heijboer H, Buller HR, DeRijk M, Jagt H, Cate JW. Acenocoumarol and heparin compared with acenocoumarol alone in the initial treatment of proximal-vein thrombosis. *N Engl J Med* 1992; **327**: 1485–9.

14 Hull RD, Raskob GE, Hirsh J, Jay RM, Leclerc JR, Geerts WH. Continuous intravenous heparin compared with intermittent subcutaneous heparin in the initial treatment of proximal-vein thrombosis. *N Engl J Med* 1986; **315**: 1109–14.

15 Hull RD, Raskob GE, Rosenbloom D, Panju AA, Brill-Edwards P, Ginsber JS. Heparin for 5 days as compared with 10 days in the initial treatment of proximal venous thrombosis. *N Engl J Med* 1990; **322**: 1260–4.

16. Elliott CG, Hiltunen SJ, Suchyta M, Hull RD, Raskob GE, Pineo GF. Physician-guided treatment compared with a heparin protocol for deep vein thrombosis. *Arch Intern Med* 1994; **154**: 999–1004.

17 Cruickshank MK, Levine MN, Hirsh J, Roberts R, Siguenza M. A standard heparin nomogram for the management of heparin therapy. *Arch Intern Med* 1991; **151**: 333–7.

18 Raschke RA, Reilly BM, Guidry JR, Fontana JR, Srinivas S. The weight-based heparin dosing nomogram compared with a 'standard care' nomogram. *Ann Intern Med* 1993; **119**: 874–81.

19 Hull RD, Raskob GE, Rosenbloom D, Lemaire J, Pineo GF, Baylis B. Optimal therapeutic level of heparin therapy in patients with venous thrombosis. *Arch Intern Med* 1992; **152**: 1589–95.

20 Hull RD, Delmore T, Carter C, Hirsh J, Genton E, Gent M. Adjusted subcutaneous heparin versus warfarin sodium in the long-term treatment of venous thrombosis. *N Engl J Med* 1982; **306**: 189–94.

21 Spiro TE. A multicenter clinical trial comparing once and twice-daily subcutaneous enoxaparin and intravenous heparin in the treatment of acute deep venous thrombosis. *Blood* 1997; **90**(Suppl. 10): 295A; AB: 1305.

22 Gallus A, Jackaman J, Tillett J, Mills W, Wycherley A. Safety and efficacy of warfarin started early after submassive venous thrombosis or pulmonary embolism. *Lancet* 1986; **2**: 1293–6.

23 Levine MN, Raskob G, Landefeld S, Kearon C. Hemorrhagic complications of anticoagulant treatment. *Chest* 1998; **114**: 511S–23S.

24 Campbell NR, Hull RD, Brant R, Hogan DB, Pineo GF, Raskob GE. Aging and heparin-related bleeding. *Arch Intern Med* 1996; **156**: 857–60.

25 Landfeld CS, Cook EF, Flatley M, Weisberg M, Goldman L. Identification and preliminary validation of predictors of major bleeding in hospitalized patients starting anticoagulant therapy. *Am J Med* 1987; **82**: 703–13.

26 Warkentin TE. Clinical presentation of heparin-induced thrombocytopenia. *Semin Hematol* 1998; **35**(Suppl. 5): 9–16.

27 Dahlman TC. Osteoporotic fractures and the recurrence of thromboembolism during pregnancy and the puerperium in 184 women undergoing thromboprophylaxis with heparin. *Am J Obstet Gynecol* 1993; **168**: 1265–70.

28 Oster JR, Singer I, Fishman L. Heparin-induced aldosterone suppression and hyperkalemia. *Am J Med* 1995; **98**: 575–86.

29 Hull RD, Raskob GE, Pineo GF, Green D, Trowbridge AA, Elliott CG. Subcutaneous low-molecular-weight heparin compared with continuous intravenous heparin in the treatment of proximal-vein thrombosis. *N Engl J Med* 1992; **326**: 975–82.

30 Levine M, Gent M, Hirsh J, Leclerc J, Anderson D, Weitz J. A comparison of low-molecular-weight heparin administered primarily at home with unfractionated heparin administered in the hospital for proximal deep-vein thrombosis. *N Engl J Med* 1996; **334**: 677–81.

31 Liezorovicz A, Simonneau G, Decousus H, Boissel JP. Comparison of efficacy and safety of low molecular weight heparins and unfractionated heparin in initial treatment of deep venous thrombosis: a meta-analysis. *BMJ* 1994; **309**: 299–304.

32 Prandoni P, Lensing SW, Buller HR, Carta M, Cogo A, Vigo M. Comparison of subcutaneous low-molecular-weight heparin with intravenous standard heparin in proximal deep-vein thrombosis. *Lancet* 1992; **339**: 441–5.

33 Simonneau G, Charbonnier B, Decousus H, Planchon B, Ninet J, Sie P. Subcutaneous low-molecular-weight heparin compared with continuous intravenous unfractionated heparin in the treatment of proximal deep vein thrombosis. *Arch Intern Med* 1993; **153**: 1541–6.

34 Columbus Investigators. Low-molecular-weight heparin in the treatment of patients with venous thromboembolism. *N Engl J Med* 1997; **337**: 657–62.

35 Simmoneau G, Sors H, Charbonnier B, et al. A comparison of low-molecular-weight heparin with unfractionated heparin for acute pulmonary embolism. *N Engl J Med* 1997; **337**: 663–9.

36 Lindmarker P, Holmstrom M, Granqvist S, et al. Comparison of once-daily subcutaneous Fragmin with continuous intravenous unfractionated heparin in the treatment of deep venous thrombosis. *Thromb Haemost* 1994; **72**: 186–90.

37 Koopman MM, Prandoni P, Piovella F, Olkelford PA, Brandjes DP, van der Meer J. Treatment of venous thromboembolism with intravenous unfractionated heparin administered in the hospital as compared with subcutaneous low-molecular-weight heparin administered at home. *N Engl J Med* 1996; **334**: 682–7.

38 Lensing AW, Prins MH, Davidson BL, Hirsh J. Treatment of deep venous thrombosis with low molecular weight heparins. A meta-analysis. *Arch Intern Med* 1995; **155**: 601–7.

39 Gould HK, Dembitzer AD, Sanders GD, Garber AM. Low-molecular-weight heparins compared with unfractionated heparin for treatment of acute venous thrombosis: a meta-analysis of randomized, controlled, trials. *Ann Intern Med* 1999; **130**: 789–99.

40 van den Belt AG, Bossuyt PM, Prins MH, et al. Replacing inpatient care by outpatient care in the treatment of deep venous thrombosis – an economic evaluation. *Thromb Haemost* 1998; **79**: 259–63.

41 Hirsh J, Dalen JE, Anderson DR, et al. Oral anticoagulants: mechanism of action, clinical effectiveness, and optimal therapeutic range. *Chest* 1998; **114**: 445S–69S.

42 Crowther MA, Ginsberg JB, Kearon C, et al. A randomized trial comparing 5-mg and 10-mg warfarin loading doses. *Arch Intern Med* 1999; **159**: 46–8.

43 Holmgrem K, Andersson G, Fagrell B. One-month versus six-month therapy with oral anticoagulants after symptomatic deep vein thrombosis. *Acta Med Scand* 1985; **218**: 279–84.

44 Petitt DB, Strom BL, Melmon KL. Duration of warfarin anticoagulant therapy and the probabilities of recurrent thromboembolism and hemorrhage. *Am J Med* 1986; **81**: 255–9.

45 Research Committee of the British Thoracic Society. Optimum duration of anticoagulation for deep-vein thrombosis and pulmonary embolism. *Lancet* 1992; **340**: 873–6.

46 Schulman S, Rhedin A, Lindmarker P, Carlsson A, Larfars G, Micol P. A comparison of six weeks with six months of oral anticoagulant therapy after a first episode of venous thromboembolism. *N Engl J Med* 1995; **332**: 1661–5.

47 Levine MN, Hirsh J, Gent M, et al. Optimal duration of oral anticoagulant therapy: a randomized trial comparing four weeks with three months of warfarin in patients with proximal deep vein thrombosis. *Thromb Haemost* 1995; **74**: 606–11.

48 Schulman S, Granqvist S, Holmstrom M, Carlsson A, Lindmarker P, Nicol P. The duration of oral anticoagulant therapy after a second episode of venous thromboembolism. *N Engl J Med* 1997; **336**: 393–8.

49 Hirsh J, Kearon C. Duration of anticoagulant therapy after first episode of venous thrombosis in patients with inherited thrombophilia. *Arch Intern Med* 1997; **157**: 2174–6.

50 Goldhaber SZ, Buring JE, Lipnick RJ, Hennekens CH. Pooled analyses of randomized trials of streptokinase and heparin in phlebographically documented acute deep venous thrombosis. *Am J Med* 1984; **76**: 393–7.

51 Arcasoy SM, Kreit JW. Thrombolytic therapy of pulmonary embolism: a comprehensive review of current evidence. *Chest* 1999; **115**: 1695–707.

52 Goldhaber SZ, Haire WD, Feldstein ML, Miller M, Toltzis R, Smith JL. Alteplase versus heparin in acute pulmonary embolism: randomised trial assessing right-ventricular function and pulmonary perfusion. *Lancet* 1993; **341**: 507–11.

53 Becker DM, Philbrick JT, Selby JB. Inferior vena cava filters, indications, safety, effectiveness. *Arch Intern Med* 1992; **152**: 1985–94.

54 Ballew KA, Philbrick JT, Becker DM. Vena cava filter devices. *Clin Chest Med* 1995; **16** (Suppl 2): 295–305.

55 Decousus H, Leizorovicz A, Parent F, et al. A clinical trial of vena caval filters in the prevention of pulmonary embolism in patients with proximal deep-vein thrombosis. *N Engl J Med* 1998; **338**: 409–15.

11

Vena cava filters

JOSEPH BONN

INTRODUCTION

Patients with deep vein thrombosis of the lower extremities most commonly present with acute swelling and pain or chronic swelling that may progress to the debilitating skin ulceration and claudication symptoms of chronic venous insufficiency. These peripheral symptoms are only a limited reminder, however, that these patients are also at risk for the more serious complications of hypoxemia, pulmonary hypertension, right heart failure, and death, which may result from pulmonary embolism.

The accepted therapy for deep vein thrombosis is systemic anticoagulation, the primary function of which is to prevent extension of existing thrombosis as well as the development of new thrombosis, while providing the opportunity for circulating lytic elements to reduce the thrombotic mass and recanalize the venous lumen. However, systemic anticoagulation has only an indirect effect on the risk of pulmonary embolism by stabilizing the thrombotic process. For those patients who have contraindications to anticoagulation, who have suffered pulmonary embolism while adequately anticoagulated, who cannot medically tolerate even the smallest pulmonary embolus, or who are at great risk for pulmonary embolism due to their specific medical condition, an alternative or additional therapy to prevent pulmonary embolism is warranted.

Vena cava interruption provides a more direct reduction in the risk of pulmonary embolism by mechanically preventing the passage of deep vein thrombi to the pulmonary arterial circulation. This chapter reviews the history of vena cava interruption, from the early surgical approaches to the current array of percutaneously inserted filtration devices. It also outlines patient selection and imaging evaluation, the characteristics of currently available filters, their complications, and their controversies, including their prophylactic use in trauma patients, their role in patients with malignancies, and the use of temporary filters.

HISTORY

For many decades, surgical ligation of the inferior vena cava provided the most definitive and complete form of vena cava interruption. Unfortunately, it had to be performed through a major surgical exploration, often in patients whose serious medical conditions placed them at greatest risk for postoperative morbidity and mortality. In addition, complete surgical occlusion of the inferior vena cava created in many patients serious lower extremity venous stasis disorders, while stimulating the formation of venous collaterals that subsequently could allow pulmonary emboli to bypass the ligated vena cava.

In response to the disadvantages of vena cava ligation, several invasive procedures were developed in the 1950s and 1960s: 'surgical weaving' and 'plication' of the vena cava were two similar suture techniques, whereas 'clipping' was the application of a circumferential clip around the vena cava.[1–3] These three procedures were designed to narrow the vena cava lumen while avoiding complete occlusion. By maintaining at least some flow through the vena cava, they were used in attempt to reduce the risk of lower extremity venous stasis disorders and the development of collateral bypasses; however, they still required a considerable surgical exploration and were eventually demonstrated to occlude at a high rate.

The first attempts to avoid a major surgical exploration by inserting a caval interruption device through a venous cutdown in a transvenous (or endovascular) manner were by Eichelter and Schenk in 1968, when they described the use in a canine model of an 'umbrella-like sieve' fashioned by cutting multiple longitudinal slits in a polyethylene catheter.[4] This was soon followed by the Pate clip, designed to narrow the vena cava by internally apposing its walls, and the Hunter–Sessions balloon, an endovascular device that was inflated in the vena cava to fill its lumen (Fig. 11.1). These devices, while avoiding the morbidity of a major surgical exploration, also proved to be excessively thrombogenic and occlusive, leading to an unacceptable risk of lower extremity venous stasis disorders.

The Mobin–Uddin umbrella, introduced in 1967, was the first endovascular caval interruption device to apply the principle that the ideal mechanical interruption is a compromise between the filtration of significant emboli and the maintenance of vena cava flow.[5] This device resembles an umbrella, with the points of its structural supports anchoring it in the vena cava wall, and its overlying latex membrane designed to trap emboli, with holes created in the membrane to maintain at least a reduced vena cava flow (Fig. 11.2). Early in the clinical experience with the Mobin–Uddin umbrella, it became evident that its design favored filtration at the expense of flow maintenance, resulting in vena cava occlusion and venous stasis complications in 70% of patients.

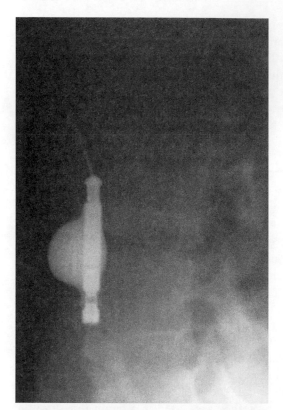

Figure 11.1 *A radiograph of a Hunter–Sessions balloon positioned in the inferior vena cava. This device was inserted in an endovascular manner and guided into the vena cava, where it was inflated and deployed, preventing emboli from passing but completely occluding flow in the vena cava as well.*

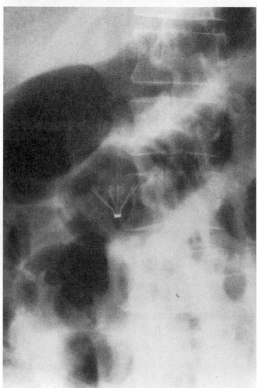

Figure 11.2 *A radiograph of a Mobin–Uddin umbrella positioned in the inferior vena cava. This was the first endovascular device to filter the vena cava, i.e., trap emboli while maintaining flow. The metal skeleton seen here was covered with a perforated latex (radiolucent) membrane. However, the perforations proved to be too small and the vena cava occlusion rate was excessive.*

The Mobin-Uddin umbrella fell out of favor soon after the introduction in 1973 of the next endovascular mechanical interruption device, the Kimray–Greenfield filter. Its original version was placed via a large delivery sheath inserted through a surgical cutdown into the internal jugular or common femoral vein, either with or without fluoroscopic visualization to guide positioning in the vena cava (Fig. 11.3).

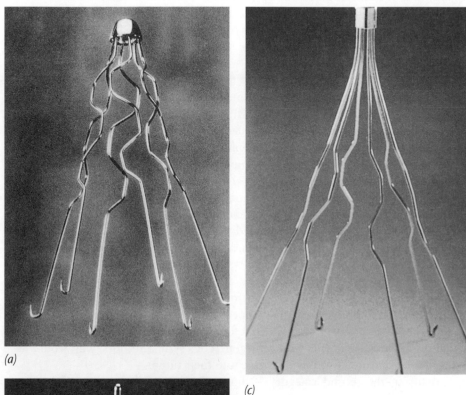

(a)

(c)

(b)

Figure 11.3 *Three versions of the Greenfield filter. (A) Original 24-French Stainless Steel Greenfield filter. (B) 12-French Titanium Greenfield filter. (C) 12-French Stainless Steel Greenfield filter. All three share a conical design, six legs with anchoring hooks, and a relative increase in filtering surface area toward the central apex. (Courtesy of Boston Scientific Corporation, Natick, MA.)*

The Greenfield filter design (Boston Scientific Corporation, Natick, MA), now available in two smaller versions for percutaneous introduction, has accumulated more than 25 years of clinical experience, and has become the standard against which other, newer filtration devices are compared. In that time, several additional filters have been approved for clinical use in the USA by the Food and Drug Administration (FDA), including the Gianturco–Roehm Bird's Nest filter (Cook, Inc., Bloomington, IN), the Simon Nitinol filter (Nitinol Medical Technologies, Inc., Boston, MA), and the Vena Tech–LGM filter (B. Braun Medical, Inc., Evanston, IL).

PATIENT SELECTION

The selection of patients for vena cava interruption with a filter can be condensed into three general criteria: (1) the patient with deep vein thrombosis who has a contraindication to standard therapy (systemic anticoagulation); (2) the patient who has failed standard therapy; and (3) prophylaxis for the patient without deep vein thrombosis who is at great risk of developing deep vein thrombosis or pulmonary embolism, or the patient who has a deep vein thrombosis treated by anticoagulation but who may suffer excessively if a pulmonary embolism were to occur.

Patients in the first category possess contraindications to systemic anticoagulation, usually as the result of recent bleeding such as a hemorrhagic stroke, recent surgery, especially involving the central nervous system and noncompressible areas such as the abdomen or chest, or recent trauma such as a closed head injury. These contraindications can also, however, be the result of complications of adequate anticoagulation, such as an acute gastrointestinal bleed from ulcer disease, or heparin antibody-induced thrombocytopenia after coronary artery bypass surgery. In addition, there can exist the potential for a contraindication to systemic anticoagulation, such as in patients with central nervous system tumors, who would have a devastating outcome from hemorrhage into their tumor.

Patients in the second category – those who have failed standard therapy – include usually the patient with a deep vein thrombosis who has incurred a pulmonary embolism while adequately systemically anticoagulated. This definition of having failed standard therapy has been broadened in some institutions to include the patient whose deep vein thrombosis worsens while adequately systemically anticoagulated without a pulmonary embolism occurring.

Patients in the third category may benefit from a vena cava filter as a prophylactic device to prevent pulmonary embolism, although this treatment indication is still somewhat controversial. These patients typically have suffered multiple trauma and are likely to be immobilized for prolonged periods of time or to undergo multiple surgical procedures. The combinations of vein and soft-tissue injury, long-bone and pelvic fractures, and slow venous flow greatly increase the risk of deep vein thrombosis and subsequent pulmonary embolism. In addition, there are patients with deep vein thrombosis who are able to be systemically anticoagulated, but, due to existing pulmonary or cardiac compromise, are considered to be at too great a risk of significant morbidity or death should they suffer a pulmonary embolism. These patients may benefit from combination therapy of both systemic anticoagulation and vena cava filtration. Another select group of patients who may benefit from a filter are those who have just undergone emergent surgical pulmonary embolectomy, and who are at great risk of significant morbidity or death should they incur a subsequent pulmonary embolism.

There are only a few contraindications to vena cava filtration, including septicemia and an uncontrolled bleeding disorder. In the former, insertion of a foreign body into the circulatory system is considered contraindicated in the presence of active septicemia, due to the risk of colonizing the foreign body with bacteria. It is possible that temporary or retrievable filters in the future may serve as a bridge device, allowing filtration until septicemia is treated, at which time the temporary device can be removed (along with the concern for foreign body colonization) and a permanent filter can be inserted.

The patient with an uncontrolled bleeding disorder, defined as a platelet count less than 50 000, or an International Normalized Ratio (INR) greater than 1.7, can usually be treated with blood products to correct these abnormalities before large-bore venous access is obtained for filter placement. Patients with these bleeding abnormalities may also benefit from the use of later-generation filter systems, such as the Simon Nitinol filter, that fit through smaller introductory sheaths (7–French diameter) which are less likely to cause postprocedure access site bleeding, and that may be inserted from upper arm veins, reducing the clinical concern about an access site hematoma.

IMAGING OF THE FILTER CANDIDATE

Following the determination that a patient is a candidate for a vena cava filter, imaging of the vena cava must be performed to define the anatomy that will guide the choice of filter and its implantation site, and to assess the presence of thrombus in the vena cava or the access veins. The vena cava anatomy to be defined includes its diameter and length at the implantation site, the location and number of renal veins (for inferior vena cava filters), and the presence of congenital anomalies such as duplicated vena cava and accessory renal veins. Filter placement should not be central to the vena cava inflow of an accessory renal vein, because many of these veins anastomose with the main renal vein in the renal hilum. This communication may potentially serve as a bypass for emboli, especially if a filter is already compromised with a large thrombus burden, and elevated pressure in the peripheral vena cava reverses flow in the accessory renal vein. Filter placement must also be planned to avoid passing the delivery system through an existing thrombus, and to position the filter central to any vena cava thrombus.

The most common vena cava imaging obtained before filter placement is the contrast vena cavogram, i.e., x-ray filming during the catheter injection of iodinated contrast into the vena cava. This is optimally done just prior to filter placement on dedicated cut film or digital recording systems to produce the detailed information required for filter choice and location decisions. Alternative contrast agents that have been shown to be safe and effective for defining the vena cava anatomy in patients with contraindications to iodinated contrast include gadolinium-based agents and carbon dioxide gas.[6,7]

An alternative imaging modality recently described is intravascular ultrasound, a catheter-based ultrasound transducer that obtains images from within the vena cava lumen, defining the presence of thrombus, vena cava dimensions, location of landmark branches such as the renal veins, and the presence of congenital vein anomalies. This modality produces the desired information without ionizing radiation and nephrotoxic iodinated contrast, making it particularly attractive for the evaluation of pregnant women and patients with pre-existing renal insufficiency or severe iodinated contrast allergies.[8]

Noninvasive imaging modalities such as external ultrasound, computed tomography, and magnetic resonance venography are usually able to produce the detailed imaging information required to guide filter selection and location, although overlying abdominal gas may limit ultrasound, and patient claustrophobia may limit magnetic resonance venography. Ultimately, filter deployment is optimally performed during the real-time imaging of X-ray fluoroscopy or intravascular ultrasound, so using these latter two modalities to image the vena cava just prior to filter placement is usually the most optimal and efficient use of resources and time.

VENA CAVA FILTERS

The currently available filter with the longest history of clinical use is the Greenfield filter, specifically the stainless-steel version placed through a 24–French delivery sheath.[9] In the last few years, a movement away from the more invasive venous cutdown typically used to insert this device and toward the less invasive percutaneous introduction method stimulated the design of smaller caliber versions of the Greenfield filter, leading to the approval of a titanium version and ultimately a smaller stainless-steel version, both of which are introduced safely through a 12–French sheath.[10,11] All three Greenfield filters share the same principles of a six-legged conical design, with six anchoring hooks at the cone's base (Fig. 11.3). The conical shape diverts trapped emboli toward the apex of the cone, where the most rapid vena cava flow is found in the center of the vena cava lumen. This design principle permits maintenance of flow around the circumferential base of the filter, even after 70% of the central, apical volume of the filter cone has been filled with thrombus. The design results in efficient emboli trapping that leads to the low incidence of 2–4% of pulmonary embolism after Greenfield filter placement, while maintaining vena cava patency in approximately 95% of patients.

The second vena cava filter to be approved for clinical use in the USA was the Gianturco–Roehm Bird's Nest filter. This multicomponent filter design relies on a somewhat random unraveling of thin, stainless-steel wires in the vena cava lumen, anchored by two apposing V-shaped barbed struts that engage the vena cava wall (Fig. 11.4). The bundle of thin wires compacted in the vena cava lumen creates interstices small enough to trap emboli to prevent pulmonary emboli in at least 96% of patients, while providing enough interstices to maintain patency of flow in approximately 95% of patients.[12,13]

Another filter approved for clinical use in the USA is the Simon Nitinol filter. This design relies on two major components: a conical body with anchoring hooks at the base of the cone secures the filter and traps emboli in the manner of the Greenfield filter, while a more central array of petal-like wires assists in centering the filter in the vena cava lumen and provides a second entrapment surface (Fig. 11.5). In

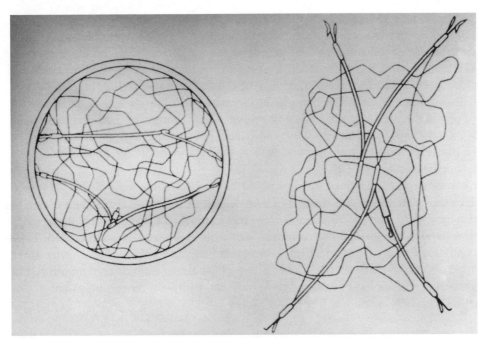

Figure 11.4 *Cross-sectional and longitudinal ex-vivo radiographs of the Gianturco–Roehm Bird's Nest filter, demonstrating its proximal and distal anchoring struts and barbs, and the array of thin wires that fill the vena cava and form the filtering surfaces. (Courtesy of Cook, Inc., Bloomington, IN.)*

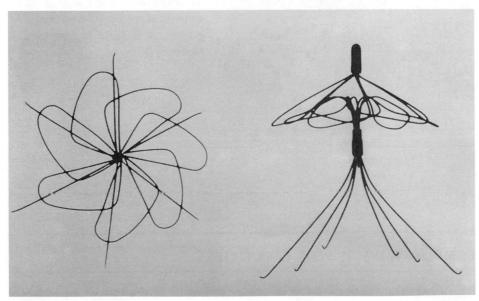

Figure 11.5 *Cross-sectional and longitudinal ex-vivo radiographs of the Simon Nitinol filter, demonstrating its six legs with anchoring hooks, and the petal-like array of seven wire loops that form its second filtering surface. (Courtesy of Nitinol Medical Technologies, Inc., Boston, MA.)*

addition, the highly elastic, thin, nitinol (nickel–titanium alloy) wire that forms the filter allows the device to be introduced through a 7–French sheath. This smaller size permits safe introduction of the filter through a greater variety of access veins, such as the upper arm, when the traditional jugular or femoral access sites are not available. These alternative access sites may be favored in patients with bleeding disorders, because effects of a hematoma in the upper arm may be less deleterious than of one in the neck or groin.[14] Clinical results with the Simon Nitinol filter have been similar to those for the previously described filters, with 95% of patients free of recurrent pulmonary embolus and 96% of patients maintaining a patent vena cava in one large study.[15]

Another filter approved for clinical use in the USA is the Vena Tech–LGM filter. This stainless-steel device consists of a six-legged cone similar in trapping design to the Greenfield filter; however, each of the legs is attached to longitudinal metal strips that parallel and engage the vena cava wall with barbs, and assist in centering the cone (Fig. 11.6). Filtering efficacy has been similar to that of the other three approved filters, with 93% of patients free of recurrent pulmonary embolism, but vena cava patency has been noted to be variable, with 94% remaining patent in one study and 80% in another.[16,17]

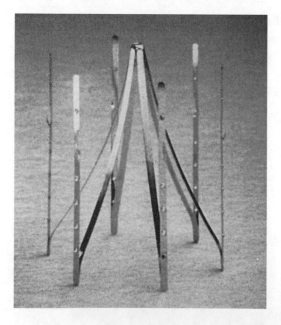

Figure 11.6 *A photograph of the Vena Tech-LGM filter, demonstrating the conical arrangement of its six ribbon-like legs attached to longitudinal barbed struts that anchor the device to the vena cava wall and assist in centering it in the vena cava lumen. (Courtesy of B. Braun Medical, Inc., Evanston, IL.)*

COMPLICATIONS OF VENA CAVA FILTERS

As with any (minimally) invasive procedure and with any implantable device, there is a variety of complications that must be considered, both by the patient in consenting to the procedure and by the physician planning and performing the procedure and following the patient postoperatively. These complications can be grouped into those that occur during filter insertion and those that occur afterwards.

Although filter introduction sheaths have been reduced in diameter to between 7-French and 12-French, the possibility of sheath-induced injury at the vein access site is still a consideration. This injury may lead to a local hematoma (that may resolve spontaneously or require surgical evacuation and repair), temporary or permanent insertion site thrombosis (and the possibility of chronic venous stasis disorder in the affected limb), or an arterial injury or arteriovenous fistula from inadvertent puncture of the adjacent artery. During the filter insertion process, there is the rare possibility of premature or incomplete release of the filter, resulting in a deformed device that may not function effectively. There are several effective endovascular techniques for manipulating deployed filters into more optimal positions or shapes.[18,19] Premature release, or release into the wrong location, can lead to inadequate filtration, for example if the filter was deployed into a common iliac vein, leaving the other extremity without protection. Premature release has also resulted in filters being placed inadvertently into the right heart chambers. Whether such malpositioned filters need to be retrieved depends on the patient's clinical status (some filters in the heart and pulmonary arteries have been well tolerated) and on the relative risk of further morbidity during the retrieval.[20] Greenfield filters released into the right atrium that cause problematic arrhythmias have been retrieved using percutaneous catheter and snare techniques.[21,22]

The most important postprocedure complications are those related to a filter's compromised function: the risks of ineffective filtration (recurrent pulmonary embolism) and overeffective filtration (filter and vena cava occlusion). The former occurs in the range of 2–7%, depending on the study and the device, whereas the latter occurs in the range of 4–6%. Recurrent pulmonary embolism is a complex issue, and may be the result of emboli finding their way through the filter interstices, thrombus forming on trapped emboli in the filter and embolizing centrally, or in-situ thrombus forming de novo on the filter metal itself before embolizing. Patients should have a second filter placed more centrally if thrombus is found to project through or have formed central to the first filter. Recurrent pulmonary embolism may also be secondary to a new and unprotected source of deep vein thrombosis, such as the upper extremity after an inferior vena cava filter is placed. In the rare patient with upper extremity deep vein thrombosis and a contraindication to anticoagulation, superior vena cava filter placement has been shown to be safe and effective in preventing pulmonary embolism in two recent reviews.[23,24]

Filter occlusion is also a complex process and can result from the trapping of an excessive volume of emboli that fill all of the device's interstices, or that so retard blood flow in the filter that in-situ thrombosis on the trapped emboli or on the filter itself completes the occlusion process. Filter occlusion, leading to vena cava occlusion, can be the source of significant lower extremity swelling and ultimately chronic venous insufficiency, but symptoms alone underestimate the incidence of filter occlusion. Of particular concern is occlusion of suprarenal inferior vena cava filters, as this process may lead to propagation of thrombus peripherally into both renal veins, leading to renal failure. This potential complication discourages routine suprarenal filter placement; however, it has been shown to be a rare event, occurring transiently in one of 22 patients in one review and in none of 73 patients in another review.[25,26] Occluded filters can recanalize, and thrombus-burdened filters can improve in patency as natural lytic factors dissolve the trapped thrombus.

In addition, a filter can malfunction by inadvertently migrating from its optimal position, penetrating the vena cava wall (filter limbs have been shown to cause complications after penetrating into the ureter and the duodenum, for example), or tilting or distorting into a less-effective filtering geometry.[27,28] An additional complication that deserves highlighting is the possibility of guidewire entrapment on a previously implanted filter during the insertion of jugular and subclavian central venous catheters. This has led to significant filter migration, distortion, and fragmentation in some cases, and underscores the importance of obtaining a complete procedure history prior to any procedure. Several endovascular techniques have been described to extract guidewires from those filters still intact and in position, and to retrieve those filters that cannot be properly repositioned.[29]

Filter complications can be diagnosed typically by imaging studies that inspect the filter itself for malposition, deformation, tilting or migration (by plain films), the access veins and vena cava for hematoma, arteriovenous fistula, thrombosis or filter penetration (by ultrasound, computed tomography or magnetic resonance venography), and the pulmonary circulation for pulmonary embolism (helical computed tomography, magnetic resonance venography, lung scintigraphy, or pulmonary angiography). Stainless-steel filters have been shown not to distort or migrate in the strong magnetic field of the magnetic resonance machine, even acutely after implantation. The Simon Nitinol filter, being nonferrous, does not possess magnetic susceptibility.

PROPHYLAXIS AFTER TRAUMA

Patients who have suffered major trauma, such as closed head injury, spinal cord injury with or without paralysis, complex pelvic fractures, lower extremity or long-bone fractures, or penetrating large vein injuries, are at high risk for thromboembolic complications, both from the injuries themselves and from the patients' prolonged immobilization. Those with pelvic fractures alone have been shown in one review to have an incidence of proximal deep vein thrombosis of 25–35% and of symptomatic pulmonary embolism of 2–10%.[30] Many major trauma patients have contraindications to anticoagulation (either prophylactic or to treat a deep vein thrombosis) due to their need for multiple surgical operations, or their higher risk of bleeding. In addition, some patients with lower extremity injuries may not be able to undergo prophylactic pneumatic compression therapy due to the location and extent of their injuries.

This patient population, many of whom are young and otherwise healthy, has been the subject of numerous prospective and retrospective trials investigating the safety and efficacy of prophylactic vena cava filter placement for the prevention of pulmonary embolism. Without standards for study design or data reporting, it is difficult to make comparisons between these trials. However, while none is both prospective and randomized, several appear to be worth examining in detail.

In one prospective, nonrandomized trial, 250 trauma patients at high risk for thromboembolic complications were studied; 151 were placed on prophylactic anticoagulation and/or compression devices and 99 received vena cava filters.[31] In comparison to a matched historical control group that had a 4.8% incidence of pulmonary embolism, the treated group had a 1.6% incidence of pulmonary embolism ($p = 0.045$), with no pulmonary embolism occurring in the subset that received vena cava filters. In a similar comparison to 216 historical matched controls, 108 patients with closed head injuries, spinal cord injuries, pelvic and/or lower extremity fractures received prophylactic filters.[32] There were 13 pulmonary embolisms, including nine which were fatal in the control group and none in the group having received filters ($p < 0.009$).

In another large study, 132 patients with similar multiple trauma received prophylactic filters and suffered only three pulmonary embolisms (one fatal), all of which were in patients whose filters had tilted > 14 degrees, or had a malpositioned filter strut.[33] There was a 3% incidence of filter-insertion site deep vein thrombosis, none of which was symptomatic and, at 3 years, vena cava patency was 97%. In a similar group of 75 patients receiving prophylactic filters, only one non-fatal pulmonary embolism was detected; there were no filter migrations, and the vena cava patency (by ultrasound imaging) was 100% at a mean follow-up period of 19 months (range 7–60 months).[34]

Identification of the patient at risk for thromboembolic complications after multiple trauma remains the subject of reasonable debate. An alternative approach to the empiric placement of filters in all multiple trauma patients, or to a clinical classification system based on type, location, and extent of injury, is the use of routine surveillance ultrasound of the deep venous system to identify deep vein thrombosis before it progresses or embolizes, and to tailor therapy based on this information. In one such study, surveillance ultrasound was found to be more cost effective than routine prophylactic vena cava filter placement, unless the patient was to be hospitalized for at least 2 weeks, and if the filter was placed in the interventional radiology suite (where costs have frequently been shown to be less than in the operating room).[35]

Not all studies have demonstrated a benefit of prophylactic vena cava filter placement in trauma patients. In a retrospective study of 248 trauma patients who received filters during a period either with liberal criteria for vena cava filter placement or with more limited, strict criteria, the authors found no significant difference in the incidence of pulmonary embolism between the two groups.[36] In a different retrospective study of 280 high-risk trauma patients with closed head injuries, spinal cord injuries, pelvic or lower extremity fractures, or venous injuries, most of whom received only compression device therapy, the authors found a 5% incidence of deep vein thrombosis and a 1.4% incidence of pulmonary embolism.[37] These findings were without significant difference compared to a low-risk trauma group of 2249 patients who had a 0.1% incidence of deep vein thrombosis and no pulmonary embolism. The authors concluded that 'aggressive screening and prophylactic inferior vena cava filters would not have benefited 95% of "high risk" patients without deep vein thrombosis and would not have prevented any deaths.'

Clearly, trials studying prophylactic vena cava filter placement to prevent pulmonary embolism in trauma patients have produced mixed results. However, the greater number of trials appear to describe a beneficial effect, although without examining the more complex issue of cost–benefit ratio. Until a well-designed, large, prospective, randomized clinical trial is conducted (which may be difficult to fund and accomplish in the USA), the issue of prophylactic vena cava filter use in trauma patients may remain controversial.

DEEP VEIN THROMBOSIS ASSOCIATED WITH MALIGNANCY

An additional debate still being conducted concerns the role of vena cava filtration in patients with a malignancy who are at an increased risk of deep vein thrombosis and often possess contraindications to anticoagulation due to the location of their tumor, bleeding complications of their tumor, and repeated requirements for invasive procedures or surgery. These apparent indications for vena cava filtration must be balanced against the hypercoagulable state many of these patients are in (which increases the risk of thrombosis at the insertion site, in the filter, and in the vena cava) and their shortened life expectancy (which limits the survival benefit they will experience from this expensive device, which is not without potential complications).

Several retrospective reviews of patients who have received vena cava filters during treatment for coexistent malignancies demonstrate the complexities of this issue. Short-term (1–3 months) mortality rates after filter placement were 18% and 26% in two studies and were as high as 65% at 1 year in another study.[38-40] In this latter study, serious life-threatening and limb-threatening complications developed in 17% of patients with filters;[40] however, in another group, 14% of patients with filters were able to undergo invasive therapeutic and palliative procedures without concern about interrupting anticoagulation.[39] Although survival and complication rates are important indicators, larger studies focusing on quality-of-life issues and more complex analyses of safety, efficacy, and cost are still needed to define the role of vena cava filters in patients with malignancies.

ELECTIVE TEMPORARY FILTRATION

Because filter insertion and the presence of a filter in the vena cava are associated with a finite risk of complications, the indications for filter placement have always been influenced by the permanence of the device. Filter placement in those with a long life expectancy raises concerns, because the device will be in place for many decades (and only the large version of the stainless-steel Greenfield has over 20 years of placement data). Concerns are also raised with female patients of child-bearing age, because only minimal data are available on the interaction between the enlarging uterus and the adjacent inferior vena cava filter. (In a series of eight pregnant women with Greenfield filters, none suffered pulmonary embolism or filter-related complications.)[41]

Those patients who might benefit from temporary filtration include those thought to be at a transient risk of pulmonary embolism, because of either a transient risk of deep vein thrombosis or a transient risk of pulmonary embolism from an existing deep vein thrombosis. There remains to be defined, however, the duration of pulmonary embolism risk and the duration of contraindications to anticoagulation for various patients and disease states.

One group that might qualify as having only a transient risk of pulmonary embolism comprises those patients whose only medical problem is closed head, spinal cord, or skeletal trauma, including long-bone and pelvic fractures. These patients do not have deep vein thrombosis, but are at an increased risk of deep vein thrombosis and significant pulmonary embolism due to their trauma and to their prolonged immobilization. However, the duration of this risk is difficult to quantify and needs to be contrasted to the poorly defined risk of a long-term permanent filter, because many of these patients are also young.

Another group that may have a transient risk of pulmonary embolism comprises those patients who have deep vein thrombosis and are adequately anticoagulated, but who need to have their anticoagulation interrupted for an invasive procedure. These patients have a transient risk of embolizing their deep vein thrombosis if their anticoagulation is removed for the period of the invasive procedure. Patients in a similar group with deep vein thrombosis and adequate anticoagulation may be at such a high risk for pulmonary embolism or its effects that they would benefit from additional mechanical protection, even if only for the brief duration of their greatest risk.

One response to this clinical dilemma has been the development of vena cava filters designed either to be temporary and removable, or to be convertible from temporary to permanent. Several of these are currently in clinical use outside the USA, whereas in the USA none has yet received approval from the FDA. Several technical issues help define the development and design of these devices. One consideration is that the anchoring points of any filter with the vena cava wall endothelialize to a relatively secure attachment within several weeks of placement, possibly limiting the window of opportunity for filter removal. One design response has been the development of filter-anchoring hooks of a configuration that allows the hooks to be removed, even from a mature vena cava endothelial covering. Therefore, these filters can either be temporary or converted to a permanent device. Another design response has been to secure the filter in place by a relatively rigid tether, rather than rely on permanent fixation points. Without anchors, however, one does not have the option of converting these filters to permanent devices.[42]

An additional issue with those filters that are only temporary in design is the management of trapped thromboemboli in a device that must be removed before a certain deadline. The time required for natural circulating factors to lyse the clot is likely to exceed the deadline at which the device must be removed before it is fixated to the vena cava wall. In many of these patients, the filter is placed because of a contraindication to anticoagulation, and most also have a contraindication to regional thrombolysis with exogenous plasminogen activators such as urokinase. Some practitioners remove the device and allow the trapped thrombus to embolize to the pulmonary circulation, but the clot burden may be a significant risk to many patients. One additional option (which has been described only in flow models) may be to mechanically fragment or remove the trapped clot, using one of several catheter-based devices recently approved in the USA.[43,44] These devices either use a spinning rotor to aspirate and macerate clot adjacent to the catheter tip, or rely on a rapidly flowing liquid across a window in the catheter tip to create a negative pressure, via the Venturi principle, that aspirates the thrombus into the catheter lumen.

Temporary filters have potential complications similar to their permanent analogues: migration, vena cava occlusion, and pulmonary embolism. Pulmonary embolism, as described above, can occur when the temporary device is removed after having trapped thrombus.[45-7] Those temporary filters that rely on a tethering device that protrudes for up to several weeks through the skin at the vein access site have a slightly increased risk of infection, noted to be 1% in one trial of three devices in 67 patients.[46] Some tethered filters also have a greater risk of migration, because filter position is dependent on the relative rigidity of the tether, not on hooks that anchor into the vena cava wall. Significant migration was found to be 7.5% in one study of 66 patients with one device, including 3% that migrated into the right atrium.[47]

CONCLUSION

In little more than two decades after clinical introduction, vena cava filters have come to play an important role in the prevention of pulmonary embolism, and are a critical advance over the previous surgical options for vena cava interruption. New technical modifications continue to improve upon the basic device designs that strive to achieve a balance between filtering efficiency and vena cava patency. Uncertainty still remains, however, regarding patient selection, especially for young patients, multiple trauma patients, and those patients with malignancies. Even greater uncertainty exists regarding the role of temporary filters, both retrievable and convertible. Large, well-designed clinical trials are needed to answer many of these lingering questions before statistically inadequate studies serve only to further confuse an already complex issue.

REFERENCES

1 Moretz WH, Rhode CM, Shepherd MH. Prevention of pulmonary emboli by partial occlusion of the inferior vena cava. *Am Surg* 1959; **25**: 617–26.
2 Spencer FC, Quattlebaum JR, Quattlebaum JK, et al. Plication of the inferior vena cava for pulmonary embolism: a report of 20 cases. *Ann Surg* 1962; **155**: 827–37.
3 DeWeese M, Hunter DC. A vena caval filter for the prevention of pulmonary emboli. *Bull Soc Int Chir* 1958; **17**: 17.
4 Eichelter P, Schenk W. Prophylaxis of pulmonary embolism: a new experimental approach with initial results. *Arch Surg* 1968; **97**: 348.
5 Mobin-Uddin K, Smith PE, Martinez LO, Lombardo CR, Jude JR. A vena cava filter for the prevention of pulmonary embolus. *Surg Forum* 1967; **18**: 209–11.
6 Kaufman JA, Geller SC, Bazari H, Waltman AC. Gadolinium-based contrast agents as an alternative at vena cavography in patients with renal insufficiency – early experience. *Radiology* 1999; **212**: 280–4.
7 Boyd-Kranis R, Sullivan KL, Eschelman DJ, Bonn J, Gardiner GA. Accuracy and safety of carbon dioxide inferior vena cavography. *J Vasc Interv Radiol* 1999; **10**: 1183–9.
8 Bonn J, Liu JB, Eschelman DJ, Sullivan KL, Pinheiro LW, Gardiner GA Jr. Intravascular ultrasound as an alternative to positive-contrast vena cavography prior to filter placement. *J Vasc Interv Radiol* 1999; **10**: 843–9.
9 Greenfield LJ, Proctor MC. Twenty-year clinical experience with the Greenfield filter. *Cardiovasc Surg* 1995; **3**: 199–205.

10 Greenfield LJ, Proctor MC, Cho JK, et al. Extended evaluation of the titanium Greenfield vena caval filter. *J Vasc Surg* 1994; **20**: 458–64.

11 Cho KJ, Greenfield LJ, Proctor MC, et al. Evaluation of a new percutaneous stainless steel Greenfield filter. *J Vasc Interv Radiol* 1997; **8**: 181–7.

12 Wojtowycz MM, Stoehr T, Crummy AB, McDermott JC, Sproat IA. The Bird's Nest inferior vena caval filter: review of a single-center experience. *J Vasc Interv Radiol* 1997; **8**: 171–9.

13 Nicholson AA, Ettles DF, Paddon AJ, Dyet JF. Long-term follow-up of the Bird's Nest IVC filter. *Clin Radiol* 1999; **54**: 759–64.

14 Engmann E, Asch MR. Clinical experience with the antecubital Simon nitinol IVC filter. *J Vasc Interv Radiol* 1998; **9**: 774–8.

15 Poletti PA, Becker CD, Prina L, et al. Long-term results of the Simon nitinol inferior vena cava filter. *Eur Radiol* 1998; **8**: 289–94.

16 Ricco JB, Dubreuil F, Reynaud P, et al. The LGM Vena-Tech caval filter: results of a multicenter study. *Ann Vasc Surg* 1995; **9**(Suppl.): S89–100.

17 Crochet DP, Brunel P, Trogrlic S, Grossetete R, Auget JL, Dary C. Long-term follow-up of Vena Tech-LGM filter: predictors and frequency of caval occlusion. *J Vasc Interv Radiol* 1999; **10**: 137–42.

18 Moore BS, Valji K, Roberts AC, Bookstein JJ. Transcatheter manipulation of asymmetrically opened titanium Greenfield filters. *J Vasc Interv Radiol* 1993; **4**: 687–90.

19 Isaacson S, Gray RR, Pugash RA. Manipulation by catheter of unopened LGM filter. *Can Assoc Radiol J* 1993; **44**: 217–20.

20 Gelbfish GA, Ascer E. Intracardiac and intrapulmonary Greenfield filters: a long-term follow-up. *J Vasc Surg* 1991; **14**: 614–17.

21 Patterson R, Fowl RJ, Lubbers DJ. Repositioning of partially dislodged Greenfield filters from the right atrium by use of a tip deflection wire. *J Vasc Surg* 1990; **12**: 70–2.

22 Queiroz R, Waldman DL. Transvenous retrieval of a Greenfield filter lodged in the tricuspid valve. *Cathet Cardiovasc Diagn* 1998; **44**: 310–12.

23 Ascer E, Gennaro M, Lorensen E, Pollina RM. Superior vena caval Greenfield filters: indications, techniques, and results. *J Vasc Surg* 1996; **23**: 498–503.

24 Spence LD, Gironta MG, Malde HM, Mickolick CT, Geisinger MA, Dolmatch BL. Acute upper extremity deep venous thrombosis: safety and effectiveness of superior vena caval filters. *Radiology* 1999; **210**: 53–8.

25 Matchett WJ, Jones MP, McFarland DR, Ferris EJ. Suprarenal vena caval filter placement: follow-up of four filter types in 22 patients. *J Vasc Interv Radiol* 1998; **9**: 588–93.

26 Greenfield LJ, Proctor MC. Suprarenal filter placement. *J Vasc Surg* 1998; **28**: 432–8.

27 Berger BD, Jafri SZH, Konczalski M. Symptomatic hydronephrosis caused by inferior vena cava penetration by a Greenfield filter. *J Vasc Interv Radiol* 1996; **7**: 99–101.

28 Al Zahrani HA. Bird's Nest inferior vena caval filter migration into the duodenum: a rare cause of upper gastrointestinal bleeding. *J Endovasc Surg* 1995; **2**: 372–5.

29 Andrews RT, Geschwind JF, Savader SJ, Venbrux AC. Entrapment of J-tip guidewires by Venatech and stainless-steel Greenfield vena cava filters during central venous catheter placement: percutaneous management in four patients. *Cardiovasc Intervent Radiol* 1998; **21**: 424–8.

30 Montgomery KD, Geerts WH, Potter HG, Helfet DL. Thromboembolic complications in patients with pelvic trauma. *Clin Orthop* 1996; **329**: 68–87.

31 Gosin JS, Graham AM, Ciocca RG, Hammond JS. Efficacy of prophylactic vena cava filters in high-risk trauma patients. *Ann Vasc Surg* 1997; **11**: 100–5.

32 Khansarinia S, Dennis JW, Veldenz HC, Butcher JL, Hartland L. Prophylactic Greenfield filter placement in selected high-risk trauma patients. *J Vasc Surg* 1995; **22**: 231–6.

33 Rogers FB, Strindberg G, Shackford SR, et al. Five-year follow-up of prophylactic vena cava filters in high-risk trauma patients. *Arch Surg* 1998; **133**: 406–11.

34 Langan EM, Miller RS, Casey WJ, Carsten CG, Graham RM, Taylor SM. Prophylactic inferior vena cava filters in trauma patients at high risk: follow-up examination and risk/benefit assessment. *J Vasc Surg* 1999; **30**: 484–8.

35 Brasel KJ, Borgstrom DC, Weigelt JA. Cost-effective prevention of pulmonary embolus in high-risk trauma patients. *J Trauma* 1997; **42**: 456–60.

36 McMurtry AL, Owings JT, Anderson JT, Battistella FD, Gosselin R. Increased use of prophylactic vena cava filters in trauma patients failed to decrease overall incidence of pulmonary embolism. *J Am Coll Surg* 1999; **189**: 314–20.

37 Spain DA, Richardson JD, Polk HC, Bergamini TM, Wilson MA, Miller FB. Venous thromboembolism in the high-risk trauma patient: do risks justify aggressive screening and prophylaxis? *J Trauma* 1997; **42**: 463–7.

38 Lossef SV, Barth KH. Outcome of patients with advanced neoplastic disease receiving vena caval filters. *J Vasc Interv Radiol* 1995; **6**: 273–7.

39 Rosen MP, Porter DH, Kim D. Reassessment of vena caval filter use in patients with cancer. J Vasc Interv Radiol 1994; **5**: 501–6.

40 Ihnat DM, Mills JL, Hughes JD, Gentile AT, Berman SS, Westerband A. Treatment of patients with venous thromboembolism and malignant disease: should vena cava filter placement be routine? *J Vasc Surg* 1998; **28**: 800–7.

41 Thomas LA, Summers RR, Cardwell MS. Use of Greenfield filters in pregnant women at risk for pulmonary embolism. *South Med J* 1997; **90**: 215–17.

42 Millward SF. Temporary and retrievable inferior vena cava filters: current status. *J Vasc Interv Radiol* 1998; **9**: 381–7.

43 Buecker A, Neuerburg J, Schmitz-Rode T, Vorwerk D, Gunther RW. In vitro evaluation of a rheolytic thrombectomy system for clot removal from five different temporary vena cava filters. *Cardiovasc Intervent Radiol* 1997; **20**: 448–51.

44 Dick A, Neuerburg J, Schmitz-Rode T, Alliger H, Gunther RW. Declotting of embolized temporary vena cava filter by ultrasound and the Angiojet: comparative experimental in vitro studies. *Invest Radiol* 1998; **33**: 91–7.

45 Linsenmaier U, Rieger J, Schenk F, Rock C, Mangel E, Pfeifer KJ. Indications, management, and complications of temporary inferior vena cava filters. *Cardiovasc Intervent Radiol* 1998; **21**: 464–9.

46 Zwaan M, Lorch H, Kulke C, et al. Clinical experience with temporary vena caval filters. *J Vasc Interv Radiol* 1998; **9**: 594–601.

47 Bovyn G, Gory P, Reynaud P, Ricco JB. The Tempofilter: a multicenter study of a new temporary caval filter implantable for up to six weeks. *Ann Vasc Surg* 1997; **11**: 520–8.

12

Heparin-related bleeding

RICHARD H WHITE

INTRODUCTION

Heparin is one of the most widely used anticoagulants in the world. It is a potent inhibitor of thrombosis and is the anticoagulant of choice for essentially all medical conditions that require prompt, effective inhibition of the clotting system, such as acute venous thromboembolism, acute arterial thrombosis, prophylaxis of clotting during cardiopulmonary bypass surgery, and prophylaxis of venous thrombosis in high-risk patients.[1] Unfortunately, inhibition of thrombosis carries with it a risk of hemorrhage.[2]

PHARMACOLOGY OF HEPARIN AND BLEEDING

Standard heparin is a highly anionic glycosaminoglycan that inhibits active thrombosis, in part, by enhancing the action of certain serine protease inhibitors (particularly antithrombin III), which in turn inactivate critical enzymes in the coagulation cascade (particularly thrombin). In a matter of seconds after the administration of an intravenous bolus dose as small as 2000 IU, plasma levels sufficient to inhibit activated factor II (thrombin) and activated factor Xa are achieved.[1] Whereas standard heparin is structurally heterogeneous, with a molecular weight ranging from 5000 to 30 000 daltons, 'low molecular weight' heparin (LMWH) preparations have recently been developed and made commercially available, which have a molecular weight in the range of 4000–8000.[3] Compared to regular heparin, LMWH preparations are touted as possessing equal or stronger antithrombotic properties, with perhaps a modestly lower incidence of bleeding complications compared to regular heparin.[4] The antithrombotic effect of heparin, its ability to inhibit the growth of a thrombus, cannot be easily measured. Instead, physicians measure either the anticoagulant effect of heparin, which is its effect on a specific coagulation test, most commonly the activated partial thromboplastin time (aPTT), or the plasma level of heparin, as determined by neutralization using titration of protamine sulfate or inhibition of clotting factor Xa activity.

BLEEDING DURING HEPARIN TREATMENT

Theoretically a hemorrhagic event during heparin therapy could be (1) definitely caused by the drug, with bleeding occurring at a site normally not commonly associated with bleeding (e.g., nontraumatic acute hemarthrosis); (2) possibly caused by the drug, with bleeding occurring at a pathologic site normally associated with a low risk of bleeding (e.g., gastritis); or (3) not caused by the drug, with bleeding coming from a pathologic bleeding site that would have bled regardless of the use of heparin (e.g., acute stress ulcer). Because most bleeding occurs at sites of pathologic changes (wounds, ulcers, cancers, etc.), in order to determine the excess risk of bleeding associated with the use of heparin, one has to have an estimate of the incidence of bleeding in a comparison control population not treated with heparin. For example, a clear estimate of the bleeding risk associated with heparin could be obtained from a double-blind clinical trial of heparin treatment versus placebo among patients with an active thrombotic disorder.

Unfortunately, there have been very few placebo-controlled studies of patients with acute thrombotic conditions, such as acute venous thrombosis or acute arterial embolism. However, there have been numerous retrospective observational studies describing the incidence of bleeding among patients treated with heparin, as well as several prospective, placebo-controlled trials of patients with stroke and coronary artery disease. Some studies have compared the incidence of bleeding using different routes of heparin administration, and many studies have compared the safety of different heparin preparations among patients with venous thrombosis and coronary artery disease.

Differences in the clinical study design (i.e., inception versus noninception cohorts) and patient comorbidity are likely to account for differing rates of bleeding between studies, and these differences make direct comparisons problematic.

DEFINITION OF MAJOR AND MINOR BLEEDING

Perhaps the biggest problem in comparing the incidence of bleeding among different studies is the lack of a universally accepted definition of major and minor bleeding. As a generalization, most studies of hospitalized patients use the following definition for major bleeding:

- a fall in the hemoglobin of 2 g/dL with signs or symptoms of bleeding;
- bleeding leading to transfusion (often 2 or more units) or death;
- intracranial or retroperitoneal bleeding (sometimes intra-articular);
  and in clinical trials:
- bleeding leading to discontinuation of treatment.

All other bleeding is usually considered minor. Thus, acute hematuria or acute hematemesis is considered minor if it does not lead to a substantial fall in the hemoglobin or transfusion. Landefeld has developed a carefully constructed and validated bleeding severity index, but it requires very detailed scrutiny of clinical data, which is tedious and time consuming.[5]

HEPARIN-ASSOCIATED BLEEDING IN PLACEBO-CONTROLLED STUDIES

Prophylactic subcutaneous heparin compared to placebo following major surgery

Numerous trials have compared the use of small prophylactic doses of heparin (10 000–15 000 IU/day) to placebo among patients undergoing major surgery. The findings provide strong evidence that heparin therapy does increase the incidence of bleeding in postoperative patients. These trials were conducted in patients at high risk for developing venous thrombosis following major orthopedic, general, or urologic surgery. In a major meta-analysis of these studies, Collins and colleagues noted the cumulative incidence of bleeding (criteria varying with the trials) was 4.4% in heparin-treated patients ($n = 6563$), compared to 2.8% in placebo-treated patients ($n = 6093$), an absolute difference of only 1.6%, but a 66% increase in the odds of bleeding (relative risk (RR) = 1.6).[6] These findings were consistent, irrespective of the dose of heparin used, as excess bleeding was observed among patients given either 10 000 IU/day or 15 000 IU/day. The study by Collins noted that, in the studies that reported a high incidence of bleeding in the placebo arm, bleeding occurred in 27% of heparin-treated patients compared to18% of placebo-treated patients, which means the odds of bleeding were increased by 62%.

Overall, fatal bleeding is rare among patients given a prophylactic dose of heparin. In Collins' study, death attributed to bleeding occurred in only seven of 6776 heparin-treated patients and six of 6838 placebo-treated patients (both ~ 0.1%). It is reasonable to conclude that low-dose heparin prophylaxis, when given preoperatively or postoperatively, is associated with a small increase in risk of bleeding, with an excess incidence of nonfatal bleeding of the order of 2%.

Subcutaneous heparin compared to placebo among patients with cerebral vascular disease

A recent large multicenter trial compared subcutaneous dosing of heparin (5000 IU twice daily or 12 500 IU twice daily) to aspirin (300 mg/day), aspirin plus heparin, and placebo.[7] Use of 10 000 IU of heparin each day was associated with the same incidence of bleeding as with aspirin alone (~1%), but use of 25 000 IU of heparin each day was associated with an approximately 2.5% higher incidence of bleeding compared with placebo, and this was true with or without aspirin (see Table 12.1). In this study, patients with atrial fibrillation had the highest incidence of intracranial bleeding (2.1%) when treated with 5000 IU twice daily or 12 500 IU twice daily. In a different study that evaluated the efficacy of LMWH and placebo among 207 patients with acute ischemic stroke, bleeding or hemorrhagic transformation of the stroke was comparable in the LMWH and placebo cohorts (~6%).[8]

Table 12.1 *Results of the International Stroke Trial*[7]

Treatment	N	Bleeding (%) Total	Intracranial	Extracranial	Fatal
Heparin 12 000 b.i.d. + aspirin 300 mg	2430	3.1	1.7	1.4	0.4
Heparin 5000 b.i.d. + aspirin 300 mg	2431	1.6	0.8	0.8	0.4
Heparin 12 000 b.i.d.	2426	3.2	1.8	1.4	0.5
Heparin 5000 b.i.d.	2429	1.1	0.7	0.4	0.4
Aspirin 300 mg/day	4858	1.0	0.5	0.5	0.4
Placebo	4859	0.6	0.3	0.3	0.1

b.i.d. = twice a day.

Subcutaneous heparin versus placebo among patients receiving thrombolytic therapy

The safety of heparin given in therapeutic doses subcutaneously (25 000 IU/day in two doses) after administration of thrombolytic therapy has been studied in two large, multicenter trials of patients with acute myocardial infarction. In both the GISSI-2 and ISIS-3 studies,[9–11] major bleeding occurred in 102 of 10 361 (1%) heparin-treated patients and in 57 of 10 407 (0.5%) patients treated with thrombolytic therapy alone, a relative risk of 1.8 and an excess risk of 0.5%.

Continuous intravenous heparin compared to placebo

There have been no large, prospective clinical trials that have compared the efficacy and safety of heparin to placebo among patients with active venous or peripheral arterial embolism. In a small study of 120 patients with symptomatic venous thrombosis, Brandjes and coworkers randomized patients to either intravenous heparin for 5–7 days followed by oral anticoagulation, or oral anticoagulation alone.[12] Interestingly, both major and minor bleeding were more common in the oral anticoagulation-alone cohort – 9 of 60 (15%) – compared to the heparin-oral anticoagulation cohort – 5 of 60 (8.3%) – possibly due to chance alone.

Subcutaneous low molecular weight heparin compared to placebo

There have been several controlled studies that have evaluated the efficacy of LMWH among patients with unstable angina.[13–15] In a study that compared LMWH to placebo among patients with unstable angina, the incidence of major bleeding over the first 6 days was 6 of 746 (0.8%) in the LMWH group, and 4 of 760 (0.5%) in the placebo group (p = NS).[13] However, minor bleeding occurred in 61 of 746 (8.2%) of the LWMH-treated patients, compared to in only 2 of 760 (0.3%) placebo-treated patients. In studies of patient with ischemic coronary artery disease, use of heparin did not appear to be associated with a significant increase in the incidence of bleeding.[16,17]

COMPARISON OF DIFFERENT ROUTES OF DELIVERY OF HEPARIN

Studies comparing the safety of different types and routes of administration of heparin have provided important information. In making such comparisons it is important to keep in mind that the safety profile (bleeding risk) of a particular route of administration or type of heparin (e.g., LMWH) can be judged to be superior to standard heparin only if the efficacy of the route or type is equivalent to or better than standard heparin. For example, if the efficacy of a LMWH preparation was shown to be substantially below the efficacy of standard heparin, it would be no surprise to observe a lower incidence of bleeding among the patients treated with the less-effective heparin.

Continuous intravenous heparin compared to intermittent bolus administration

Until the mid-1970s, heparin was administered as a series of intravenous bolus doses which were given every 3, 4, or 6 hours. This was done because of the absence of the technology necessary to deliver a constant infusion.[18] A number of studies performed in the 1970s and 1980s looked at the incidence of bleeding associated with continuous intravenous heparin compared to either intermittent bolus regimens or subcutaneously administered heparin. These studies have been reviewed in detail by Levine and Hirsh.[19] To summarize their findings: among 647 patients given therapeutic doses of heparin, the incidence of heparin-associated bleeding was 28 of 237 (12%) when given by intermittent bolus, 4 of 112 (3.6%) when given subcutaneously, and 9 of 288 (3.1%) when given intravenously. Their analysis suggested that the incidence of bleeding increased as the total daily dose increased, and that intermittent bolus dosing was associated with a higher cumulative incidence of bleeding compared to continuous intravenous heparin. These findings led to the widespread use of continuous intravenous heparin in the USA and the use of subcutaneously administered heparin in Europe.

Continuous intravenous heparin compared to subcutaneous regular heparin

Several clinical trials have compared subcutaneous standard heparin to continuously infused intravenous heparin in the treatment of venous thrombosis. In a large meta-analysis of eight of these trials, Hommes and colleagues reported no difference in the relative risk of major hemorrhage (RR = 0.78, 95% confidence interval (CI) = 0.42–1.48) despite greater efficacy associated with the subcutaneous route of administration (RR = 0.62, CI = 0.4–1.0).[20]

Subcutaneously administered LMWH compared to intravenously administered standard heparin

Numerous studies have compared the incidence of bleeding associated with therapeutic or prophylactic doses of LMWH (always given subcutaneously) and standard heparin given intravenously.

TREATMENT OF VENOUS THROMBOSIS

There have been many small clinical trials that have compared LMWH to standard intravenous heparin in the treatment of acute venous thrombosis, and there have been four formal meta-analyses of these trials.[21–4] In all of the trials, warfarin overlapped with the period of heparin treatment. Among the three early meta-analyses performed before 1996,[21–3] there was agreement that the relative risk of major bleeding is reduced among patients treated with LMWH. Lensing's analysis suggested a 68% reduction in the relative risk of bleeding, and Leizorovicz found a similar 65% risk reduction. However, a recent meta-analysis by Gould et al., which included recent large, randomized clinical trials, reported only a 43% risk reduction, which was only of borderline statistical significance ($p = 0.047$).[24] In fact, using a different method of modeling the data, Gould found no statistically significant difference in the incidence of bleeding complications.

Focusing on the two largest clinical trials, which randomized over 1600 patients with venous thrombosis or pulmonary embolism, the incidence of bleeding in the first 2 weeks of treatment was no different in the patients given standard heparin – 13 of 819 (1.6%) – and patients given LMWH – 13 of 814 (1.6%).[25,26] In these studies, it is possible that the anticipated beneficial effects of LMWH were not observed either because both treatment groups were started on warfarin on the first or second day of heparin therapy, or because the patients randomized to receive regular heparin were dosed more appropriately using a heparin-dosing nomogram.

TREATMENT OF ACCELERATED ANGINA

In a study of over 3000 patients with unstable angina, the use of LMWH was compared to intravenous standard heparin (1000 IU/hour). The results indicated that the use of LMWH was associated with a lower incidence of adverse coronary outcomes, an equal incidence of major bleeding, and a slightly higher incidence of minor bleeding (18% versus 14%).[14]

SUBCUTANEOUSLY ADMINISTERED LMWH COMPARED TO SUBCUTANEOUS STANDARD HEPARIN

PROPHYLAXIS OF VENOUS THROMBOSIS

A recent meta-analysis summarized the findings of clinical trials comparing LMWH (variable but lower doses) to standard heparin (5000 IU twice daily or 7500 IU twice daily) in the prophylaxis of venous thromboembolism after general or orthopedic surgery.[27] For all studies combined, there was a trend for LMWH to be associated with a lower risk of bleeding complications (odds ratio, OR = 0.88, 95% CI = 0.76–1.03), with an unimpressive difference in overall efficacy (OR = 0.92, 95% CI = 0.80–1.05). Among patients undergoing orthopedic surgery, there was a trend toward slightly better efficacy in preventing venous thrombosis (OR = 0.83, 95% CI = 0.68–1.02), with no difference in bleeding (OR = 0.96, 95% CI = 0.68–1.4). Among patients undergoing general surgery, low-dose LMWH (< 3500 anti-Xa units/day, 19 studies) was associated with a significantly lower risk of bleeding compared to standard heparin (5.4% versus 3.8%, OR = 0.68, 95% CI = 0.56–0.82), without any improvement in efficacy. When higher doses of LMWH were administered, a significantly higher incidence of bleeding complications was noted (OR =1.47, 95% CI = 1.07–2.01, seven studies). Thus, it appears that the use of prophylactic LMWH is associated with a modest reduction in the incidence of bleeding complications.

Chronic LMWH therapy compared to chronic warfarin therapy

The standard of practice in the treatment of venous thrombosis is to use intravenous heparin or subcutaneously administered LMWH followed by oral warfarin for 6–12 weeks for patients following trauma, surgery, or other temporary risk factors, or for up to 6 months for 'idiopathic' cases without any apparent risk factors.[28] One study compared long-term (3-month) treatment with a LMWH (enoxaparin 40 mg/day) to standard warfarin.[29] Bleeding rates were lower in the LMWH group, occurring in 4 of 93 (4%) compared to in 12 of 94 (12.8%) in the warfarin group (p = 0.04). Efficacy appeared to be comparable, with 6 of 93 (6.5%) in the LMWH group developing recurrent thromboembolism compared to 4 of 94 (4.3%) in the warfarin group (p = 0.5). Further studies comparing once-daily LWMH to warfarin certainly appear warranted, together with cost–benefit analyses and studies to determine the long-term effect of LMWH on the incidence of osteoporosis.

RELATIONSHIP BETWEEN THE ANTICOAGULANT EFFECT OF HEPARIN AND BLEEDING

The relationship between the anticoagulant response, measured using the aPTT, and the outcomes of thrombosis and bleeding is controversial and far from clear.[30] The most widely accepted 'therapeutic range' for the aPTT is 1.5–2.5 times the laboratory control value.[1] Whereas the lower limit of this suggested range is based on one study completed in the early 1970s, which evaluated clinical outcomes in patients with venous thrombosis,[31] there have been no methodologically rigorous clinical trials that have evaluated higher intensity (higher aPTT) treatment compared to lower intensity (lower aPTT) therapy for any condition.

With regard to bleeding, it is not clear if there is an upper limit to the aPTT response, above which the risk of bleeding increases significantly. Extremely large doses, which lead to unmeasurable aPTT values > 150 seconds, are routinely given to patients undergoing cardiopulmonary bypass, and these doses appear to be safe, at least for a few hours. Moreover, one nonrandomized, unblinded, retrospective study that compared extremely high-dose intravenous heparin therapy for venous thrombosis (~60 000 IU/day) with high-dose intravenous heparin (~40 000 IU/day) reported a low rate of major bleeding in both cohorts – 8% in the extremely high-dose group and 12% in the high-dose group.[32]

More recently, Hull and colleagues have championed the idea that patients should be started on high doses of heparin (40 000 IU/day) and allowed to achieve a supratherapeutic aPTT response before tapering the dose to achieve an aPTT between 1.5 and 2.5 times the laboratory control value.[33] In a subgroup analysis of a study designed to compare 10 days of heparin, starting warfarin on the fifth day, and 5 days of heparin, starting warfarin on the first day, 3 of 93 patients (3.2%) who achieved an aPTT > 85 seconds had major bleeding, compared to 10 of 103 patients (9.7%) who did not achieve an aPTT > 85 seconds ($p = 0.09$).[33,34]

Several lines of evidence suggest that the achievement of a higher aPTT is associated with an increased risk of bleeding. Landefeld and colleagues completed a careful retrospective study of 617 cases from a single hospital, with the aim of determining risk factors for bleeding during the start of anticoagulation therapy, which included warfarin as well as heparin in most cases.[35] The cumulative incidence of major plus minor bleeding increased linearly to 20% over the first 7 days of heparin treatment, and multivariate analysis indicated that an excessive anticoagulant response (measured using either the prothrombin time or the aPTT) was an independent predictor of major bleeding. In the Global Utilization of Streptokinase and Tissue Plasminogen Activator for Occluded Coronary Arteries Study (GUSTO-I) trial, the incidence of bleeding complications was significantly lower among patients who achieved an aPTT between 50 and 70 seconds compared to patients who had higher aPTT values.[36] Interestingly, in this analysis, higher aPTT values were associated with lower weight, older age, female sex, and smoking. Each of these factors is known to be associated with lower heparin requirements.[37] This suggests that, in studies that do not include aPTT data, age and female sex may be a proxy for an excessive anticoagulant effect.

In summary, it is likely that the incidence of bleeding does increase as the aPTT rises, but that short periods of time (i.e., 24 hours) with an elevated aPTT are associated with a negligible increase in risk.[38] More protracted time with the aPTT value greater than 2.5–3.0 times the control value appears to be a risk factor for major bleeding. Lighter individuals, women, and older individuals are at risk of being transiently over-anticoagulated if they started on the same dose of heparin as younger, larger individuals.

CLINICAL RISK FACTORS FOR HEPARIN-ASSOCIATED BLEEDING

A number of studies have tried to identify clinical risk factors associated with bleeding during anticoagulant therapy, but very few have focused strictly on intravenous

Table 12.2 *Risk factors for heparin-related bleeding*

1   Age > 60 years
2   Female sex
3   Prior history of bleeding
4   Serious comorbid disease
    Liver disease
    Renal disease
    Malignancy
    Anemia
    Cardiac disease
5   Activated partial thromboplastin time > 80 seconds (2.5 × control)

heparin therapy in the absence of oral anticoagulant therapy (Table 12.2). In an early study, Basu and colleagues followed 234 patients with venous thrombosis who were treated with intravenous heparin.[31] They found that older age was a predictor of bleeding among the subgroup of patients who had undergone recent surgery, but not among patients who had not had surgery. Campbell and colleagues have also provided evidence that risk of bleeding increases somewhat with age.[39] In a large study, Walker and Jick analyzed risk factors for bleeding among 2656 patients treated with regular heparin for a variety of conditions; all received intermittent bolus therapy.[40] These authors found that older age and female sex were associated with major bleeding, together with the use of alcohol, presence of renal disease, and use of aspirin. These authors did not analyze the relationship between bleeding and the aPTT response and, as noted above, it may be that older age and female sex predict bleeding simply because they are associated with higher aPTT responses.

Nelson and coworkers did a careful retrospective study of 131 patients treated with intravenous heparin, and they reported that older age, female sex, history of abnormal bleeding or peptic ulcer disease were significant predictors of major or minor bleeding.[41] These authors did not analyze the relationship between the aPTT and bleeding. Finally, Juergens et al. recently reported the incidence of bleeding complications in 1253 patients with coronary artery disease who were treated with intravenous heparin.[42] Independent risk factors for bleeding were female sex, recent thrombolytic therapy, and anemia. The use of aspirin was not a risk factor, and the mean aPTT values of patients who bled and patients who did not bleed were not significantly different. Although Landefeld's comprehensive study of patients starting anticoagulant therapy did not report risk factors for heparin-associated bleeding, independent risk factors for anticoagulant related bleeding included: (1) the presence of comorbid conditions (cardiac disease, liver disease, renal disease, and cancer or severe anemia); (2) older age; and (3) an elevated prothrombin time or aPTT and severe liver disease.[35]

Although the absence of a control population in any of these studies makes it very difficult to know which clinical factors are truly associated with heparin-related bleeding, the data suggest that bleeding may be more common in: (1) patients older than 60 years, (2) women, (3) patients with a prior history of bleeding (especially gastrointestinal bleeding), and (4) patients with serious comorbid diseases including liver disease, renal disease, malignancy, anemia, and cardiac disease. To the extent that chronic use of aspirin and nonsteroidal anti-inflammatory agents is associated with gastric erosions, it is likely that the use of these drugs increases the risk of bleeding. It is certainly plausible that older age and female sex are associated with bleeding, because these same factors are associated with reduced heparin requirements, putting these patients at greater risk of being excessively anticoagulated.[39] Older age is also likely to be associated with a greater burden of comorbidity.

Summary of the risks of bleeding during heparin treatment

In summary, placebo-controlled trials suggest that prophylactic doses of standard heparin are associated with an increased risk of bleeding complications among postoperative patients undergoing orthopedic, urologic, or general surgery (odds ratio, (OR) = 1.6, 95% CI= 1.4–1.9).[6] The absolute risk of major bleeding appears to be of the order of 1–2%, but this varies depending on the specific cohort studied, because of differences in the prevalence of risk factors for bleeding. Among patients with acute stroke, prophylactic doses of heparin are associated with only an 0.5% increase in the incidence of bleeding. Among general medical patients without stroke, myocardial infraction or cancer, the incidence of bleeding is comparable to that with placebo, but there is little evidence of any benefit either.[44]

Among patients treated with therapeutic doses of heparin, there are no placebo-controlled trials for those with acute venous thrombosis. The absolute incidence of major bleeding during hospitalization is 2–3%. Use of LMWH is associated with a modest reduction in absolute risk of bleeding of 0.6% compared with standard heparin.[24] In a large placebo-controlled trial that evaluated the efficacy of LMWH among patients with stroke, patients randomized to receive therapeutic doses of heparin each day had a 2.5% higher incidence of bleeding compared to placebo.[7] Among patients with coronary artery disease treated with LMWH, the incidence of major bleeding appears to be comparable to placebo, but more studies are needed.[13,16,17]

TREATMENT OF BLEEDING DURING HEPARIN THERAPY

Standard intravenous heparin

In the event that major bleeding occurs during treatment with standard heparin, steps that should be taken depend on the site and severity of the bleeding. If intravenous heparin is stopped immediately, the anticoagulant effect should be gone in 4–5 hours (several half-lives).

If bleeding is life threatening, protamine sulfate can be given. If bleeding occurs within minutes of a bolus injection of heparin, the amount of protamine sulfate required for neutralization is 1 mg for every 100 IU of heparin.[19,43] If the patient is on a constant infusion of heparin with a therapeutic aPTT, the dose of protamine sulfate should be about 6 mg, because it only takes approximately 1200 IU of heparin to achieve an aPTT of 50–60 seconds in most patients. Protamine sulfate is cleared more rapidly than heparin, and a repeat dose may be necessary. Protamine sulfate must be given slowly over 10 minutes to avoid hypotension.

Low molecular weight heparin

Little information is published in the literature regarding the use of protamine sulfate to reverse the effect of subcutaneously administered LMWH. In experimental systems, protamine sulfate only reverses approximately 60% of the anti-Xa activity of LMWH. If bleeding is profuse and reversal necessary, 6–10 mg of intravenous protamine sulfate should be given, monitoring the aPTT and giving repeated doses over 12 hours. In one case report of a patient given an excessive dose of LWWH, the aPTT and anti-Xa activity normalized after the administration of protamine sulfate. Seventeen hours after the administration of protamine sulfate, the anti-Xa activity was in the high-normal therapeutic range (0.6–0.8 IU/ml).

REFERENCES

1 Hirsh J, Raschke R, Warkentin TE, Dalen JE, Deykin D, Poller L. Heparin: mechanism of action, pharmacokinetics, dosing considerations, monitoring, efficacy, and safety. *Chest* 1995; **108**(Suppl. 4): 258S–75S.

2 Landefeld CS, Beyth RJ. Anticoagulant-related bleeding: clinical epidemiology, prediction, and prevention (see comments). *Am J Med* 1993; **95**: 315–28.

3 Weitz JI. Low-molecular-weight heparins. *N Engl J Med* 1997; **337**: 688–98.

4 Nurmohamed MT, ten Cate H, ten Cate JW. Low molecular weight heparin(oid)s. Clinical investigations and practical recommendations. *Drugs* 1997; **53**: 736–51.

5 Landefeld CS, Anderson PA, Goodnough LT, et al. The bleeding severity index: validation and comparison to other methods for classifying bleeding complications of medical therapy. *J Clin Epidemiol* 1989; **42**: 711–18.

6 Collins R, Scrimgeour A, Yusuf S, Peto R. Reduction in fatal pulmonary embolism and venous thrombosis by perioperative administration of subcutaneous heparin. Overview of results of randomized trials in general, orthopedic, and urologic surgery. *N Engl J Med* 1988; **318**: 1162–73.

7 The International Stroke Trial (IST): a randomised trial of aspirin, subcutaneous heparin, both, or neither among 19 435 patients with acute ischaemic stroke. International Stroke Trial Collaborative Group (see comments). *Lancet* 1997; **349**: 1569–81.

8 Kay R, Wong KS, Yu YL, et al. Low-molecular-weight heparin for the treatment of acute ischemic stroke (see comments). *N Engl J Med* 1995; **333**: 1588–93.

9 GISSI-2: a factorial randomised trial of alteplase versus streptokinase and heparin versus no heparin among 12 490 patients with acute myocardial infarction. Gruppo Italiano per lo Studio della Sopravvivenza nell'Infarto Miocardico (see comments). *Lancet* 1990; **336**: 65–71.

10 The International Study Group. In-hospital mortality and clinical course of 20 891 patients with suspected acute myocardial infarction randomised between alteplase and streptokinase with or without heparin. *Lancet* 1990; **336**: 71–5.

11 ISIS-3: a randomised comparison of streptokinase vs tissue plasminogen activator vs anistreplase and of aspirin plus heparin vs aspirin alone among 41 299 cases of suspected acute myocardial infarction. ISIS-3 (Third International Study of Infarct Survival) Collaborative Group. *Lancet* 1992; **339**: 753–70.

12 Brandjes DP, Heijboer H, Buller HR, de Rijk M, Jagt H, ten Cate JW. Acenocoumarol and heparin compared with acenocoumarol alone in the initial treatment of proximal-vein thrombosis. *N Engl J Med* 1992; **327**: 1485–9.

13 Group CADFs. Low-molecular-weight heparin during instability in coronary artery disease, Fragmin during Instability in Coronary Artery Disease (FRISC) study group. *Lancet* 1996; **347**: 561–8.

14 Cohen M, Demers C, Gurfinkel EP, et al. A comparison of low-molecular-weight heparin with unfractionated heparin for unstable coronary artery disease. Efficacy and Safety of Subcutaneous Enoxaparin in Non-Q-Wave Coronary Events Study Group. *N Engl J Med* 1997; **337**: 447–52.

15 Klein W, Buchwald A, Hillis SE, et al. Comparison of low-molecular-weight heparin with unfractionated heparin acutely and with placebo for 6 weeks in the management of unstable coronary artery disease. Fragmin in Unstable Coronary Artery Disease Study (FRIC). *Circulation* 1997; **96**: 61–8.

16 Theroux P, Ouimet H, McCans J, et al. Aspirin, heparin, or both to treat acute unstable angina. *N Engl J Med* 1988; **319**: 1105–11.

17 Neri Serneri GG, Rovelli F, Gensini GF, Pirelli S, Carnovali M, Fortini A. Effectiveness of low-dose heparin in prevention of myocardial reinfarction. *Lancet* 1987; **1**: 937–42.

18 Salzman EW, Deykin D, Shapiro RM, Rosenberg R. Management of heparin therapy: controlled prospective trial. *N Engl J Med* 1975; **292**: 1046–50.

19 Levine MN, Hirsh J. Hemorrhagic complications of anticoagulant therapy. *Semin Thromb Hemost* 1986; **12**: 39–57.

20 Hommes DW, Bura A, Mazzolai L, Buller HR, ten Cate JW. Subcutaneous heparin compared with continuous intravenous heparin administration in the initial treatment of deep vein thrombosis. A meta-analysis. *Ann Intern Med* 1992; **116**: 279–84.

21 Siragusa S, Cosmi B, Piovella F, Hirsh J, Ginsberg JS. Low-molecular-weight heparins and unfractionated heparin in the treatment of patients with acute venous thromboembolism: results of a meta-analysis. *Am J Med* 1996; **100**: 269–77.

22 Lensing AW, Prins MH, Davidson BL, Hirsh J. Treatment of deep venous thrombosis with low-molecular-weight heparins. A meta-analysis. *Arch Intern Med* 1995; **155**: 601–7.

23 Leizorovicz A, Simonneau G, Decousus H, Boissel JP. Comparison of efficacy and safety of low molecular weight heparins and unfractionated heparin in initial treatment of deep venous thrombosis: a meta-analysis. *BMJ* 1994; **309**: 299–304.

24 Gould MK, Dembitzer AD, Doyle RL, Hastie TJ, Garber AM. Low-molecular-weight heparins compared with unfractionated heparin for treatment of acute deep venous thrombosis. A meta-analysis of randomized, controlled trials. *Ann Intern Med* 1999; **130**: 800–9.

25 The Columbus Investigators. Low-molecular-weight heparin in the treatment of patients with venous thromboembolism. *N Engl J Med* 1997; **337**: 657–62.

26 Simonneau G, Sors H, Charbonnier B, et al. A comparison of low-molecular-weight heparin with unfractionated heparin for acute pulmonary embolism. The THESEE Study Group. Tinzaparine ou Heparine Standard: Evaluations dans l'Embolie Pulmonaire. *N Engl J Med* 1997; **337**: 663–9.

27 Koch A, Bouges S, Ziegler S, Dinkel H, Daures JP, Victor N. Low molecular weight heparin and unfractionated heparin in thrombosis prophylaxis after major surgical intervention: update of previous meta-analyses. *Br J Surg* 1997; **84**: 750–9.

28 Schulman S, Rhedin AS, Lindmarker P, et al. A comparison of six weeks with six

months of oral anticoagulant therapy after a first episode of venous thromboembolism. Duration of Anticoagulation Trial Study Group. *N Engl J Med* 1995; **332**: 1661–5.

29 Pini M, Aiello S, Manotti C, et al. Low molecular weight heparin versus warfarin in the prevention of recurrences after deep vein thrombosis. *Thromb Haemost* 1994; **72**: 191–7.

30 Ginsberg JS. Management of venous thromboembolism. *N Engl J Med* 1996; **335**: 1816–28.

31 Basu D, Gallus A, Hirsh J, Cade J. A prospective study of the value of monitoring heparin treatment with the activated partial thromboplastin time. *N Engl J Med* 1972; **287**: 324–7.

32 Conti S, Daschbach M, Blaisdell FW. A comparison of high-dose versus conventional-dose heparin therapy for deep vein thrombosis. *Surgery* 1982; **92**: 972–80.

33 Hull RD, Raskob GE, Rosenbloom D, et al. Optimal therapeutic level of heparin therapy in patients with venous thrombosis. *Arch Intern Med* 1992; **152**: 1589–95.

34 Hull RD, Raskob GE, Rosenbloom D, et al. Heparin for 5 days as compared with 10 days in the initial treatment of proximal venous thrombosis. *N Engl J Med* 1990; **322**: 1260–4.

35 Landefeld CS, Cook EF, Flatley M, Weisberg M, Goldman L. Identification and preliminary validation of predictors of major bleeding in hospitalized patients starting anticoagulant therapy. *Am J Med* 1987; **82**: 703–13.

36 Granger CB, Hirsh J, Califf RM, et al. Activated partial thromboplastin time and outcome after thrombolytic therapy for acute myocardial infarction: results from the GUSTO-I trial. *Circulation* 1996; **93**: 870–8.

37 White RH, Zhou H, Woo L, Mungall D. Effect of weight, sex, age, clinical diagnosis, and thromboplastin reagent on steady-state intravenous heparin requirements. *Arch Intern Med* 1997; **157**: 2468–72.

38 Hirsch DR, Lee TH, Morrison RB, Carlson W, Goldhaber SZ. Shortened hospitalization by means of adjusted-dose subcutaneous heparin for deep venous thrombosis. *Am Heart J* 1996; **131**: 276–80.

39 Campbell NR, Hull RD, Brant R, Hogan DB, Pineo GF, Raskob GE. Aging and heparin-related bleeding. *Arch Intern Med* 1996; **156**: 857–60.

40 Walker AM, Jick H. Predictors of bleeding during heparin therapy. *JAMA* 1980; **244**: 1209–12.

41 Nelson PH, Moser KM, Stoner C, Moser KS. Risk of complications during intravenous heparin therapy. *West J Med* 1982; **136**: 189–97.

42 Juergens CP, Semsarian C, Keech AC, Beller EM, Harris PJ. Hemorrhagic complications of intravenous heparin use. *Am J Cardiol* 1997; **80**: 150–4.

43 Penner JA. Managing the hemorrhagic complications of heparin therapy. *Hematol Oncol Clin North Am* 1993; **7**: 1281–9.

13

Warfarin-related bleeding

REBECCA J BEYTH

INTRODUCTION

Oral anticoagulant therapy is used for the prevention and treatment of many thromboembolic disorders, particularly for patients with venous thromboembolism,[1–11] acute myocardial infarction,[12–18] mechanical heart valves,[11,19–22] and chronic or paroxysmal atrial fibrillation.[23–7] The findings of recent studies are likely to increase the use of anticoagulants for conditions that are especially common in older patients, such as atrial fibrillation and myocardial infarction. Unfortunately, the use of anticoagulant therapy is a double-edged sword. It can prevent disabling and potentially life-threatening thromboembolism (e.g., stroke), but it can also endanger the health of patients by causing serious bleeding. It is estimated that annually 1–5% of patients treated chronically with oral anticoagulant therapy will suffer a major bleeding event that warrants hospitalization. Physicians' concerns about the safety of anticoagulant therapy may outweigh compelling evidence about the beneficial effects of anticoagulant therapy. This chapter reviews the risk factors associated with warfarin-related bleeding, the assessment of risk and preventive strategies, and the management of warfarin-related bleeding.

RISK FACTORS ASSOCIATED WITH WARFARIN-RELATED BLEEDING
(Table 13.1)

The risk of warfarin-induced bleeding is influenced primarily by: (1) the intensity of the anticoagulant effect as measured by the International Normalized Ratio

Table 13.1 *Examples of risk factors associated with warfarin-related bleeding*

Intensity of the anticoagulant effect
   Warfarin dose
   Vitamin K intake
   Liver dysfunction
Comorbid conditions
   History of gastrointestinal bleeding
   Cerebrovascular disease
   Liver disease
   Renal insufficiency
Length of therapy
   Variance in INR over time
Patient compliance
Use of interacting medications

(INR); (2) the presence of comorbid conditions that increase the likelihood of bleeding; (3) the length of therapy; (4) patient compliance; and (5) the use of drugs that interfere with warfarin increase the likelihood of gastrointestinal bleeding.[28–30]

The intensity of the anticoagulant response to warfarin is affected by the dose of warfarin, the patient's intake of vitamin K, and other factors (e.g., liver dysfunction, concomitant medications) that alter the pharmacokinetics and pharmacodynamics of warfarin. Different intensities of therapy with warfarin have been compared in six randomized trials,[8,14,20,21,31,32] which provide convincing evidence that lower intensity therapy (INR 2.0–3.0) is associated with a reduced incidence of bleeding without an increase in the incidence of thromboembolic complications. Bleeding is about three times more likely in patients with an INR of 3.0–4.5 compared with those with an INR of 2.0–3.0.

Although lower intensity warfarin decreases the risk of bleeding, the limit of how low is just beginning to be defined. A recent trial[33] tested whether aspirin plus low-intensity, fixed-dose warfarin (INR 1.2–1.5) or standard adjusted-dose warfarin (INR 2.0–3.0) would be safe and effective in preventing stroke in atrial fibrillation. The trial was stopped after 1 year because the embolization rate was significantly greater in the aspirin with the low-intensity, fixed-dose warfarin group (7.9% per year) than in the standard adjusted-dose group (1.9% per year), despite similar bleeding rates. Similarly, Hylek et al.[34] reported that as the INR decreased (using an INR of 2.0 as the referent), the adjusted odds ratio for stroke increased dramatically. For example, the odds ratio was 6.0 (95% confidence interval (CI) 3.6–9.8) for an INR of 1.3, compared to an odds ratio of 1.2 (95% CI 1.2–1.3) for an INR of 1.9. Thus, the lowest effective intensity of warfarin for atrial fibrillation appears to be an INR of 2.0.

Two small studies have reported that fixed 'low-dose' warfarin regimens may be effective in specific situations. Levine et al.[35] conducted a double-blind, randomized trial of either low-dose warfarin (mean INR 1.52; target range 1.3–1.9) or placebo with 300 women with stage IV breast cancer who were receiving chemotherapy, and found it effective ($p = 0.03$) in the prevention of thromboembolism. Similarly, Bern et al.[36] found a fixed dose of 1 mg of warfarin daily was effective in the prevention of thromboembolism associated with central venous catheters. However, it should be stressed that many studies have found that 'mini'-dose warfarin (e.g., 1 mg/day) or 'fixed low-dose' warfarin is no more effective than placebo or aspirin alone.[37,38]

The risk of bleeding during warfarin therapy is also related to baseline patient characteristics other than the indication for therapy. Although studies have not consistently identified the same independent predictors of major bleeding, it is generally agreed that past history of gastrointestinal bleeding, cerebrovascular disease, liver disease, and renal insufficiency are factors that increase the risk of bleeding from warfarin. Other comorbid conditions, such as atrial fibrillation, hypertension, and malignancy, have also been reported as risk factors, but not consistently.[39–51]

Older patients may be at increased risk for anticoagulant-related bleeding, in part because they have an increased incidence of adverse drug reactions compared with younger patients.[52] They are more likely to be taking more than one type of medication,[53,54] thereby increasing the likelihood of drug interactions and adverse reactions. Chronic diseases, which are more common in older patients,[55–7] may also increase the risk for bleeding during anticoagulant therapy. Furthermore, the dose of warfarin required to achieve a given anticoagulant effect decreases in older patients, because they metabolize warfarin more slowly.[58] Toohey[59] observed that older patients required smaller doses of anticoagulants, and others have shown that the anticoagulant response to warfarin increases with age.[54,60,61] Lastly, vascular integrity may become impaired with age.[62–4] Increased vascular or endothelial fragility may make older patients more susceptible to anticoagulant-related bleeding, especially intracranial bleeding.[65,66]

Although the role of age in bleeding during warfarin therapy remains controversial, substantial and compelling evidence indicates that the risk of bleeding may be approximately twice as high in older patients.[39,40,42–4,46,47,67,68] The second Stroke Prevention in Atrial Fibrillation Study[67] was designed specifically to examine the benefits and risks of warfarin in patients with atrial fibrillation, according to age. Although the results are controversial, patients over 75 years of age had a significantly higher rate of major bleeding complications (4.2% per year) when compared with patients aged less than 75 years (1.6% per year; $p = 0.008$), despite similar anticoagulant intensity and control. Similarly, Fihn et al.[46] found that the combined, unadjusted incidence of life-threatening or fatal complications was significantly higher among the oldest patients. Patients older than 80 years of age had a relative risk of 4.5 (95% CI 1.3–15.6) compared with patients aged 50 years or younger.

In contrast, other studies, such as those by Fihn et al.[45] and Gurwitz et al.,[69] showed no association between age and the risk of major bleeding. Although reasons for this discrepancy are not entirely clear, likely factors include: chance; differences in measurement methods (especially in the classification of major bleeding); and biases inherent in observational studies, especially those that used noninception cohorts (i.e., those that enrolled patients who had already been treated with warfarin for some time).

The cumulative risk of bleeding has been shown to be directly related to the length of warfarin therapy, but the risk of bleeding also appears to vary during the course of warfarin therapy. Specifically, frequencies of bleeding have been noted to be substantially higher early in the course of therapy,[40] probably due to a high prevalence of poorly controlled anticoagulant therapy and bleeding from pre-existing pathologic lesions.[41,45] Landefeld et al.[40] noted that the monthly risk of bleeding decreased from 3% in the first month to 0.8% per month during the rest of the first year, and 0.3% per month thereafter. Fihn et al.[45] reported similar findings, noting that serious bleeding complications were more common in the first 3 months of therapy, with a rate of 21 episodes per 100 patient-years. The relative risks for serious bleeding during the first 3 months of treatment, compared with the rest of the first year, the second year, and thereafter, were 1.9 (95% CI 1.3–3.0), 3.0 (95% CI 1.8–4.8), and 5.9 (95% CI 3.8–9.3), respectively.

An additional characteristic that appears to be important, but that has only been studied recently,[45] is the variability of the INR over time. Fihn et al.[45] reported that the incidence of serious bleeding was significantly related to the variance in the INR over time, with the relative risk for serious bleeding being highest among patients with the highest INR variability, compared with those with the lowest INR variability, (relative risk 1.6; 95% CI 1.2–2.7). Other characteristics of the course of therapy that may be important in predicting anticoagulant-related bleeding include interaction with comorbid conditions, intercurrent illnesses, and the addition of new medications to the treatment regimen. Unfortunately, there is little information regarding any of these characteristics. Even though these factors associated with bleeding may be present in a given patient, they should not be seen as an absolute contraindication to warfarin therapy. Rather, they should be weighed against the benefits of warfarin in the context of individual patient preferences and values.

ASSESSMENT OF RISK AND PREVENTIVE STRATEGIES

Although most warfarin-related bleeding is not life threatening and does not result in permanent morbidity, intracerebral hemorrhage and death do occasionally occur, with a rate of approximately 0.6 events/100 patients-year. The decision about whether to initiate warfarin therapy in a particular patient hinges on the balance between the efficacy of warfarin in preventing a morbid or fatal thromboembolic event, such as a major stroke, and its likelihood of precipitating a life-threatening hemorrhagic event. This assessment is further compounded by the fact that the risks of both thromboembolic and hemorrhagic events vary over time.

Patients can be categorized into low, middle, or high risk for warfarin-related bleeding (Table 13.2). The estimated risk for major bleeding during warfarin therapy at 3 months has been reported to be 2% in low-risk patients, 5% in medium-risk patients, and 23% in high-risk patients.[70] Whereas these risk factors need to be

Table 13.2 *Risk categories for warfarin-related bleeding*

Low risk	< 65 years of age
	No comorbid conditions
	No concomitant therapy that interferes with hemostasis (e.g., aspirin, nonsteroidal anti-inflammatory agents)
Medium risk	One or two risk factors for bleeding (e.g., history of gastrointestinal bleeding and renal insufficiency)
High risk	Three or more risk factors for bleeding (e.g., 80-year-old patient with a history of stroke, past gastrointestinal bleeding, and recent myocardial infarction who develops a deep vein thrombosis)

considered when starting warfarin therapy, they are not static; rather, the physician and the patient must continually re-evaluate the risks and benefits of warfarin therapy throughout its course.

Among high-risk patients in whom the risk of warfarin-related bleeding is felt to outweigh the potential benefit of treatment, consideration should be given to the use of other alternative antithrombotic agents. For example, chronic once-daily LMWH or adjusted-dose heparin may be a more reasonable alternative for the treatment of a deep vein thrombosis in a medium-risk or high-risk patient.[71,72] Likewise, aspirin during the first 3 months after a bioprosthetic valve replacement in aortic position for high-risk patients may be more prudent. Other steps, such as avoiding aspirin or other drugs that interfere with hemostasis, may also help reduce the risk of bleeding in high-risk patients. Similarly, consideration of alternative antithrombotic agents, along with risk reduction, may be appropriate in certain patients. Also, if a trial of warfarin therapy determines that the patient may not be able to comply with taking warfarin as prescribed, and the risk of bleeding is great, discontinuation of the warfarin may be reasonable.

For all patients starting long-term therapy with warfarin, an assessment of the risks that can be modified should be made to reduce even further the individual patient's risk of warfarin-related bleeding. The concomitant use of drugs like aspirin or nonsteroidal anti-inflammatory agents that interfere with hemostasis should be avoided or discontinued while the patient is being treated with warfarin. Closer and more frequent monitoring of the INR may be warranted in older patients considered at high risk for bleeding, or in patients in whom a drug that is known to potentiate the anticoagulant effect of warfarin needs to be prescribed.

MANAGEMENT OF WARFARIN-RELATED BLEEDING

Contemporary rates of warfarin-related bleeding have been reported to range from 1% to 7% per year, depending on the indication for anticoagulant therapy and the classification of bleeding.[28] Although most bleeding is not life threatening, it does causes short-term morbidity and inconvenience to patients, as well as possibly diminishing their quality of life to some degree. Prompt recognition of warfarin-related bleeding and early treatment of life-threatening bleeding can reduce the associated morbidity.

When a patient presents with evidence suggesting warfarin-related bleeding, factors that may be contributing to the bleeding need to be considered. For example, if a patient presents with guaiac-positive stools while on warfarin therapy, it should also be determined if the patient has been using aspirin or other nonsteroidal anti-inflammatory drugs that may be a contributing cause. Elimination of other contributing causes may resolve or minimize the bleeding episode.

If the patient has *active, life-threatening bleeding* that cannot be stopped by the simple application of pressure, one must immediately hospitalize the patient and obtain consultation with a surgical specialist if it appears that surgical, endoscopic, or angiographic intervention is needed. One can transiently reverse the anticoagulant effect, because such reversal is associated with a low risk of thromboembolism in the ensuing few days.[73] The most immediate way of reversing the anticoagulant effect is to administer 3 units of fresh frozen plasma (administering a second dose if the INR is not corrected), although clotting factor concentrate is far superior.[74] A large dose of vitamin K can be administered intravenously, but one will not see a substantial fall in the INR for approximately 12–24 hours. For full reversal, a single dose of 10 mg of vitamin K given intravenously over 10 minutes in 50 ml of 5% dextrose in water is recommended. The appropriate dose of vitamin K for partial reversal is not known. For individuals with very high INR values, giving 0.5 mg intravenously or 1.0 mg intravenously usually brings the INR down to the range of 2.0–3.0 without complete reversal. If the INR is normalized, one can simply institute intravenous heparin therapy as soon as bleeding is stopped and the risk of further bleeding is felt to be low, restarting oral warfarin at the same time.

If the INR is > 6.0 and there is minor bleeding, such as epistaxis, the patient may respond to local measures plus a reduction in warfarin dosage. The INR starts to fall approximately 30 hours after the last dose of warfarin, with a half-life of about 1 day (slightly longer for older individuals; shorter for younger individuals).[75] Thus, if bleeding starts on Monday morning with an INR of 5.0 (i.e., 4 units above a value of 1.0), and the last dose of warfarin was given on Sunday evening, then the INR will start to fall at about midnight on Monday. The INR will fall 2 units by midnight on Tuesday (i.e., the INR will now be 3.0) and will fall 1 unit by midnight on Wednesday (i.e, the INR will now be 2.0), etc.

If the INR is > 6.0 and there is serious bleeding, such as gross hematuria, the INR should be promptly reduced using low-dose vitamin K (0.5 or 1.0 mg intravenously), with immediate consultation with a surgeon. It must be stressed that in patients at high risk for thromboembolism, such as patients with a Starr–Edwards mitral valve, heart failure, atrial fibrillation, and history of prior stroke, full reversal of the warfarin therapy can result in a thromboembolic event. Therefore, heparin must be started in these patients when their risk of bleeding falls.[76]

If the INR is < 3.0 and there is minor bleeding, it is frequently associated with an obvious underlying cause or occult gastrointestinal or renal lesion.[77] Local measures should be undertaken to control the bleeding and monitor the patient. If the bleeding stops, warfarin can be continued and diagnostic studies can be undertaken to determine the cause so that possible treatments (e.g., anti-ulcer therapy) may be instituted. If the bleeding continues or becomes major, the steps outlined above should be taken, with administration of fresh frozen plasma, coagulation concentrate and/or vitamin K, together with discontinuation of warfarin.

ACKNOWLEDGMENT

The author is a recipient of a NIA Mentored Career Department Award (K08 AG00712).

REFERENCES

1 Sevitt S, Gallagher NG. Prevention of venous thrombosis and pulmonary embolism in injured patients. *Lancet* 1959; **2**: 981–9.

2 Francis CW, Marder VJ, Evarts CM, et al. Two-step warfarin therapy; prevention of postoperative venous thrombosis without excessive bleeding. *JAMA* 1983; **249**: 374–8.

3 Powers PJ, Gent M, Jay RM, et al. A randomized trial of less intense postoperative warfarin or aspirin therapy in the prevention of venous thromboembolism after surgery for fractured hip. *Arch Intern Med* 1989; **149**: 771–4.

4 Taberner DA, Poller L, Burslem RW, et al. Oral anticoagulants controlled by the British comparative thromboplastin versus low-dose heparin in prophylaxis of deep vein thrombosis. *BMJ* 1978; **1**: 272–4.

5 Poller L, McKernan A, Thomson JM, et al. Fixed minidose warfarin: a new approach to prophylaxis against venous thrombosis after major surgery. *BMJ* 1987; **295**: 1309–12.

6 NIH Consensus Conference. Prevention of venous thrombosis and pulmonary embolism. *JAMA* 1986; **256**: 744–9.

7 Hull R, Delmore T, Genton E, et al. Warfarin sodium versus low-dose heparin in the long-term treatment of venous thrombosis. *N Engl J Med* 1979; **302**: 855–8.

8 Hull R, Hirsh J, Jay R, et al. Different intensities of oral anticoagulant therapy in the treatment of proximal-vein thrombosis. *N Engl J Med* 1982; **307**: 1676–81.

9 Lagerstedt CI, Fagher BO, Albrechtsson U, et al. Need for long-term anticoagulant treatment in symptomatic calf- vein thrombosis. *Lancet* 1985; **2**: 515–18.

10 Hull RD, Raskob GE, Rosenbloom D, et al. Heparin for 5 days as compared with 10 days in the initial treatment of proximal venous thrombosis. *N Engl J Med* 1990; **322**: 1260–4.

11 Gallus AS, Jackaman J, Tillett J, et al. Safety and efficacy of warfarin started early after submassive venous thrombosis or pulmonary embolism. *Lancet* 1986; **2**: 1293–6.

12 Resnikov L, Chediak J, Hirsh J, et al. Antithrombotic agents in coronary artery disease. *Chest* 1989; **95**: 52–72.

13 Goldberg RJ, Gore JM, Dalen JE, et al. Long term anticoagulant therapy after acute myocardial infarction. *Am Heart J* 1985; **109**: 616–62.

14 Medical Research Council Group. Assessment of short-term anticoagulant administration after cardiac infarction: report of the working party on anticoagulant therapy in coronary thrombosis. *BMJ* 1969; **1**: 335–42.

15 Veterans Administration Cooperative Study. Anticoagulants in acute myocardial infarction: results of a cooperative clinical trial. *JAMA* 1973; **225**: 724–9.

16 Drapkin A, Merskey C. Anticoagulant therapy after acute myocardial infarction. *JAMA* 1972; **222**: 541–8.

17 Sixty-Plus Reinfarction Study Group. A double-blind trial to assess long-term oral anticoagulant therapy in elderly patients after myocardial infarction. *Lancet* 1980; **2**: 989–94.

18 Smith P, Arnesen H, Lome I. The effect of warfarin on mortality and reinfarction after myocardial infarction. *N Engl J Med* 1990; **323**: 147–51.

19 Mok CK, Boey J, Wang R, et al. Warfarin versus dipyridamole-aspirin and pentoxifylline-aspirin for the prevention of prosthetic heart valve thromboembolism: a prospective clinical trial. *Circulation* 1985; **72**: 1059–63.

20 Turpie AGG, Gunstensen J, Hirsh J, et al. Randomized comparison of two intensities of oral anticoagulant therapy after tissue heart valve replacement. *Lancet* 1988; **1**: 1242–5.

21 Saour JN, Sieck JO, Mamo LAR, et al. Trial of different intensities of anticoagulant therapy in patients with substitute heart valves. *N Engl J Med* 1990; **322**: 427–32.

22 Fuster V, Pumphrey CW, McGoon MD, et al. Systemic thromboembolism in mural and aortic Starr–Edwards prosthesis: a long-term follow-up (10–19 years). *Circulation* 1982; **66**: 157–61.

23 Petersen P, Boysen G, Godtfredsen J, Andersen ED, Andersen B. Placebo-controlled, randomised trial of warfarin and aspirin for prevention of thromboembolic complications in chronic atrial fibrillation. *Lancet* 1989; **1**: 175–9.

24 Boston Area Anticoagulation Trial for Atrial Fibrillation Investigators. The effect of low-dose warfarin on the risk of stroke in patients with nonrheumatic atrial fibrillation. *N Engl J Med* 1990; **323**: 1505–11.

25 Connolly SJ, Laupacis A, Gent M, Roberts RS, Cairns JA, Joyner C. Canadian atrial fibrillation anticoagulation (CAFA) study. *J Am Coll Cardiol* 1991; **18**: 349–55.

26 Ezekowitz MD, Bridgers SL, James KE, et al. Warfarin in the prevention of stroke associated with nonrheumatic atrial fibrillation. *N Engl J Med* 1992; **327**: 1406–12.

27 Stroke Prevention in Atrial Fibrillation Study Group Investigators. Stroke prevention in atrial fibrillation study. Final results. *Circulation* 1991; **84**: 527–39.

28 Levine MN, Raskob G, Landefeld CS. Hemorrhagic complications of anticoagulant treatment. *Chest* 1995; **108**: 276s-90s.

29 Younossi ZM, Strum WB, Teirstein PS, Cloutier DA, Spinks TJ. Effect of combined anticoagulation and low-dose aspirin treatment on upper gastrointestinal bleeding. *Dig Dis Sci* 1997; **47**: 79–82.

30 Blackshear JL, Baker VS, Holland A, et al. Fecal hemoglobin excretion in elderly patients with atrial fibrillation: combined aspirin and low-dose warfarin vs conventional warfarin therapy. *Arch Intern Med* 1996; **156**: 658–60.

31 Hill AG, Marshall J, Shaw DA. Cerebrovascular disease: trial of long-term anticoagulant therapy. *BMJ* 1962; **2**: 1003–6.

32 Altman R, Rouvier J, Gurfinkel E. Comparison of two levels of anticoagulant therapy in patients with substitute heart valves. *J Thorac Cardiovasc Surg* 1991; **101**: 427–31.

33 Stroke Prevention in Atrial Fibrillation Investigators. Adjusted-dose warfarin versus low-intensity, fixed-dose warfarin plus aspirin for high-risk patients with atrial fibrillation: stroke prevention in atrial fibrillation III randomised clinical trial. *Lancet* 1996; **348**: 633–8.

34 Hylek EM, Skates SJ, Sheehan MA, Singer DE. An analysis of the lowest effective intensity of prophylactic anticoagulation for patients with nonrheumatic atrial fibrillation. *N Engl J Med* 1996; **335**: 540–6.

35 Levine M, Hirsh J, Gent M, et al. Double-blind randomized trial of very low dose warfarin for prevention of thromboembolism in stage IV breast cancer. *Lancet* 1994; **343**: 886–9.

36 Bern MM, Lokich JJ, Wallach SR, et al. Very low doses of warfarin can prevent thrombosis in central vein catheters: a randomized prospective trial. *Ann Intern Med* 1990; **112**: 423–8.

37 Coumadin Aspirin Reinfarction Study (CARS) Investigators. Randomised double-blind trial of fixed low-dose warfarin with aspirin after myocardial infarction. *Lancet* 1997; **350**: 389–96.

38 Dale C, Gallus A, Wycherley A, Langlois S, Howie D. Prevention of venous thrombosis with mini-dose warfarin after joint replacement. *BMJ* 1991; **303**: 224.

39 Pollard JW, Hamilton MJ, Christensen NA, et al. Problems associated with long-term anticoagulant therapy. *Circulation* 1962; **25**: 311–17.

40 Landefeld CS, Goldman L. Major bleeding in outpatients treated with warfarin: incidence and prediction by factors known at the start of outpatient therapy. *Am J Med* 1989; **87**: 144–52.

41 Petitti DB, Strom BL, Melmon KL. Duration of warfarin anticoagulant therapy and the probabilities of recurrent thromboembolism and hemorrhage. *Am J Med* 1986; **81**: 255–9.

42 van der Meer FJM, Rosendaal FR, Vandenbroucke JP, et al. Bleeding complications in oral anticoagulant therapy: an analysis of risk factors. *Arch Intern Med* 1993; **153**: 1557–62.

43 Launbjerg J, Egeblad H, Heaf J, et al. Bleeding complications to oral anticoagulant therapy: multivariate analysis of 1010 treatment years in 551 outpatients. *J Intern Med* 1991; **229**: 351–5.

44 Coon WW, Willis PWI. Hemorrhagic complications of anticoagulant therapy. *Arch Intern Med* 1974; **133**: 386–92.

45 Fihn SD, McDonell M, Martin D, et al. Risk factors for complications of chronic anticoagulation. A multicenter study. *Ann Intern Med* 1993; **118**: 511–20.

46 Fihn SD, Callahan CM, Martin DC, McDonnell MB, Henikoff JG, White RH. The risk and severity of bleeding complications in elderly patients treated with warfarin. *Ann Intern Med* 1996; **124**: 970–9.

47 Palareti G, Leali N, Coccheri S, et al. Bleeding complications of oral anticoagulant treatment: an inception-cohort, prospective collaborative study (ISCOAT). *Lancet* 1996; **348**: 423–8.

48 Lundstrom T, Ryden L. Hemorrhagic and thromboembolic complications in patients with atrial fibrillation on anticoagulant prophylaxis. *J Intern Med* 1989; **225**: 137–42.

49 Peyman MA. The significance of haemorrhage during the treatment of patients with the coumarin anticoagulants. *Acta Med Scand* 1958; **339**: 1–62.

50 Landefeld CS, Beyth RJ. Anticoagulant-related bleeding: clinical epidemiology, prediction and prevention. *Am J Med* 1993; **95**: 315–28.

51 Gitter MJ, Jaeger TM, Petterson TM, Gersh BJ, Silverstein MD. Bleeding and thromboembolism while receiving anticoagulation therapy: a population-based study in Rochester, Minnesota. *Mayo Clin Proc* 1995; **70**: 725–33.

52 Nolan L, O'Malley K. Prescribing for the elderly. Part II. Prescribing patterns: difference due to age. *J Am Geriatr Soc* 1988; **36**: 245–54.

53 Nolan L, O'Malley K. Prescribing for the elderly. Part I. Sensitivity of the elderly to adverse drug reactions. *J Am Geriatr Soc* 1988; **36**: 142–9.

54 Gurwitz JH, Avorn J, Ross-Degnan D, Choodnovskiy I, Ansell J. Aging and the anticoagulant response to warfarin therapy. *Ann Intern Med* 1992; **116**: 901–4.

55 Seeman TE, Guralnik J, Kaplan GA, et al. The health consequences of multiple morbidity in the elderly. The Alameda County Study. *J Aging Health* 1989; **1**: 50–66.

56 Guralnik JM, LaCroix AZ, Everett DF, Kovar MG. Aging in the eighties: the prevalence of comorbidity and association with disability. *Advance Data from Vital and Health Statistics*, No. 170. Hyattsville, MD: National Center for Health Statistics; 1989.

57 US Senate Special Committee on Aging (1987–88). *Aging America, 1988: trends and projections*. Washington, DC: US Department of Health and Human Services; 1991.

58 Mungall D, White RH. Aging and warfarin therapy (letter). *Ann Intern Med* 1992; **117**: 878–9.

59 Toohey M. Clinical trial of phenylindanedione as an anticoagulant. *BMJ* 1953; **1**: 650–62.

60 Shepherd AMM, Hewick DS, Moreland TA, Stevenson IH. Age as a determinant of sensitivity to warfarin. *Br J Clin Pharmacol* 1977; **4**: 315–20.

61 O'Malley K, Stevenson IH, Ward CA, Wood AJJ, Crooks J. Determinants of anticoagulant control in patients receiving warfarin. *Br J Clin Pharmacol* 1977; **4**: 309–14.

62 Friedman SA. Organ systems: cardiovascular disorders. In: Abrams WB, Berkow R, eds *The Merck manual of geriatrics*. Rahway, NJ: Merck Sharp and Dohme Research Laboratories; 1990: 408.

63 Masuda J, Tanak K, Ueda K, et al. Autopsy study of incidence and distribution of cerebral amyloid angiopathy in Hisayama, Japan. *Stroke* 1988; **19**: 205–10.

64 Vonsattel JP, Myers RH, Hedley-Whyte ET, et al. Cerebral amyloid angiopathy without and with cerebral hemorrhages: a comparative histological study. *Ann Neurol* 1991; **30**: 637–49.

65 Hylek EM, Singer DE. Risk factors for intracranial hemorrhage in outpatients taking warfarin. *Ann Intern Med* 1994; **120**: 897–902.

66 Case records of the Massachusetts General Hospital. Weekly clinicopathological exercises. Case 22–1996. Cerebral hemorrhage in a 69-year-old woman receiving warfarin (clinical conference). *N Engl J Med* 1996; **335**: 189–96.

67 Stroke Prevention in Atrial Fibrillation Study Group Investigators. Warfarin versus aspirin for prevention of thromboembolism in atrial fibrillation: stroke prevention in atrial fibrillation II study. *Lancet* 1994; **343**: 687–91.

68 Petitti DB, Strom BL, Melmon KL. Prothrombin time ratio and other factors associated with bleeding in patients treated with warfarin. *J Clin Epidemiol* 1989; **42**: 759–64.

69 Gurwitz JH, Goldberg RJ, Holden A, Knapic N, Ansell J. Age-related risks of long-term oral anticoagulant therapy. *Arch Intern Med* 1988; **148**: 1733–6.

70 Beyth RJ, Landefeld CS. Anticoagulants in older patients: a safety perspective. *Drugs Aging* 1995; **6**: 45–54.

71 Das SK, Cohen AT, Edmondson RA, Melissari E, Kakkar VV. Low-molecular-weight heparin versus warfarin for prevention of recurrent venous thromboembolism: a randomized trial. *World J Surg* 1996; **20**: 521–6.

72 Pini M, Aiello S, Manotti C, et al. Low molecular weight heparin versus warfarin in the prevention of recurrences after deep vein thrombosis. *Thromb Haemost* 1994; **72**: 191–7.

73 White RH, McKittrick T, Takakuwa J, Callahan C, McDonell M, Fihn S. Management and prognosis of life-threatening bleeding during warfarin therapy. *Arch Intern Med* 1996; **156**: 1197–201.

74 Markis M, Greaves M, Phillips WS, Kitchen S, Rosendaal FR, Preston EF. Emergency oral anticoagulant reversal: the relative efficacy of infusions of fresh frozen plasma and clotting factor concentrate on correction of the coagulopathy. *Thromb Haemost* 1997; **77**: 477–80.

75 White RH, McKittrick T, Hutchinson R, Twitchell J. Temporary discontinuation of warfarin therapy: changes in the international normalized ratio. *Ann Intern Med* 1995; **122**: 40–2.

76 Shetty HG, Backhouse G, Bentley DP, et al. Effective reversal of warfarin-induced excessive anticoagulation with low dose vitamin K1. *Thromb Haemost* 1992; **67**: 13–15.

77 Landefeld CS, Rosenblatt MW, Goldman L. Bleeding in outpatients treated with warfarin: relation to the prothrombin time and important remediable lesions. *Am J Med* 1989; **87**: 153–9.

14

Nonhemorrhagic complications of antithrombotic therapy

THEODORE E WARKENTIN

INTRODUCTION

Two important drugs in any therapeutic armamentarium are heparin and warfarin. Ironically, these two widely used anticoagulant agents are both capable of triggering paradoxical thrombotic and other unusual nonhemorrhagic adverse events (Table 14.1). The most common of these adverse reactions is heparin-induced thrombocytopenia (HIT). Characterized by in-vivo platelet activation caused by a heparin-dependent IgG antibody, HIT has been implicated in a diverse spectrum of thrombotic complications that typically involve large veins or arteries. Less commonly, skin lesions at heparin injection sites result from HIT antibodies. In contrast, thrombosis caused by warfarin and other oral anticoagulants (coumarins) typically involves the skin and subcutaneous tissues, and is characterized pathologically by thrombosis of small subdermal venules. Immune mechanisms are not responsible for warfarin-induced skin necrosis; rather, a warfarin-induced reduction – or exacerbation of a pre-existing congenital deficiency – of the natural anticoagulant protein C usually contributes to the small vessel thrombosis seen in this syndrome. Recently, it has been recognized that the catastrophic syndrome of venous limb gangrene can be caused by the *combination* of HIT and a severe warfarin-induced reduction in protein C activity.[1–3] This complication arises from a distur-

Table 14.1 *Major nonhemorrhagic complications of heparin and warfarin*

	Heparin (unfractionated and low-molecular-weight preparations)	Warfarin (and other coumarin anticoagulants)
Prothrombotic syndromes	Heparin-induced thrombocytopenia (HIT)	Coumarin-induced skin necrosis; coumarin-induced venous limb gangrene
Miscellaneous dermatologic syndromes	Heparin-induced skin lesions (secondary to HIT antibodies)	Purple (blue) toe syndrome? Dermatitis Alopecia
Bone syndromes	Osteoporosis	Chondrodysplasia punctata (fetal warfarin syndrome)

Heparin-induced skin lesions are believed to be caused by HIT antibodies; however, this syndrome is listed separately in the table to highlight the observation that most patients with heparin-induced skin lesions do not develop thrombocytopenia.[25] Although coumarin anticoagulants have been implicated in the 'purple toe' syndrome, it is unclear whether coumarin anticoagulation is causal or coincidental, and whether this syndrome is identical to the 'blue toe' syndrome ascribed to cholesterol microembolization.

bance in procoagulant/anticoagulant balance: increased thrombin generation (caused by HIT or cancer), together with a severe reduction in protein C (resulting from warfarin).

Both heparin and warfarin also have clinically important effects on bone metabolism, which are also summarized briefly.

HEPARIN-INDUCED THROMBOCYTOPENIA

HIT is one of the most important adverse drug reactions in clinical medicine, because of its relatively high frequency and its strong association with venous and arterial thrombosis.[4] The key role for coagulation system activation in HIT has led to a recent emphasis on treatments that reduce thrombin generation in patients with HIT (e.g., danaparoid, lepirudin, argatroban).[5–7]

Pathogenesis

Figure 14.1 summarizes the pathogenesis of HIT. It is now widely accepted that HIT is caused by an immunoglobulin – usually IgG – that activates platelets via their Fc receptors.[6] However, the antigen is not heparin alone; rather, a multimolecular complex of heparin and platelet factor 4 (PF4) triggers the pathogenic antibody.[8,9] PF4 is a positively charged, normal constituent of platelet α granules.

Several features of HIT explain its prothrombotic nature (Fig. 14.1): (i) the potent platelet-activating properties of the HIT antibodies, including generation of procoagulant, platelet-derived microparticles;[10,11] (ii) activation of endothelium – including surface expression of tissue factor – by HIT antibodies that recognize PF4 bound

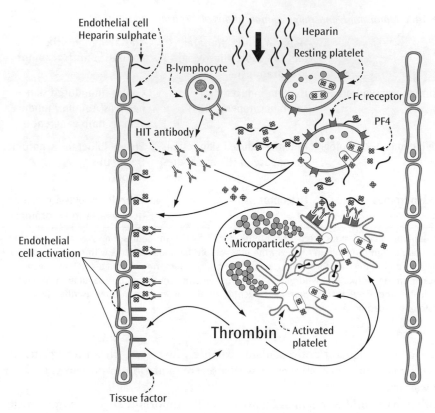

Figure 14.1 *Pathogenesis of heparin-induced thrombocytopenia (HIT). (PF4 = platelet factor 4).*

to endothelial heparin-like molecules (heparan sulfate);[12] and, (iii) neutralization of the anticoagulant effects of heparin by PF4 released from activated platelets. Thus, greatly increased thrombin generation in vivo occurs in most patients with HIT.[1]

Comorbid clinical factors play an important role in the types of thrombosis that patients with HIT develop. For example, postoperative orthopedic patients with HIT have at least a 50% chance of developing venous thromboembolism; arterial thrombosis results less often.[4] In contrast, medical patients are about as likely to develop arterial as venous thrombi.[13,14] The location of upper limb deep vein thrombosis complicating HIT is almost always associated with the use of a central venous catheter.

Clinical syndromes

HIT differs considerably on clinical and pathological grounds from other 'typical' drug-induced, immune-mediated thrombocytopenic syndromes (Table 14.2).

TIMING

The typical patient with HIT develops a platelet count fall that begins between days 5 and 10 (inclusive) of heparin treatment (first day of heparin use = day zero). It is

Table 14.2 *Comparison between heparin-induced thrombocytopenia and 'typical' drug-induced immune thrombocytopenia*

	Heparin-induced thrombocytopenia (HIT)	'Typical' drug-induced immune thrombocytopenic purpura (DITP)
Implicated drugs	Unfractionated heparin, low molecular weight heparin	Quinine, quinidine, sulfa antibiotics, vancomycin, rifampin, many others
Frequency	~1–3% for unfractionated heparin, and < 1% for low molecular weight heparin, when heparin is given for at least 1 week	Rare (e.g., frequency approximately 1/10 000 for sulfa antibiotics)
Mechanism	Heparin-dependent IgG-mediated platelet activation (target antigen usually platelet factor 4–heparin complex)	Drug-dependent binding of IgG to platelet glycoproteins, resulting in platelet removal by reticuloendothelial system
Temporal features	Platelet fall typically begins between days 5 and 10, inclusive	Platelet fall typically begins > 7 days after starting the drug
Severity of thrombo-cytopenia	Mild to moderate: most patients have platelet counts between 20 and 150 × 10^9/L; also, the platelet count may fall but remain > 150; rarely the platelet count is <20	Severe (less than 20 × 10^9/L in >90% of affected patients)
Sequelae	Thrombosis, numerous other sequelae (see Table 14.3); absence of petechiae (even when the platelet count is less than 20 × 10^9/L)	Mucocutaneous bleeding, especially petechiae and oral mucosal ('wet') purpura

often stated that the thrombocytopenia can occur earlier in patients who have been previously exposed to heparin. In my experience, this is unlikely, except in one circumstance: in patients who have been *recently* exposed to heparin (within the past 100 days), there can be an *immediate* fall in the platelet count upon re-exposure to heparin. It is likely that this abrupt recurrence of thrombocytopenia is caused by circulating HIT antibodies triggered by the recent prior heparin exposure, rather than representing a true anamnestic HIT antibody response.[15]

SEVERITY

The thrombocytopenia is usually mild-to-moderate in severity, usually between 20–150 × 10^9/L (the median platelet count nadir is about 55–60 × 10^9/L).[16,17] This is in marked contrast to other *typical* drug-induced immune thrombocytopenic syndromes, e.g., caused by quinine, quinidine, or sulfa antibiotics. In these disorders, the platelet count is generally less than 20 × 10^9/L, and the patient presents with petechiae and purpura. In contrast, even when the platelet count is less than 20 × 10^9/L in a patient with severe HIT, thrombosis rather than petechiae usually results. Patients with HIT can also develop thrombosis even when their platelet count remains greater than $150 \times 10^9/L$.[4,16] However, there is usually an associated fall in the platelet count that is greater than 30%, e.g., a 50% fall from 400 to $200 \times 10^9/L$.

SEQUELAE

Table 14.3 summarizes the adverse clinical events that can complicate HIT. The wide spectrum of reported sequelae means that clinicians should consider HIT in all patients who develop unexpected and unusual events in association with thrombocytopenia or a falling platelet count during – or shortly after stopping – heparin therapy. Some of the life-threatening and limb-threatening complications of HIT that should be suspected on clinical grounds include: bilateral adrenal hemorrhagic infarction and adrenal failure (flank pain and hypotension), pulmonary embolism (dyspnea, pleuritic chest pain, hemoptysis), warfarin-induced venous limb gangrene (progressive swelling, cyanosis, and acral ischemia during warfarin treatment of a deep vein thrombosis complicating HIT), and acute systemic inflammatory reactions (fever, chills, flushing, hypertension, tachycardia, and acute thrombocytopenia within 5–30 minutes of receiving an intravenous heparin bolus in a patient

Table 14.3 *Clinical sequelae associated with heparin-induced thrombocytopenia syndrome*

Isolated thrombocytopenia
Limb thrombosis syndromes
    Deep vein thrombosis (can affect both lower and upper limbs)
        May progress to phlegmasia cerulea dolens or venous limb gangrene during
        warfarin treatment
    Arterial thromboembolism
        Large vessel thrombosis
        Microvascular ischemia
Neurologic syndromes
    Cerebrovascular accident (CVA) secondary to arterial thrombosis or cerebral sinus
    thrombosis
    Ischemic paralysis (myelopathy, radiculopathy)
    Transient global amnesia
    Headache
Cardiac syndromes
    Myocardial infarction
    Intracardiac thrombosis (intra-atrial, intraventricular)
Adrenal hemorrhagic infarction (bilateral infarction can cause acute or chronic adrenal insufficiency)
Heparin-induced skin lesions (at heparin injection sites)
    Erythematous plaques
    Skin necrosis
Acute systemic reactions within 30 minutes after intravenous heparin bolus
    Symptoms/signs can include: fever, chills, hypertension, tachycardia, flushing,
    diaphoresis, cyanosis, tachypnea, dyspnea, chest pain, nausea, vomiting, diarrhea,
    transient global amnesia
Hemodialysis complications
    Clotting in hemodialysis machine
    Thrombosis of arteriovenous shunt

See Warkentin (1997a)[5] for references.

with HIT antibodies). Heparin-induced skin lesions are discussed later in this chapter.

Laboratory testing

There are two general types of assay to detect HIT antibodies: (i) functional, and (ii) antigen assays.[6,18] Unfortunately, no single test is ideal for confirming HIT.

FUNCTIONAL ASSAYS

Functional assays exploit the platelet-activating properties of the pathogenic HIT antibodies. HIT sera will activate normal donor platelets in the presence of therapeutic concentrations of heparin, optimally at 0.1–0.3 U/mL. The most sensitive functional assays are those that use normal donor platelets that have been washed and resuspended in buffer, e.g., the ^{14}C-platelet serotonin release assay (SRA) and the heparin-induced platelet activation assay (HIPA). A number of technical maneuvers are helpful in confirming the presence of HIT antibodies, including: (i) the demonstration that high concentrations of heparin (e.g., 100 U/mL) inhibit the ability of the HIT serum to activate platelets; (ii) showing that a monoclonal antibody that blocks the platelet FcγII receptor inhibits platelet activation by the HIT antibodies; and (iii) the use of negative, 'weak,' and 'strong' HIT control sera to confirm that the test platelets selected are adequate to detect HIT antibodies of varying strength. When performed by experienced laboratories, the sensitivity and specificity of washed platelet assays for HIT are at least 90%.

Unfortunately, the most widely used functional assay – the platelet aggregation assay using normal donor platelets suspended in citrated plasma – may have a sensitivity for HIT as low as 50%. Specificity is also less than optimal, because heparin can sometimes produce nonspecific activation of platelets in citrated plasma.

ANTIGEN ASSAYS

Antigen assays using the enzyme-linked immunosorbent assay (ELISA) technique have been developed using PF4–heparin as target antigen,[8,19] as well as PF4 bound to polyvinylsulfonate.[18] Although these assays may be more convenient for the routine laboratory, disadvantages include occasional false-negative and false-positive results. The former problem may result when the pathogenic HIT antibodies recognize 'minor' antigens other than heparin–PF4 complex; the latter problem may relate to the high sensitivity of ELISA for detecting weak, clinically insignificant HIT antibodies. Nonetheless, sometimes, inconclusive test results are obtained using functional assays for HIT, and in these instances the ELISA assay is required to diagnose HIT.

Overall, the concordance between functional and antigen assays for HIT is approximately 90%. Because functional and antigen assays for HIT complement one another, it is recommended that both types of assay be available in reference laboratories.[6] HIT antibodies usually remain detectable in patient serum or plasma for only 4–12 weeks (by functional assay), and therefore only acute serum or plasma should be used for diagnostic testing.

Treatment

Heparin should be discontinued in patients with clinically suspected HIT. However, two retrospective studies of patients with serologically confirmed HIT suggest that these patients are at relatively high risk for subsequent thrombosis (approximately 38–53%), even if there is no clinical evidence of HIT-associated thrombosis at the time heparin is discontinued.[17,20] Moreover, early discontinuation of heparin (within 48 hours of onset of thrombocytopenia) was not associated with more favorable clinical outcomes compared with later heparin cessation.[17] Therefore, the use of an alternative anticoagulant for a patient with clinically suspected HIT is recommended,[6,7] particularly if the patient is otherwise at a relatively high risk for thrombosis (e.g., an immobile, postoperative patient).

The management of HIT complicated by thrombosis should include an alternative anticoagulant agent that either reduces thrombin generation or directly inactivates thrombin.[6,7] Currently, there are three such agents that appear to be clinically effective: danaparoid, recombinant hirudin (lepirudin), and argatroban. Each agent has advantages and disadvantages.

DANAPAROID (ORGARAN®)

Danaparoid sodium is a mixture of anticoagulant glycosaminoglycans with predominant anti-factor Xa activity, including low-sulfated heparan sulfate (84%) and dermatan sulfate (12%). One or more of these constituents may interact weakly with PF4, because – depending upon the sensitivity of the assay – approximately 10–40% of HIT sera will show some degree of in-vitro cross-reactivity for danaparoid. However, studies suggest that such laboratory detection of cross-reactivity is usually clinically insignificant.[21] In my opinion, treatment with danaparoid should not be delayed to perform in-vitro cross-reactivity studies.

I usually avoid starting warfarin until the patient's platelet count has nearly recovered to normal during anticoagulation with danaparoid. The half-life of danaparoid is quite long (approximately 25 hours for its anti-factor Xa activity), and I therefore stop or taper danaparoid when the International Normalized Ratio (INR) begins to increase during warfarin treatment. The risk of warfarin-induced venous limb gangrene appears to be negligible when warfarin is given together with danaparoid. Anticoagulant monitoring of danaparoid can be performed via the measurement of anti-factor Xa activity (using a danaparoid calibration curve); however, this assay is generally not available in routine laboratories. This is usually not a major limitation, however, because the anticoagulant effects of danaparoid are largely predictable, and there is a high likelihood of obtaining therapeutic anticoagulant levels using an empirically derived standard treatment protocol (Table 14.4). However, because danaparoid can accumulate in renal failure, this is a clinical situation in which the anti-factor Xa activity should be monitored, if possible. I also recommend monitoring patients with life-threatening or limb-threatening HIT.

A prospective, open-label, randomized clinical trial demonstrated improved clinical outcomes with danaparoid, compared with dextran, for the treatment of HIT complicated by thrombosis.[22] Overall, approximately 90% of patients are successfully treated with danaparoid, as defined by platelet count recovery without the development of a new thrombotic event during treatment. Although danaparoid has been approved for the treatment of HIT in some countries (e.g., Great Britain, Germany, Netherlands, Belgium, and New Zealand), it may be available to physicians for off-label use in other countries in which it has been approved for the prevention of deep vein thrombosis (Ireland, Australia, Canada, and USA).

LEPIRUDIN (REFLUDAN®)

Lepirudin is a recombinant hirudin (r-hirudin) derivative that inhibits thrombin via a high-affinity, noncovalent interaction. Based upon a favorable experience in treating HIT in Germany – compared with a historical control population[23] – lepirudin has been approved both in the European Union (since May 1997) and in the USA (since March 1998) to treat HIT complicated by thrombosis (Table 14.4). An advantage of lepirudin is that its anticoagulant effect can be monitored readily using activated partial thromboplastin times (aPTT). However, this agent is renally eliminated, and should be used cautiously – if at all – in patients with renal failure. Antihirudin antibodies are commonly generated in patients treated with lepirudin; in a minority of patients, this, paradoxically, can lead to a greater anticoagulant effect of lepirudin.[24]

ARGATROBAN (NOVASTAN®)

Argatroban is a synthetic, small-molecule antithrombin that has been evaluated for HIT in North America (Table 14.4). Like lepirudin, argatroban's anticoagulant effect is readily monitored using the aPTT. Unlike lepirudin, however, argatroban is predominantly metabolized by the liver, and so may be safer in HIT patients with renal failure. Argatroban was recently approved by the US Food and Drug Administration to treat and prevent HIT-associated thrombosis.

The decision about whether to use danaparoid, lepirudin, or argatroban to treat HIT depends upon several factors, including whether the drug is available to the physician, as well as various pharmacologic and pharmacokinetic considerations.

Table 14.4 *Treatment protocols for heparin-induced thrombocytopenia complicated by thrombosis*

Danaparoid	*Loading dose*: 2250 U intravenous bolus,[a] followed by 400 U/hr × 4 hours, then 300 U/hour × 4 hours; then *maintenance:* 150–200 U/hour, with subsequent dose adjustments made using anti-factor Xa levels (target range 0.5–0.8 anti-Xa U/mL), if assay available[b]
Lepirudin	*Loading dose*: 0.4 mg/kg bolus, followed by *maintenance*: 0.15 mg/kg per hour infusion, with dose adjustments to maintain the aPTT 1.5–3.0 times the mean of the normal laboratory aPTT range
Argatroban	Infusion rate of 2 µg/kg per minute, with dose adjustments to maintain the aPTT 1.5–3.0 times the control value

[a]Adjust bolus for body weight: < 60 kg, 1500 U; 60–75 kg, 2250 U; 75–90 kg, 3000 U; > 90 kg, 3750 U. The recommendations are based on 750-U ampule availability; for 1250-U ampules, the loading dose would be 2500 U, etc.
[b]The calibration curve for anti-factor Xa testing must be derived using danaparoid rather than low molecular weight heparin.
aPTT, activated partial thromboplastin time.

Regarding danaparoid, its predictable dose-dependent anticoagulant effects and long half-life, its availability for both intravenous and subcutaneous administration, and its lack of interference with the INR make it a convenient option in patients in whom a gradual overlap with warfarin is anticipated, e.g., the majority of HIT patients who have deep vein thrombosis or pulmonary embolism and will therefore require several months of oral anticoagulation. However, the long half-life may be a comparative disadvantage in patients in whom surgery or invasive procedures are planned, or who develop bleeding. Although there is no antidote for danaparoid, bleeding complications are uncommon. For patients with limb-threatening arterial thrombosis, or in whom urgent surgery may be required, either lepirudin or argatroban may be preferred, as their short half-lives (1.3 and 0.9 hours, respectively) mean that their anticoagulant effects will disappear quickly following cessation. There are no known antidotes for either antithrombin agent.

Prevention

HIT is potentially preventable: there is a lower frequency of HIT, associated thrombosis, and HIT antibody formation in patients treated with low molecular weight heparin (LMWH), compared with unfractionated heparin (UFH).[4] However, the lower frequency of HIT does *not* mean that LMWH should be used to treat HIT: this is because HIT antibodies activate platelets equally well in the presence of either LMWH or UFH when sensitive washed platelet assays are used for testing. Further, the risk of worsening thrombocytopenia or triggering thrombosis is too high to justify the use of LMWH to treat acute HIT.[5,7]

It is unknown whether frequent routine platelet count measurements lead to earlier clinical recognition of HIT and improved patient outcomes. Nevertheless, frequent platelet count monitoring – at least once every second day – is recommended for patients at relatively high risk for HIT, such as postoperative orthopedic and cardiovascular patients receiving unfractionated heparin.[6] Irrespective of the frequency of platelet count monitoring, however, it is important that physicians suspect HIT quickly in the appropriate clinical context, e.g., symptoms or signs of thrombosis or other characteristic sequelae of HIT that develop during, or shortly after stopping, heparin therapy. In such patients, physicians must order a complete blood count, and compare the platelet count with recent previous values. For patients with thrombocytopenia or a falling platelet count, physicians must usually institute an appropriate management strategy for presumptive HIT, even prior to laboratory confirmation of the diagnosis.

HEPARIN-INDUCED SKIN LESIONS

Heparin-induced skin lesions (Plates 1 and 2) develop at heparin injection sites, typically beginning 5–10 days after starting subcutaneous injections of unfractionated heparin or LMWH.[25] They range in appearance from erythematous plaques to actual skin necrosis. Although the formation of HIT antibodies is strongly associated with these skin lesions, only about one-quarter of patients with heparin-induced skin lesions develop thrombocytopenia.[26] However, the risk for thrombosis is much

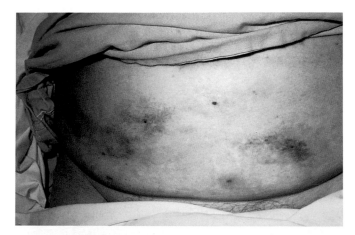

Plate 1 *Heparin-induced skin lesions: erythematous plaques. (Reprinted with permission from Warkentin TE. Heparin-induced skin lesions. Br J Haematol 1996; **92**: 494–7.)*

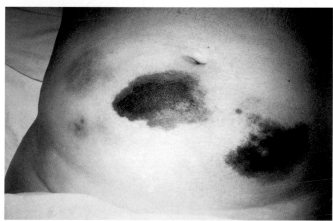

Plate 2 *Heparin-induced skin lesions: skin necrosis. (Reprinted with permission from Warkentin TE. Heparin-induced skin lesions. Br J Haematol 1996; **92**: 494–7.)*

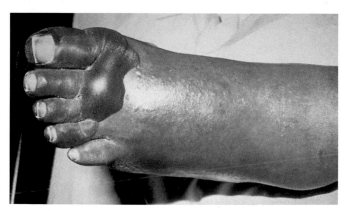

Plate 3 *Venous limb gangrene. This patient developed limb gangrene necessitating below-knee amputation during warfarin treatment of deep vein thrombosis and heparin-induced thrombocytopenia. Palpable pulses were observed at the onset of necrosis. (Reprinted with permission from Warkentin TE, Elavathil LJ, Hayward CPM et al. The pathogenesis of venous limb gangrene associated with heparin-induced thrombocytopenia. Ann Intern Med 1997; **127**: 804–12.)*

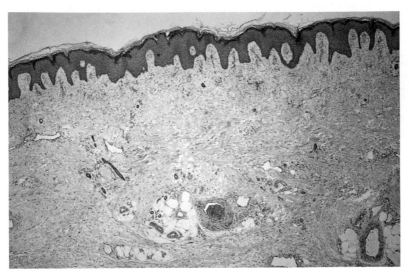

Plate 4 *An occluding thrombus can be seen in a subcutaneous venule (original magnification, × 40); this is a characteristic pathologic feature of warfarin-associated necrosis. (Reprinted with permission from Warkentin TE, Elavathil LJ, Hayward CPM et al. The pathogenesis of venous limb gangrene associated with heparin-induced thrombocytopenia.* Ann Intern Med *1997; **127**: 804–12.)*

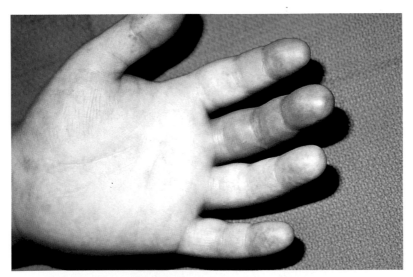

Plate 5 *Phlegmasia cerulea dolens. This patient's hand ischemia was attributed to warfarin treatment of an upper limb deep vein thrombosis complicating heparin-induced thrombocytopenia, as there was evidence for marked deficiency of the functional protein C level (INR = 4.0; prothrombin = 31%; factor VII = 12%; functional protein C = 4%). The ischemia resolved with reversal of warfarin anticoagulation, using vitamin K and plasma given by apheresis. (See patient #4 in Warkentin TE, Elavathil LJ, Hayward CPM et al. The pathogenesis of venous limb gangrene associated with heparin-induced thrombocytopenia.* Ann Intern Med *1997; **127**: 804–12.)*

greater in the subgroup of patients who do develop thrombocytopenia. Platelet monitoring should be performed for several days, even after stopping the heparin injections, because of the skin lesions; this is because thrombocytopenia and thrombosis can occur shortly after the discontinuation of heparin.

HEPARIN-INDUCED OSTEOPOROSIS

Long-term UFH heparin use has been associated with osteoporosis and skeletal fractures.[27] A case-control study of 61 women who had previously received at least 1 month of UFH during pregnancy did not identify any women with symptomatic fractures (upper 95% confidence interval (CI), 5.9%); however, a greater proportion of these women had osteopenia, compared with controls, as shown by bone density measurements.[28] Thus, there could be long-term health implications of prolonged heparin treatment in certain patients.

Animal studies indicate that UFH decreases cancellous bone volume, both by decreasing the rate of bone formation and by increasing the rate of bone resorption.[29] In contrast, LMWH causes less osteopenia in animals, because it decreases the rate of bone formation without any effect upon bone resorption. Monreal and colleagues[30] observed that LMWH was less likely than UFH to be associated with symptomatic spinal fractures when used for 3–6 months (15% vs 2.5%; $p = 0.054$).

COUMARIN-INDUCED SKIN NECROSIS

Coumarin-induced skin necrosis, characterized by necrosis of the skin and underlying subcutaneous tissues, is the most important nonhemorrhagic side-effect of warfarin and other coumarin anticoagulants.[31,32] These drugs interfere with post-translational modification of four procoagulant and two anticoagulant vitamin K-dependent factors (Table 14.5), by way of their action in vitamin K antagonism. Vitamin K is the cofactor required for the action of an enzyme (vitamin K-dependent γ-glutamylcarboxylase) that adds a carboxyl group to each member of a cluster

Table 14.5 *Vitamin K-dependent procoagulant and anticoagulant factors*

Procoagulant factors (half-life)	Anticoagulant factors (half-life)
Factor II, or prothrombin (60 hours)	Protein C (9 hours)
Factor X (40 hours)	Protein S (60 hours)
Factor IX (24 hours)	
Factor VII (4–6 hrs)	

There are six vitamin K-dependent hemostatic factors, four with procoagulant activity, and two with anticoagulant activity. Treatment with coumarin anticoagulants reduces functional levels of these factors. The paradoxical procoagulant effect of warfarin can be explained by the different half-lives[57] of these factors following onset of action of coumarin: the time to a therapeutically significant reduction of the major procoagulant factor, prothrombin (half-life ~60 hours), is much longer than the time to a clinically important reduction in the major anticoagulant factor, protein C (half-life 9 hours). Thus, within the first few days of coumarin anticoagulation, and under certain clinical circumstances (see text), there can arise transient, but clinically important, procoagulant effects that can result in skin necrosis.

of glutamyl residues, thereby forming γ-carboxyglutamyl (Gla) residues that are crucial for the ability of these hemostatic factors to interact with phospholipid membranes in a calcium-dependent fashion. During this γ-carboxylation reaction, the reduced form of the cofactor (vitamin KH_2) is oxidized to vitamin K epoxide; coumarins inhibit the two enzymes (vitamin K epoxide reductase and vitamin K reductase) that act in sequence to regenerate the reduced form of vitamin K.

Warfarin (Coumadin®), a 4-hydroxycoumarin derivative, is the most widely used oral anticoagulant in North America because of its high bioavailability, leading to predictable onset and duration of action.[31] Thus, most examples of coumarin necrosis on this continent are 'warfarin-induced skin necrosis'. However, the syndrome can be caused by other coumarin congeners (e.g., phenprocoumon, acenocoumarol, nicoumalone), as well as the rarely used phenindione group of oral anticoagulants.[33] Phenprocoumon (Marcumar®) is widely used in continental Europe. As its half-life is substantially longer than that of warfarin (6 vs. 1.5 days), relatively large loading doses are often given; however, whether this results in a greater frequency of skin necrosis, compared with warfarin, is unknown.

Pathogenesis

Several lines of evidence suggest that a transient disturbance in procoagulant/anticoagulant balance during the initial stages of coumarin anticoagulation, which is related to significant differences in the half-lives of the major procoagulant and anticoagulant vitamin K-dependent factors (Table 14.5), underlies the pathogenesis of coumarin-induced skin necrosis. First, coumarin-induced necrosis typically occurs 3–6 days after initiating oral anticoagulant therapy, i.e., prior to achieving a therapeutically effective reduction in the level of the most important procoagulant factor (prothrombin), and during a time when the major anticoagulant factor (protein C) can be markedly reduced. Protein C levels typically fall to a greater extent, compared with prothrombin levels, during the first few days of warfarin use.[34] Second, the pathology of coumarin-induced necrosis is that of predominantly noninflammatory, small vessel thrombosis affecting the subcutaneous postcapillary venules and small veins.[35] This is consistent with the established role of the protein C anticoagulant pathway to downregulate thrombin in these vessels. Third, a relatively high proportion of patients with coumarin-induced necrosis have a hereditary abnormality of the protein C anticoagulant pathway (discussed subsequently). Such an abnormality predisposes to skin necrosis by increasing the risk for a transient imbalance in procoagulant/anticoagulant processes during early warfarin therapy. Finally, the clinical and pathologic appearance of coumarin-induced necrosis closely resembles that of neonatal purpura fulminans, which is usually caused by severe congenital protein C deficiency.

Clinical syndromes

'CENTRAL' SKIN NECROSIS

Coumarin-induced skin necrosis can be divided into central and peripheral syndromes (Fig. 14.2); the peripheral syndrome is more commonly recognized as

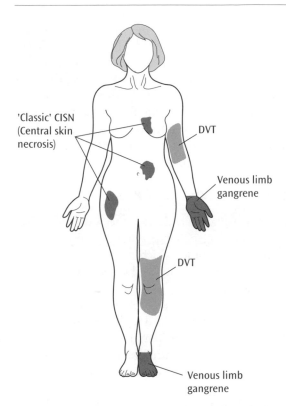

'Classic' CISN
(Central skin
necrosis)

DVT

Venous limb
gangrene

DVT

Venous limb
gangrene

Figure 14.2 *Coumarin-induced skin necrosis (CISN) syndromes. Central skin necrosis tends to occur in patients with congenital abnormalities of the protein C anticoagulant pathway who are treated with warfarin. In contrast, peripheral (acral) skin necrosis (venous limb gangrene) tends to occur distal to an active deep vein thrombosis (DVT) in a patient who develops a very low protein C level (correlating with a 'supratherapeutic' INR) during warfarin treatment of an acute thrombocytopenic process associated with increased thrombin generation, e.g., heparin-induced thrombocytopenia or cancer-associated disseminated intravascular coagulation. (Reprinted, with permission, from Warkentin.[58])*

venous limb gangrene (discussed subsequently). *Central* coumarin-induced necrosis most commonly involves areas of skin with substantial underlying fatty tissues, such as the female breast, buttocks, hips, and thighs. Less common sites include the anterior abdomen, flank, back, penis, legs, arms, and face.[2,36] About one-third of patients have multiple lesions, which are sometimes symmetric. The majority (approximately 75%) of patients are women. Coumarin-induced necrosis is rare: a survey of approximately 20 000 hospital inpatients who received warfarin identified only two possible cases of skin necrosis, i.e., a frequency of 0.01%.[32]

The typical onset between days 3 and 6 of oral anticoagulant therapy is observed for more than 90% of patients.[36] The earliest symptoms and signs of skin necrosis include localized pain, induration, and erythema in one or more of the characteristic sites; over the next few hours, the skin lesions progress to central purplish or black discoloration, often with associated blistering, with subsequent well-demarcated, full-thickness necrosis involving the skin and subdermal tissues. With or without surgical debridement, there is usually a permanent region of depressed skin that reflects the loss of underlying tissues.

It can be difficult to distinguish the earliest stages of coumarin-induced necrosis from subcutaneous hemorrhage. The clinician should strongly suspect incipient central coumarin-induced skin necrosis when: (i) coumarin treatment has been recently initiated; (ii) one of the characteristic tissue sites is involved; (iii) there is no history of local trauma; and (iv) the INR does not indicate excess anticoagulation (cf. peripheral coumarin-induced necrosis, discussed below).

A relatively high proportion of patients with coumarin-induced necrosis are subsequently shown to have congenital protein C deficiency.[32] Congenital deficiencies of protein S and antithrombin have also been observed in some patients.[32,37,38] Factor V Leiden – a relatively common mutation that renders factor V less susceptible to proteolytic degradation by activated protein C – has also been implicated.[39] Most patients with coumarin-induced necrosis are receiving the oral anticoagulant because of an underlying thrombosis such as deep vein thrombosis or pulmonary embolism, rather than for anticoagulant prophylaxis (e.g., chronic atrial fibrillation).[32] The explanation for this observation is unknown.

VENOUS LIMB GANGRENE ('PERIPHERAL' SKIN NECROSIS)

Venous limb gangrene involves the acral (peripheral) regions of the body, most often the toes/feet/legs, but sometimes also the fingers/hands/arms. Usually, there is associated deep vein thrombosis of the affected limb, which may be an important component in the pathogenesis (see above). The severity of the necrosis can range from bluish discoloration without necrosis (Plates 3–5), to distal necrosis with tissue sloughing not requiring amputation, to extensive venous limb gangrene requiring limb amputation. The syndrome of phlegmasia caerulea dolens (i.e., the 'swollen blue painful' limb) typically precedes the progression to venous limb gangrene.

Two disorders appear to predispose to coumarin-induced venous limb gangrene: HIT[1,2] and chronic disseminated intravascular coagulation associated with malignancy.[3,40]

The clinician should suspect anticoagulation with coumarin as the paradoxical explanation for acral ischemia or necrosis when this complication occurs in temporal relation to oral anticoagulant use, and particularly when there is laboratory evidence for apparent 'overanticoagulation,' i.e., an INR that is 3.5 or greater.[1–3] The supratherapeutic INR results from severe reduction in the vitamin K-dependent procoagulant factor, factor VII; a parallel severe reduction in protein C activity explains the microvascular thrombosis underlying this syndrome. Thus, the coumarin critically interferes with the protein C anticoagulant pathway, while being unable to control the increased thrombin generation characteristic of HIT or cancer-associated disseminated intravascular coagulation.[1–3]

Treatment and prevention

Reversal of anticoagulation with vitamin K may prevent incipient coumarin-induced necrosis if it is recognized in its earliest stages.[41] Unfortunately, the diagnosis is usually not made until some necrosis is established; at this point, it is unknown whether discontinuation of warfarin, administration of vitamin K, or use of plasma or protein C concentrates[42] alters the natural history of tissue injury. In patients without HIT who require further anticoagulation, heparin is usually substituted for warfarin. Approximately half of affected patients ultimately require surgical treatment, such as skin grafting or tissue amputation.

Because coumarin-induced skin necrosis is probably attributable to several dynamic interacting factors, including the rate of coumarin-induced reductions in anticoagulant and procoagulant factors, it may be acceptable to reintroduce warfarin in patients with a history of this complication. Some authors recommend starting with relatively low doses of warfarin (e.g., 1–2 mg/day for 3–4 days), followed by an attempt gradually to increase the INR into the therapeutic range over 1.5–2 weeks. Published experience indicates that doses between 2 and 5 mg/day may also be relatively safe.[43] Concurrent use of therapeutic-dose heparin is recommended in these patients,[44] provided there is no evidence for concomitant HIT, as heparin reduces thrombin generation that could contribute to the pathogenesis of skin necrosis. Some physicians have administered plasma to patients with known congenital protein C deficiency during repeat initiation of warfarin anticoagulation. The risk of recurrence of coumarin-induced skin necrosis using these precautions is unknown, but is believed to be low.

Harrison and associates[34] performed a randomized clinical trial comparing 5 mg and 10 mg warfarin as an initial 'loading' dose for patients undergoing initial warfarin anticoagulation. These investigators showed that the probability of achieving therapeutic anticoagulation (target INR, 2.0–3.0) at 5 days was similar in both patient groups (approximately 70%). However, the group of patients who received the lower dose of warfarin had significantly higher levels of protein C at 36 and 60 hours after the initiation of warfarin, and they were less likely to have early excess anticoagulation, as measured by the INR. Thus, there are no clinical advantages to giving a relatively high initial dose of warfarin, but there may be advantages to using a lower dose, i.e., there is less risk for precipitating a hypercoagulable state related to low protein C levels.

Warfarin should be used cautiously – if at all – in patients who have uncontrolled thrombin generation. This includes patients with acute disseminated intravascular coagulation (e.g., secondary to septicemia), chronic disseminated intravascular coagulation (e.g., secondary to metastatic cancer), or acute HIT. As a corollary, some physicians routinely administer vitamin K to patients with disseminated intravascular coagulation.[45]

COUMARIN-ASSOCIATED 'PURPLE TOE' AND CHOLESTEROL EMBOLISM SYNDROMES

Feder and Auerbach[46] reported six patients who developed 'dark blue-tinged bilateral purple discolouration of the feet, especially the plantar surfaces and the sides of the first two toes' that began 3–8 weeks after starting coumarin anticoagulants. They noted that the color blanched completely on moderate pressure, and that the patients usually had pain and tenderness of the toes. The abnormalities tended to persist despite stopping coumarin. All of their patients were male, with evidence for peripheral vascular disease. Subsequently, it was suggested that this syndrome might be caused by cholesterol microembolization,[47,48] a concept that is meeting with growing acceptance.[49] However, some patients with purple toe syndrome do not have other clinical features of cholesterol embolism syndrome.

Classically, cholesterol (or atheromatous) embolism syndrome is characterized by a variety of peripheral ischemic signs (livedo reticularis, 'blue' toes, sometimes with progression to focal digital necrosis) and organ dysfunction (most frequently renal failure).[48] Pedal pulses are usually palpable, consistent with the pathologic findings of biconvex clefts in small arteries and arterioles that indicate prior embolism of cholesterol crystals. Patients with cholesterol embolism syndrome have advanced atherosclerosis, usually with a recent injury to a large artery (e.g., cardiac surgery or arteriography) or disruption of an adherent thrombus (e.g., post-thrombolytic therapy).[48]

Only a minority of patients diagnosed as having cholesterol embolism syndrome are receiving concomitant coumarin anticoagulation.[50] Nevertheless, some have suggested that oral anticoagulants could contribute to this syndrome in these patients, by causing a gradual loss of the protective fibrin layer that overlies an ulcerated atherosclerotic plaque, thereby facilitating cholesterol microembolization.[51] However, any such pathogenic role for coumarin anticoagulation – whether causal or coincidental – is usually unclear in an individual patient. Therefore, physicians need to balance carefully the potential risks and benefits of oral anticoagulation, as well as the available therapeutic options, before deciding whether to stop oral anticoagulants in a patient who develops cholesterol embolism syndrome. For example, aspirin reduces the frequency of strokes in elderly patients with chronic atrial fibrillation, and could be substituted for warfarin in a patient who develops cholesterol embolism syndrome during oral anticoagulant use.

MISCELLANEOUS CUTANEOUS EFFECTS OF ORAL ANTICOAGULANTS

In addition to ecchymotic purpura related to the anticoagulant effects of warfarin and other oral anticoagulants, a few patients may develop macular, papular, vesicular, or urticarial lesions that are presumably of an allergic origin.[52] Alopecia of varying severity in relation to oral anticoagulant usage has also been described. The use of a different oral anticoagulant agent may permit further anticoagulation with resolution of these adverse effects.

FETAL WARFARIN SYNDROME

Three vitamin K-dependent, γ-carboxyglutamate-containing proteins found in bone are synthesized by osteoblasts: osteocalcin, matrix γ-carboxyglutamate protein, and protein S.[53] Impaired γ-carboxylation of one or more of these proteins because of coumarin anticoagulation of mothers during their first trimester of pregnancy is believed to explain the occurrence of chondrodysplasia punctata (fetal warfarin syndrome) in affected offspring. This embryopathy is characterized by nasal bridge hypoplasia (resulting in a flattened, upturned appearance of the nose), finger shortening, and stippling of the epiphyses and vertebrae evident on radiography performed during the first year of life.[54-6] The critical period of exposure to warfarin appears to be between 6 and 9 weeks of gestation. The risk for fetal warfarin syndrome may also be dose dependent: the highest reported frequencies of fetal warfarin syndrome were observed in North America during a time when oral anticoagulation was consistently more intense than in Europe. The availability of long-term anticoagulants that can be given as an outpatient (e.g., subcutaneous injections of UFH or LMWH or heparinoid) means that few women are compelled to receive warfarin or other oral anticoagulants during the first trimester of pregnancy. It remains unresolved whether oral anticoagulants have clinically significant effects on the bones of children and adults.[53]

ACKNOWLEDGMENTS

Several studies described in this chapter were funded by the Heart & Stroke Foundation of Ontario. Dr Warkentin was supported by a Research Scholarship of the Heart and Stroke Foundation of Canada.

REFERENCES

1 Warkentin TE, Elavathil LJ, Hayward CPM, Johnston MA, Russett JI, Kelton JG. The pathogenesis of venous limb gangrene associated with heparin-induced thrombocytopenia. *Ann Intern Med* 1997; **127**: 804–12.

2 Warkentin TE, Sikov WM, Lillicrap DP. Multicentric warfarin-induced skin necrosis complicating heparin-induced thrombocytopenia. *Am J Hematol* 1999; **62**: 44–8.

3 Warkentin TE. Venous limb gangrene (VLG) complicating warfarin treatment of deep-vein thrombosis (deep vein thrombosis) in metastatic carcinoma. *Blood* 1999; **94**(Suppl. 1): 1146 (abstract).

4 Warkentin TE, Levine MN, Hirsh J, et al. Heparin-induced thrombocytopenia in patients treated with low-molecular-weight heparin or unfractionated heparin. *N Engl J Med* 1995; **332**: 1330–5.

5 Warkentin TE. Heparin-induced thrombocytopenia: pathogenesis, frequency, avoidance and management. *Drug Saf* 1997; **17**: 325–41.

6 Warkentin TE, Chong BH, Greinacher A. Heparin-induced thrombocytopenia: towards consensus. *Thromb Haemost* 1998; **79**: 1–7.

7 Greinacher A, Warkentin TE. Treatment of heparin-induced thrombocytopenia: an overview. In: Warkentin TE, Greinacher A, eds *Heparin-induced thrombocytopenia*. New York: Marcel Dekker, 2000: 261–90.

8 Amiral J, Bridey F, Dreyfus M, et al. Platelet factor 4 complexed to heparin is the target for antibodies generated in heparin-induced thrombocytopenia (letter). *Thromb Haemost* 1992; **68**: 95–6.

9 Greinacher A, Pötzsch B, Amiral J, Dummel V, Eichner A, Mueller-Eckhardt C. Heparin-associated thrombocytopenia: isolation of the antibody and characterization of a multimolecular PF4–heparin complex as the major antigen. *Thromb Haemost* 1994; **71**: 247–51.

10 Warkentin TE, Hayward CPM, Boshkov LK, et al. Sera from patients with heparin-induced thrombocytopenia generate platelet-derived microparticles with procoagulant activity: an explanation for the thrombotic complications of heparin-induced thrombocytopenia. *Blood* 1994; **84**: 3691–9.

11 Warkentin TE, Sheppard JI. Generation of platelet-derived microparticles and procoagulant activity by heparin-induced thrombocytopenia IgG/serum and other IgG

platelet agonists: a comparison with standard platelet agonists. *Platelets* 1999; **10**: 319–26.

12 Visentin GP, Ford SE, Scott JP, Aster RH. Antibodies from patients with heparin-induced thrombocytopenia/thrombosis are specific for platelet factor 4 complexed with heparin or bound to endothelial cells. *J Clin Invest* 1994; **93**: 81–8.

13 Boshkov LK, Warkentin TE, Hayward CPM, Andrew M, Kelton JG. Heparin-induced thrombocytopenia and thrombosis: clinical and laboratory studies. *Br J Haematol* 1993; **84**: 322–8.

14 Lee DH, Warkentin TE. Frequency of heparin-induced thrombocytopenia. In: Warkentin TE, Greinacher A, eds *Heparin-induced thrombocytopenia*. New York: Marcel Dekker, 2000: 81–112.

15 Warkentin TE, Kelton JG. Timing of heparin-induced thrombocytopenia (HIT) in relation to previous heparin use: absence of an anamnestic immune response, and implications for repeat heparin use in patients with a history of HIT. *Blood* 1998; **92**(Suppl. 1): 182a.

16 Warkentin TE. Clinical presentation of heparin-induced thrombocytopenia. *Semin Hematol* 1998; **35**(Suppl. 5): 9–16.

17 Wallis DE, Workman DL, Lewis BE, Steen L, Pifarre R, Moran JF. Failure of early heparin cessation as treatment for heparin-induced thrombocytopenia. *Am J Med* 1999; **106**: 629–35.

18 Warkentin TE, Greinacher A. Laboratory testing for heparin-induced thrombocytopenia. In: Warkentin TE, Greinacher A, eds *Heparin-induced thrombocytopenia*. New York: Marcel Dekker, 2000: 211–44.

19 Greinacher A, Amiral J, Dummel V, Vissac A, Kiefel V, Mueller-Eckhardt C. Laboratory diagnosis of heparin-associated thrombocytopenia and comparison of platelet aggregation test, heparin-induced platelet activation test, and platelet factor 4/heparin enzyme-linked immunosorbent assay. *Transfusion* 1994; **34**: 381–5.

20 Warkentin TE, Kelton JG. A 14-year study of heparin-induced thrombocytopenia. *Am J Med* 1996; **101**: 502–7.

21 Newman PM, Swanson RL, Chong BH. Heparin-induced thrombocytopenia: IgG binding to PF4–heparin complexes in the fluid phase and cross-reactivity with low molecular weight heparin and heparinoid. *Thromb Haemost* 1998; **80**: 292–7.

22 Chong BH. Low molecular weight heparinoid and heparin-induced thrombocytopenia (abstract). *Aust NZ J Med* 1996; **26**: 331.

23 Greinacher A, Völpel H, Janssens U, et al. Recombinant hirudin (lepirudin) provides safe and effective anticoagulation in patients with heparin-induced thrombocytopenia: a prospective study. *Circulation* 1999; **99**: 73–80.

24 Greinacher A. Recombinant hirudin for the treatment of heparin-induced thrombocytopenia: an overview. In: Warkentin TE, Greinacher A, eds *Heparin-induced thrombocytopenia*. New York: Marcel Dekker, 2000: 313–38.

25 Warkentin TE. Heparin-induced skin lesions. *Br J Haematol* 1996; **92**: 494–7.

26 Warkentin TE. Heparin-induced thrombocytopenia, heparin-induced skin lesions, and arterial thrombosis (abstract). *Thromb Haemost* 1997; **77**(Suppl.): 562.

27 Jaffe MD, Willis PW III. Multiple fractures associated with long-term sodium heparin therapy. *JAMA* 1965; **193**: 152–4.

28 Ginsberg JS, Kowalchuk G, Hirsh J, et al. Heparin effect on bone density. *Thromb Haemost* 1990; **64**: 286–9.

29 Muir JM, Hirsh J, Weitz JI, Andrew M, Young E, Shaughnessy SG. A histomorphometric comparison of the effects of heparin and low-molecular-weight heparin on cancellous bone in rats. *Blood* 1997; **89**: 3236–42.

30 Monreal M, Lafoz E, Olive A, del Rio L, Vedia C. Comparison of subcutaneous unfractionated heparin with a low molecular weight heparin (Fragmin®) in patients with venous thromboembolism and contraindications to coumarin. *Thromb Haemost* 1994; **71**: 7–11.

31 Hirsh J. Oral anticoagulant drugs. *N Engl J Med* 1991; **324**: 1865–75.

32 Comp PC. Coumarin-induced skin necrosis. Incidence, mechanisms, management and avoidance. *Drug Saf* 1993; **8**: 128–35.

33 Nalbandian RM, Mader IJ, Barrett JL, Pearce JP, Rupp EC. Petechiae, ecchymoses, and necrosis of skin induced by coumarin congeners. *JAMA* 1965; **192**: 603–8.

34 Harrison L, Johnston M, Massicotte MP, Crowther M, Moffat K, Hirsh J. Comparison of 5-mg and 10-mg loading doses in initiation of warfarin therapy. *Ann Intern Med* 1997; **126**: 133–6.

35 Comp PC, Elrod JP, Karzenski S. Warfarin-induced skin necrosis. *Semin Thromb Hemost* 1990; **16**: 293–8.

36 Cole MS, Minifee PK, Wolma FJ. Coumarin necrosis – a review of the literature. *Surgery* 1988; **103**: 271–7.

37 Anderson DR, Brill-Edwards P, Walker I. Warfarin-induced skin necrosis in 2 patients with protein S deficiency: successful reinstatement of warfarin therapy. *Haemostasis* 1992; **22**: 124–8.

38 Gailani D, Reese EP Jr. Anticoagulant-induced skin necrosis in a patient with hereditary deficiency of protein S. *Am J Hematol* 1999; **60**: 231–6.

39 Makris M, Bardhan G, Preston FE. Warfarin induced skin necrosis associated with activated protein C resistance (letter). *Thromb Haemost* 1995; **75**: 523–4.

40 Campbell R, Clanton TO, Heckman JD. Necrosis and gangrene as a complication of coumarin therapy. *J Bone Joint Surg* 1980; **62A**: 1016–17.

41 Van Amstel WJ, Boekhout-Mussert MJ, Loeliger EA. Successful prevention of coumarin-induced hemorrhagic skin necrosis by timely administration of vitamin K$_1$. *Blut* 1978; **36**: 89–93.

42 Schramm W, Spannagl M, Bauer KA, et al. Treatment of coumarin-induced skin necrosis with a monoclonal antibody purified protein C concentrate. *Arch Dermatol* 1993; **129**: 753–6.

43 Jillella AP, Lutcher CL. Reinstituting warfarin in patients who develop warfarin skin necrosis. *Am J Hematol* 1996; **52**: 117–19.

44 Zauber NP, Stark MW. Successful warfarin anticoagulation despite protein C deficiency and a history of warfarin necrosis. *Ann Intern Med* 1986; **104**: 659–60.

45 Baglin T. Disseminated intravascular coagulation: diagnosis and treatment. *BMJ* 1996; **312**: 683–7.

46 Feder W, Auerbach R. 'Purple toes': an uncommon sequela of oral coumarin drug therapy. *Ann Intern Med* 1961; **55**: 911–17.

47 Hyman BT, Landas SK, Ashman RF, Schelper RL, Robinson RA. Warfarin-related purple toes syndrome and cholesterol microembolization. *Am J Med* 1987; **82**: 1233–7.

48 Colt HG, Begg RJ, Saporito JJ, Cooper WM, Shapiro AP. Cholesterol emboli after cardiac catheterization. Eight cases and a review of the literature. *Medicine* 1988; **67**: 389–400.

49 Sallah S, Thomas DP, Roberts HR. Warfarin and heparin-induced skin necrosis and the

purple toe syndrome: infrequent complications of anticoagulant treatment. *Thromb Haemost* 1997; **78**: 785–90.

50 Fine MJ, Kapoor W, Falanga V. Cholesterol crystal embolization: a review of 221 cases in the English literature. *Angiology* 1987; **38**: 769–84.

51 Bols A, Nevelsteen A, Verhaughe R. Atheromatous embolization precipitated by oral anticoagulants. *Int Angiol* 1994; **13**: 271–3.

52 Kwong P, Roberts P, Prescott SM, Tikoff G. Dermatitis induced by warfarin. *JAMA* 1978; **239**: 1884–5.

53 Vermeer C, Knapen MHJ, Hamulyák K. Effects of vitamin K and oral anticoagulants on human bone metabolism. In: Poller L, Hirsh J, eds *Oral anticoagulants*. New York: Oxford University Press, 1996: 76–83.

54 Pettifor JM, Benson R. Congenital malformations associated with the administration of oral anticoagulants during pregnancy. *J Pediatr* 1975; **86**: 459–62.

55 Hall JG, Pauli RM, Wilson KM. Maternal and fetal sequelae of anticoagulation during pregnancy. *Am J Med* 1980; **68**: 122–40.

56 Letsky EA. Oral anticoagulants in pregnancy. In: Poller L, Hirsh J, eds *Oral anticoagulants*. New York: Oxford University Press, 1996: 192–215.

57 Stirling Y. Warfarin-induced changes in procoagulant and anticoagulant proteins. *Blood Coagul Fibrinolysis* 1995; **6**: 361–73.

58 Warkentin TE. Heparin-induced thrombocytopenia: IgG-mediated platelet activation, platelet microparticle generation, and altered procoagulant/anticoagulant balance in the pathogenesis of thrombosis and venous limb gangrene complicating heparin-induced thrombocytopenia. *Transf Med Rev* 1996; **10**: 249–58.

15

The management of anticoagulation before and after procedures

JOHN SPANDORFER

INTRODUCTION

Warfarin has been increasingly used to either treat or prevent thromboembolism; currently, over 1 million people are taking this anticoagulant.[1] Patients maintained on warfarin may occasionally need to stop their anticoagulation during invasive procedures. This chapter reviews the literature on bleeding risks of certain procedures; thrombosis risks of stopping anticoagulation; and heparin and warfarin pharmacokinetics. Recommendations regarding how to manage anticoagulated patients are discussed.

BLEEDING RISKS OF PROCEDURES

Although there are no randomized, prospective trials, the general consensus is that when a patient undergoes major surgery or surgery in which a body cavity is entered, the bleeding risk is high.[2] Therefore, patients undergoing these high-bleeding-risk procedures should be off warfarin and have an International Normalized Ratio (INR) of less than 1.5. For patients who are at high risk of thrombosis (see below), anticoagulation may be started in the postoperative period. However, postoperative anticoagulation may increase the rate of major bleeding by approximately 3%.[3] One area in which more caution is required is neurosurgery; most neurosurgeons recommend a normal INR prior to proceeding with surgery.[4] Restarting anticoagulation postoperatively may need to be delayed in neurosurgical patients.

There are various examples of minimally invasive procedures that have been safely performed while patients remain anticoagulated (Table 15.1). The literature, however, is limited due to the lack of prospective trials. Case reports have suggested that patients undergoing dental procedures, several types of ophthalmic procedures, and dermatologic procedures may be at low risk of bleeding while anticoagulated.

Table 15.1 *Procedures that can be performed while patients remain anticoagulated*

Ophthalmic surgery
Cataract surgery
Trabeculectomy
Vitreoretinal surgery
Dental procedures
Dental hygiene
Simple extractions
Restorations
Endodontics
Prosthetics

Routine general dental treatment, including dental hygiene treatments, restorations, endodontics, prosthetics, minor periodontal therapy, and uncomplicated extractions, poses a low risk for significant bleeding in the anticoagulated patient.[5,6] Multiple tooth extractions or other extensive surgeries may cause the patient to be at increased risk for bleeding and should be done with an INR less than 1.5.[5] Anticoagulated patients who have dental surgery and have prolonged bleeding may benefit from tranexamic acid mouthwash.[7] Tranexamic acid inhibits the proteolytic degradation of fibrin by preventing the attachment of plasminogen and plasmin.

Most ophthalmic procedures can be safely performed while the patient remains anticoagulated.[8] Case reports have shown that cataract surgery, trabeculectomy, and vitreoretinal surgery can be performed safely in anticoagulated patients.[8-12] Bleeding risk, however, is increased in patients undergoing complex lid, lacrimal, and orbital surgery.

Transurethral resection of the prostate has been reported to have been safely performed in anticoagulated patients.[13] Other clinicians remain skeptical and feel that it may only be safe when using laser therapy.[14]

There are no data examining the safety of performing endoscopies, with or without biopsies, among anticoagulated patients. A survey of 1269 gastroenterologists found that, depending on the indication for anticoagulation, 51–60% of physicians stopped warfarin before upper endoscopy, and 71–82% of physicians stopped warfarin before colonoscopies. The authors of the survey found a wide variation in the management of anticoagulation around endoscopies and argue that a consensus statement is needed.[15]

Very few data are available on the safety of cutaneous surgery among anticoagulated patients. One report reviewed 26 patients who required dermatologic surgery and were on warfarin.[16] Only one patient had a complication, and the authors concluded that cutaneous surgery can often be performed while patients are anticoagulated, although further studies were needed. No statements were made on the type of surgery that may increase the risk of bleeding.

Although no studies of anticoagulated patients undergoing podiatric procedures are available, one group of authors feel that it may be safe to perform minor procedures (nail avulsions, phenol matrixectomies) without stopping anticoagulation.[17] They recommended that more invasive procedures should be done off anticoagulation.

THROMBOSIS RISKS OF STOPPING ANTICOAGULATION (Table 15.2)

In order to determine the relative safety of discontinuing either warfarin or heparin for a specific duration, it is necessary to understand the risks of thrombosis when patients are off anticoagulants. Estimated below are the predicted thrombosis rates when patients with specific conditions are taken off anticoagulation. Variables that are difficult to account for include the thrombotic effect of surgery and a possible 'rebound' phenomenon off warfarin. Postoperatively, patients may develop a prothrombotic state. Elevated levels of fibrin degradation products (elevated fibrinogen degradation products, thrombin–antithrombin complexes, prothrombin F1+2 complexes), indicating increased fibrin formation, have been shown among trauma patients and patients undergoing elective hip surgery.[18] The discontinuation of warfarin may cause a rebound increase in clotting factors.[19] Although this theoretical effect may increase the likelihood of thrombotic complications, there has been no evidence that this occurs clinically.[20] There is no known rebound phenomenon when patients are taken off heparin.

Table 15.2 *Estimated risk of thromboembolic complication of anticoagulation in perioperative period*

Condition	Risk of thromboembolism (%)
Atrial fibrillation	0.012–0.3
Prosthetic valve	0.08–0.36
Deep vein thrombosis	
1st month	4–6
2nd–3rd month	0.8–1.2
3rd month	0.16–0.24

See text for details.

Atrial fibrillation

Patients who have atrial fibrillation and additional risk factors for stroke, such as mitral stenosis, prosthetic heart valves, heart failure, age greater than 65, hypertension, diabetes, previous stroke or transient ischemic attack, or thyrotoxicosis, and have no contraindications to anticoagulation have a decreased risk of stroke when placed on warfarin.[21] The use of warfarin decreases the risk of embolism among patients with nonvalvular atrial fibrillation by approximately 68%.[22] The annual risk of stroke without anticoagulation varies from 1% to 20%, depending on the number of risk factors for atrial fibrillation-associated stroke.[22] Therefore, the approximate risk of stroke per day while a patient has a subtherapeutic INR may be between 0.003% and 0.05%. A patient requiring discontinuation of warfarin during a procedure may have a subtherapeutic INR 2–3 days before the procedure and 2–3 days after the procedure, totaling 4–6 days. Therefore, the approximate risk of stroke during the temporary discontinuation of warfarin may be between 0.012% and 0.3%.

Prosthetic valves

Patients with mechanical prosthetic heart valves are at increased risk for thromboembolic complications, and anticoagulation, therefore, is the standard of care to prevent stroke. Patients with older, first-generation aortic mechanical valves (Ball, Bjork–Shiley, Lillehei–Kaster) and mechanical valves in the mitral position are at higher risk than those who have the newer generation valves and valves in the aortic position. Nevertheless, all patients should be anticoagulated. It is estimated that patients off anticoagulation have between an 8% and 22% risk per year of stroke.[23,24] Therefore, the approximate risk of stroke per day while a patient has a subtherapeutic INR may be between 0.02% and 0.06%. If a patient has a subtherapeutic INR for 4–6 days during a procedure, the approximate risk of stroke during the temporary discontinuation of warfarin may be between 0.08% and 0.36%.

Venous thromboembolic disease

Patients with deep vein thrombosis are also at increased risk for thrombotic complications off anticoagulants. Guidelines that recommend the duration of anticoagulation have recently been published.[25] Patients with deep vein thrombosis and who do not have ongoing risk factors for thrombosis may generally be anticoagulated for 3 months; patients with deep vein thrombosis and ongoing risk factors for thrombosis should be anticoagulated for at least 6 months. It has been estimated that stopping anticoagulation in the first month after an acute event is associated with up to a 1% per day absolute increase in the risk of recurrent venous thromboembolism.[3] Stopping anticoagulation during the second and third month after an acute event may be associated with up to a 0.2% per day absolute increase in the risk of recurrent venous thromboembolism. Following the third month, the risk decreases further, to a 0.04% per day absolute increase in the risk of recurrent venous thromboembolism.

Hypercoagulable states

Patients who have had a thrombotic event may be found to have a hypercoagulable state such as factor V Leiden mutation, prothrombin gene mutation, anticardiolipin antibody, protein C deficiency, protein S deficiency, or antithrombin III deficiency. The risk of a thrombotic event while these patients have anticoagulation briefly discontinued is not known. Probable factors for increased risk for thrombosis while briefly off anticoagulation include recent thrombotic event, recurrent thrombosis, and life-threatening thrombotic complication.

WARFARIN AND HEPARIN PHARMACOKINETICS

When anticoagulation is discontinued prior to a procedure, it is preferable to maintain the patient off anticoagulation for the shortest possible time that would allow for an INR low enough to perform the procedure safely. In order to know how many days prior to a procedure warfarin and heparin should be discontinued, it is necessary to understand the pharmacokinetics of both of these agents.

Warfarin

There is only one study published which has examined the decrease in INR over time after the discontinuation of warfarin. White et al. studied 22 patients receiving warfarin who required a discontinuation of warfarin prior to a procedure.[26] They found that the INR decreased exponentially, with a wide variation in the rate of decrease (Fig. 15.1). Increased age was associated with a slower rate of decrease. They

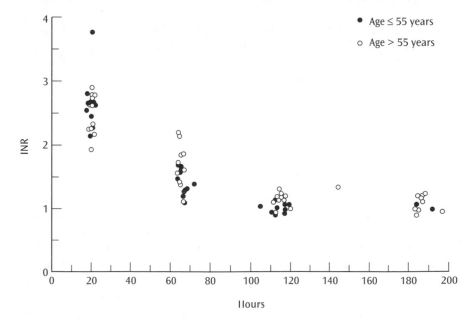

Figure 15.1 *Decrease in the International Normalized Ratio (INR) over time after discontinuation of warfarin therapy. The measured INR is depicted as a function of time after the last dose of warfarin. (After White, 1995 reprinted with permission.[26])*

recommended that, among patients who had a steady-state INR between 2.0 and 3.0, warfarin should be held between 96 and 115 hours (4–5 days). Warfarin should be held for a longer duration for patients with a higher INR.

Patients restarted on warfarin take about 4–5 days to reach a therapeutic INR.[27] They should be started on their previous dose of warfarin; there does not appear to be any advantage in giving a higher initial 'loading dose.'[28]

Heparin

Patients receiving standard heparin intravenously may have their anticoagulant effect reversed after 2–3 hours off heparin, the precise time varying with the dose of heparin. The biologic half-life of standard heparin is 30 minutes with an intravenous bolus of 25 U/kg, and 60 minutes with an intravenous bolus of 100 U/kg.

Low molecular weight heparins (LMWHs) have variable half-lives. Enoxaparin (Lovenox), given at 4000 anti-Xa inhibitory units (IU aXa) should have insignificant antifactor Xa levels 12–15 hours following injection.[29,30] Dalteparin (Fragmin), given at 2500 IU aXa, and nadroparin (Fraxiparin), at 3000 IU aXa, should also have an insignificant antifactor Xa level 15 hours following injection.[29] Therefore, invasive procedures may be carried out without an increase in the hemorrhagic risk after 15 hours following the last dose of these LMWHs. The half-life of all heparin products may be longer in patients with impaired renal function.

ANTICOAGULATION AND ANESTHESIA

General anesthesia can be administered safely to the anticoagulated patient. However, the following precautions have been recommended.[31]

1. Ideally, administration of the anesthesia should be oral or intravenous rather than intramuscular or subcutaneous.
2. If central venous access is needed, inserting the line through the brachial vein in the antecubital fossa is preferred over the internal jugular or subclavian vein.
3. Laryngoscopy and tracheal intubation should be atraumatic, and nasogastic tubes should be avoided because of the high incidence of epistaxis.

Several reports have shown that bleeding and neurologic dysfunction (including paraplegia) may occur when a spinal or epidural catheter is inserted or removed in the patient who is anticoagulated.[32–4] However, there have been ample reports demonstrating the safety of both standard heparin and LMWH after epidural and spinal anesthesia has been started.[35,36] Anticoagulation should therefore be fully reversed prior to epidural or spinal catheter placement or removal. Full reversal may be performed by discontinuing standard heparin at least 2–3 hours and LMWH at least 12 hours prior to catheter placement or removal. Standard heparin or LMWH may then be restarted 2 hours after catheter placement or removal. Restarting anticoagulation should be delayed several hours if blood appears during the insertion or withdrawal of the needle or catheter.

RECOMMENDATIONS

Patients undergoing procedures with a low bleeding risk

Procedures considered to be a low bleeding risk are cataract procedures, trabeculectomy, vitreoretinal surgery, routine dental treatment, simple extractions, and most cutaneous surgery.

These patients can proceed with their procedure with an INR on the 'low end' of the therapeutic range (approximately 2.0). Thus, if the INR is on the 'high end' of the therapeutic range (approximately 3.0), warfarin can be discontinued for 1 or 2 days and then restarted on the evening following the procedure. Restarting warfarin should be delayed if bleeding complications occur as a result of the procedure.

Patients with a low thrombosis risk undergoing procedures with a high bleeding risk

Patients considered at low risk for thrombosis are those who have atrial fibrillation without risk factors for stroke, patients with deep vein thrombosis treated at least 1 month after the acute event, and patients with a hypercoagulable state without a recent thrombotic complication, recurrent thrombosis, or history of a life-threatening thrombosis (Table 15.3).

Table 15.3 *Thrombosis risk in perioperative period*

High
Mitral mechanical valves
Older (first-generation) aortic mechanical valves (ball, Bjork–Shiley, Lillehei–Kaster)
Atrial fibrillation plus a history of stroke or multiple risk factors for stroke
Deep venous thrombosis diagnosed within the last month
Hypercoagulable state plus recent thrombosis or history of life-threatening thrombosis
Low
Newer (second-generation) aortic mechanical valve
Atrial fibrillation without multiple risk factors for stroke
Deep venous thrombosis treated for more than 1 month

See text for details.

These patients should have their warfarin stopped 4–5 days prior to the procedure. The INR should be assessed on the morning of the procedure. If the INR is above 1.5, the procedure should be delayed until 1 or 2 days later and the INR should be reassessed. If the procedure needs to be done more urgently, vitamin K at 0.5–1.0 mg can be given either orally or subcutaneously to reverse the warfarin. Higher doses of vitamin K should be avoided as they may cause resistance to warfarin anticoagulation for several days following the procedure.

After the procedure, warfarin should be restarted. Patients who are being anticoagulated for deep vein thrombosis and are at bedrest postoperatively are at increased risk for recurrent thromboembolic disease. Heparin should be started in these patients after the procedure and maintained either until the INR is greater than 2.0 or the patient is ambulatory. However, restarting anticoagulation should be delayed if bleeding complications occur as a result of the procedure.

Patients with a high thrombosis risk undergoing procedures with a high bleeding risk

Patients with a high thrombosis risk include patients with mechanical valves (particularly mechanical valves in the mitral position), patients with atrial fibrillation with multiple risk factors for stroke, and patients with a hypercoagulable state with recurrent thrombosis, recent thrombosis (within the past month), or life-threatening thrombosis (Table 15.3). When these patients require surgery that is considered to be associated with a high risk of bleeding, anticoagulation should be continued as close as possible to the procedure and started soon after the procedure to help minimize any thrombotic complications.

The following may be done to minimize the risk of both bleeding and thrombosis in these patients. Patients may have their warfarin discontinued 4–5 days preoperatively. Once the INR is subtherapeutic, patients may start on either intravenous heparin (typically requiring hospitalization) or adjusted-dose subcutaneous heparin (aPTT 6 hours after heparin injection should be approximately two times control; heparin should be dosed every 12 hours). Intravenous heparin should be discontinued at least 2 hours preoperatively; subcutaneous heparin should be discontinued 12 hours preoperatively. Heparin (intravenous or subcutaneous) along with warfarin may be started postoperatively once there are no contraindications to anticoagulation. Restarting anticoagulation may be delayed up to 48 hours if the surgeon feels the bleeding risks are too high. Heparin may then be discontinued once the INR is therapeutic.

Although not yet approved for this indication, LMWHs can probably be safely substituted for standard heparin. For instance, enoxaparin can be given at doses ranging between 30 mg every 12 hours and 1 mg/kg every 12 hours; the higher dosages are reserved for those at highest risk for thrombosis, such as mitral mechanical valve patients. Enoxaparin should be stopped at least 12 hours preoperatively and should not be used postoperatively until the surgeon feels the bleeding risk is acceptable.

REFERENCES

1 Spandorfer JM, Merli GJ. Outpatient anticoagulation issues for the primary care physician. *Med Clin N Am* 1996; **80**: 475–91.

2 Travis S, Wray R, Harrison K. Perioperative anticoagulant control. *Br J Surg* 1989; **76**: 1107–8.

3 Kearon C, Hirsh J. Management of anticoagulation before and after elective surgery. *N Engl J Med* 1997; **336**: 1506–11.

4 Allen MB, Johnston KW. Preoperative evaluation: complications, their prevention and treatment. In: Youmans JR, ed. *Neurologic surgery* Philadelphia: WB Saunders, 1990: 833–45.

5   Weibert RT. Oral anticoagulant therapy in patients undergoing dental surgery. *Clin Pharmcol* 1992; **11**: 857–64.

6   McIntyre H. Management, during dental surgery, of patients on anticoagulants. *Lancet* 1966; **2**: 99–100.

7   Sindet-Pedersen S, Ramstrom G, Bernvil S, et al. Hemostatic effect of tranexamic acid mouthwash in anticoagulated patients undergoing oral surgery. *N Engl J Med* 1989; **320**: 840–3.

8   McCormack P, Simcock PR, Tullo AB. Management of the anticoagulated patient for ophthalmic surgery. *Eye* 1993; **7**: 749–50.

9   Robinson GA, Nylander A. Warfarin and cataract extraction. *Br J Ophthalmol* 1989; **73**: 702–3.

10 Gainey SP, Robertson DM, Fay W, Ilstrup D. Ocular surgery on patients receiving long-term warfarin therapy. *Am J Ophthalmol* 1989; **108**: 142–6.

11 McMahan LB. Anticoagulants and cataract surgery. *J Cataract Refract Surg* 1988; **14**: 569–71.

12 Moll AC, Van Rij G. Anticoagulant therapy and cataract surgery. *Doc Ophthalmol* 1989; **72**: 367–73.

13 Parr NJ, Loh CS, Desmond AD. Transurethral resection of the prostate and bladder tumour without withdrawal of warfarin therapy. *Br J Urol* 1989; **64**: 623–25.

14 Bolton DM, Costello AJ. Management of benign prostatic hyperplasia by transurethral laser ablation in patients treated with warfarin anticoagulation. *J Urol* 1994; **151**: 79–81.

15 Kadakia SC, Angueira CE, Ward JA, Moore M. Gastrointestinal endoscopy in patients taking antiplatelet agents and anticoagulants: survey of ASGE memebers. *Gastrointest Endosc* 1996; **44**: 309–16.

16 Otley CC, Fewkes JL, Frank W, Olbricht SM. Complications of cutaneous surgery in patients who are taking warfarin, aspirin, or nonsteroidal anti-inflammatory drugs. *Arch Derm* 1996; **132**: 161–6.

17 Lanzat M, Danna AT, Jacobson DS. New protocols for perioperative management of podiatric patients taking oral anticoagulants. *J Foot Ankle Surg* 1994; **33**: 16–19.

18 Lassen MR, Borris LC. Prevention in orthopedic surgery and trauma. In: Hull R, Pineo G, eds *Disorders of thrombosis*. Philadelphia: WB Saunders, 1996: 209–16.

19 Genewein U, Haeberli A, Straub PW, Beer JH. Rebound after cessation or oral anticoagulant therapy: the biochemical evidence. *Br J Haematol* 1996; **92**: 479–85.

20 Palareti G, Legnani C. Warfarin withdrawal: pharmacokinetic–pharmacodynamic considerations. *Clin Pharmacokin* 1996; **30**: 300–13.

21 Laupacis A, Albers GW, Dunn MI, Feinberg WM. Antithrombotic therapy in atrial fibrillation. *Chest* 1992; **102** (Suppl.): 426S–33S.

22 Risk factors for stroke and efficacy of antithrombotic therapy in atrial fibrillation. Analysis of pooled data from five randomized controlled trials. *Arch Int Med* 1994; **154**: 1449–57.

23 Baudet EM, Oca CC, Roques XF, et al. A 5 1/2 year experience with the St. Jude medical cardiac valve prosthesis: early and late results of 737 valve replacements in 671 patients. *J Thor Cardiovasc Surg* 1985; **90**: 137–44.

24 Cannegieter SC, Rosendaal FR, Briet E. Thromboembolic and bleeding complications in patients with mechanical heart valve prostheses. *Circulation* 1994; **89**: 635–41.

25 Hirsh J. Duration of anticoagulant therapy after first episode of venous thrombosis in patients with inherited thrombophilia. *Arch Intern Med* 1997; **157**: 2174–7.

26 White RH, McKittrick T, Hutchinson R, Twitchell J. Temporary discontinuation of warfarin therapy: changes in the international normalized ratio. *Ann Intern Med* 1995; **122**: 40–2.
27 Hirsh J, Dalen JE, Deykin D, et al. Mechanisms of action, clinical effectiveness, and optimal therapeutic range. *Chest* 1995; **108**: 231S–46S.
28 Harrison L, Johnston M, Massicotte MP, et al. Comparison of 5-mg and 10-mg loading doses in initiation of warfarin therapy. *Ann Intern Med* 1997; **126**: 133–6.
29 Collignon F, Frydman A, Caplain H, et al. Comparison of the pharmacokinetic profiles of three low molecular mass heparins – dalteparin, enoxaparin and nadroparin-administered subcutaneously in healthy volunteers (doses for prevention of thromboembolism). *Thromb Haemost* 1995; **73**: 630–40.
30 Agnelli G, Iorio A, Renga C, et al. Prolonged antithrombin activity of low-molecular weight heparins. *Circulation* 1995; **92**: 2819–24.
31 Stow PJ, Burrows FA. Anticoagulants in anaesthesia. *Can J Anaesth* 1987; **34**: 632–49.
32 Vandermeulen EP, Van Aken H, Vermylen J. Anticoagulants and spinal–epidural anesthesia. *Anesth Analg* 1994; **79**: 1165–77.
33 Porterfield W, Wu C. Epidural hematoma in an ambulatory surgical patient. *J Clin Anesth* 1997; **9**: 74–7.
34 Hynson J, Katz J, Bueff H. Epidural hematoma associated with enoxaparin. *Anesth Analg* 1996; **82**: 1072–5.
35 Horlocker TT, Heit JA. Low molecular weight heparin: biochemistry, pharmacology, perioperative prophylaxis regimens and guidelines for regional anesthetic management. *Anesth Analg* 1997; **85**: 874–85.
36 Rao TLK, El-Etr AA. Anticoagulation following placement of epidural and subarachnoid catheters: an evaluation of neurologic sequelae. *Anesthesiology* 1981; **55**: 618–20.

16

Thrombosis and its treatment during pregnancy

SANJEEV D CHUNILAL, JEFF S GINSBERG

INTRODUCTION

The purpose of this review is to provide guidelines for the management of venous thromboembolism in pregnancy. This chapter is divided into three sections: first, the frequency of venous thromboembolism is discussed and the unique physiology of pregnancy and how this brings about changes which favor venous thromboembolism in pregnancy. The second section focuses on the diagnosis, discusses appropriate tests to perform for deep vein thrombosis and pulmonary embolism, and deals briefly with new technology. Finally, the management of venous thromboembolism during pregnancy is discussed, with emphasis on the side-effects, for the mother and fetus, of anticoagulation, and on guidelines for treatment and prophylaxis.

INCIDENCE

Pulmonary embolism is a common cause of maternal mortality. In a cohort study of almost 170 000 pregnancies by Rutherford et al.,[1] the incidence of venous thromboembolism was 0.055% – which includes deep vein thrombosis (0.038%) and pulmonary embolism (0.017%). In a cohort study of patients with antepartum deep vein thrombosis, Ginsberg et al.[2] reported that 21.7% occurred in the first trimester, 46.7% in the second trimester, and 31.7% in the third; they also demonstrated a remarkable predisposition to left-leg deep vein thrombosis.

PATHOPHYSIOLOGY

Virchow's triad postulates that thrombosis requires altered coagulation, blood stasis and vascular injury. Each of these factors is altered in pregnancy and may contribute to a predisposition to venous thromboembolism.

Altered coagulation

This can be further divided into changes in procoagulant proteins and anticoagulant proteins and an altered balance of fibrinolysis. Of the procoagulant proteins, fibrinogen, factors VII, VIII, X, and von Willebrand factor rise markedly throughout pregnancy.[3,4] Of the inhibitors of coagulation, free protein S levels have been shown to decrease during pregnancy; the magnitude of reduction is comparable to that seen with protein S deficiency.[5] Protein C levels fluctuate from baseline, but are not consistently lowered during pregnancy.[6] Both functional and antigenic antithrombin III levels remain normal or are slightly reduced throughout all three trimesters.

All studies show gradual increases during pregnancy of the plasminogen activators tissue plasminogen activator (t-PA) and urokinase plasminogen activator (u-PA), with corresponding increases in their inhibitors, plasminogen activator inhibitors 1 and 2 (PAI-1 and PAI-2).[7,8] The net effect of these changes is a reduction in global fibrinolysis.[3]

Blood stasis

Lower limb venous dynamic studies have shown that there is increased venous stasis when flow through the femoral vein is measured by ultrasound. There is a gradual increase in the degree of obstruction from the first trimester to the third trimester. The degree of obstruction to flow is highly position and trimester dependent. The observed venous stasis is also compounded by a decrease in venous tone.[9,10]

Vascular injury

Endothelial injury-related thrombosis is the hallmark of arterial disease, particularly unstable angina. In venous thrombosis, the contribution of vascular injury is less; whether endothelial injury occurs at the point of compression of the left iliac vein by the right iliac artery is also not established.

In summary, pregnancy appears to be associated with an increased risk of venous thromboembolism, which most ascribe to a 'hypercoagulable state' based on the increased levels of several clotting factors, reduced levels of free protein S, and, possibly, a global reduction in fibrinolysis. Elevated levels of factor VII, VIII, and fibrinogen have been identified as risk factors for arterial but not venous thrombosis, in some way implicating the elevated levels of clotting factors and/or decreased fibrinolysis.[11]

Additionally, there is altered venous tone and evidence of increasing obstruction to venous outflow in the lower limb. None of the above in isolation is sufficient to cause thrombosis, but combined with the increased anatomical compression of the left iliac vein, each of these factors probably becomes additive and has the potential to cause thrombosis in pregnancy.

DIAGNOSIS

This can be divided into the diagnosis of deep vein thrombosis and the diagnosis of pulmonary embolism, although the two comprise a continuum of venous thromboembolic disease, and the presence of one may be indicative of the other.

Deep venous thrombosis

Contrast venography is the 'gold standard,' but it is invasive, sometimes technically difficult, requires contrast, and is often not available. The diagnosis of venous thrombosis is made when a constant intraluminal filling defect on at least two views is seen; persistent nonfilling of a vessel is suspicious, but not diagnostic. Noninvasive tests such as impedance plethysmography, compression ultrasound, and, more recently, D-dimer assays have replaced venography as initial tests in symptomatic patients with suspected deep vein thrombosis.

NONINVASIVE TESTING: IMPEDANCE PLETHYSMOGRAPHY AND COMPRESSION ULTRASOUND

Impedance plethysmography
The principle of the procedure is based on the observation that changes in blood volume in the calf, produced by inflation and deflation of a pneumatic thigh cuff which alters venous return, result in changes in electrical resistance detected at the skin surface. These changes are altered in patients with obstruction of the popliteal or more proximal veins.[12]

Compression ultrasound
Compression ultrasound examines the compressibility of the common femoral vein at the level of the inguinal ligament, the popliteal vein behind the knee, and at the trifurcation of calf veins. Using this technique, the iliac vessels are not routinely visualized. If the ultrasound probe is able to completely compress the vein in the transverse plane, then the test is normal.[13]

Both impedance plethysmography and compression ultrasound are sensitive to proximal deep vein thrombosis (approximately 90% and >95%, respectively), but less sensitive for calf deep vein thrombosis.[13] Impedance plethysmography has been validated by clinical trials (in pregnant and nonpregnant patients) in which anticoagulant therapy was safely withheld in symptomatic outpatients with negative serial tests.[12,14] Similarly, clinical trials have shown that anticoagulants can be safely withheld in symptomatic nonpregnant outpatients with normal serial compression ultrasound, but this approach has not been tested in pregnant patients.[15]

Of the patients who present with symptomatic deep vein thrombosis, approximately 20% have calf deep vein thrombosis at presentation and, of these, about one-fifth are destined to extend proximally, within 1 week. It is for this reason that serial testing has evolved – to detect late extension of a calf deep vein thrombosis, because isolated calf deep vein thrombosis rarely causes pulmonary embolism in nonpregnant patients.[12,15] The natural history of calf deep vein thrombosis in pregnancy is not understood. An additional concern is the impression that isolated iliac vein thrombosis has an increased incidence in pregnancy.

How is deep vein thrombosis during pregnancy best diagnosed?

The only prospectively tested and validated approach for managing pregnant women with clinically suspected deep vein thrombosis is serial impedance plethysmography.[14] Anticoagulant therapy can be safely withheld in women with three serial negative tests. Care should be taken in the third trimester to avoid a false-positive test (due to extrinsic compression of the iliac vein by the gravid uterus) by lying women in the lateral decubitus position for 30 minutes prior to testing.

As compression ultrasound is more sensitive than impedance plethysmography in detecting proximal deep vein thrombosis,[13,15] it is reasonable to substitute serial compression ultrasound for impedance plethysmography and withhold treatment in women with serially negative tests. However, one concern is that compression ultrasound may be insensitive to isolated iliac vein thrombosis. If there is a high clinical suspicion of iliac deep vein thrombosis and compression ultrasound is negative, venography should be performed, with appropriate precautions to limit fetal radiation exposure: venography is relatively safe for the fetus in pregnancy.[16] Alternatively, if venography cannot be performed, and there is a strong clinical suspicion of iliac deep vein thrombosis, two reasonable options are: (1) magnetic resonance imaging of the pelvis and lower limb (described below), or (2) Doppler ultrasound of the iliac vessels, looking for evidence of intraluminal thrombus. Neither of these latter two methods has been prospectively validated (Fig. 16.1).

Pulmonary embolism

Venous thromboembolism is a spectrum with pulmonary embolism representing one end and deep vein thrombosis the other. This is illustrated by the fact that about one-half of patients presenting with proximal deep vein thrombosis have evidence of asymptomatic pulmonary embolism, demonstrated by a high-probability ventilation/perfusion (V/Q) scan, and many patients with pulmonary embolism have asymptomatic proximal deep vein thrombosis.[17] As the treatments for pulmonary embolism and deep vein thrombosis are essentially the same, when pulmonary embolism is suspected, it is reasonable to first look for deep vein thrombosis, and treat the patient if it is present. However, the absence of lower limb deep vein throm-

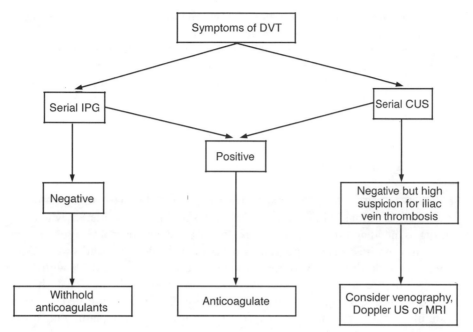

Figure 16.1. *An algorithm for diagnosis of deep vein thrombosis (DVT) in pregnant patients. (IPG = impedance plethysmography; CUS = compression ultrasound; US = ultrasound; MRI = magnetic resonance imaging.)*

bosis should not preclude performing a V/Q scan, as many patients with pulmonary embolism will have normal objective tests for deep vein thrombosis.[18]

VENTILATION/PERFUSION SCAN

Using pulmonary angiography as the 'gold standard,' the Prospective Investigation of Pulmonary Embolism Diagnosis (PIOPED) investigators found a positive predictive value of just under 90% for a high-probability lung scan and a negative predictive value of 90–96% for normal or near-normal lung scans. Over 75% of the remaining patients had intermediate-probability scans and for these patients pulmonary angiography was the only reliable method for excluding the presence of pulmonary embolism.[19] Hull and colleagues used serial impedance plethysmography to follow patients with nondiagnostic V/Q scans and normal cardiorespiratory reserve. Using this strategy, they were able to withhold anticoagulant treatment safely in patients with serially negative impedance plethysmography.[20]

Pregnant patients were excluded from the above studies; therefore, how do these studies relate to pregnant women? There are several potential differences between these patients and pregnant women.

1. The average age of patients in PIOPED was 56 years, an average 20–30 years older than pregnant women.
2. In pregnant women, lung perfusion is increased, as evidenced by decreased pulmonary vascular resistance, an unchanged pressure gradient across the pulmonary circulation, and increased cardiac output.[21]

3. There are a number of physiological changes that occur in ventilation during pregnancy, the most important of which occurs during the last month or so; this is the increased closure of small airways at normal tidal volumes, which can be reflected by a mild increase in the arterial–alveolar gradient.[21] The significance of this with respect to V/Q scanning is unclear, but is likely to leave perfusion unchanged but affect ventilation, and so potentially cause areas reverse of mismatch.

PULMONARY ANGIOGRAPHY

The diagnostic criteria of pulmonary embolism on a pulmonary angiography is a constant intraluminal filling defect. This test should be considered when V/Q scanning is nondiagnostic. So, what are the risks of angiography? From a large cohort study in which 1111 angiograms were performed, 0.5% of deaths were associated with the procedure, 1% with major nonfatal complications, and 5% with minor complications.[22] In addition, there is some radiation absorbed by the fetus when the test is performed, although it is our strong opinion that, when indicated, the small risk should not preclude its performance.[16] Our approach to pregnant women with suspected pulmonary embolism is shown in Fig. 16.2.

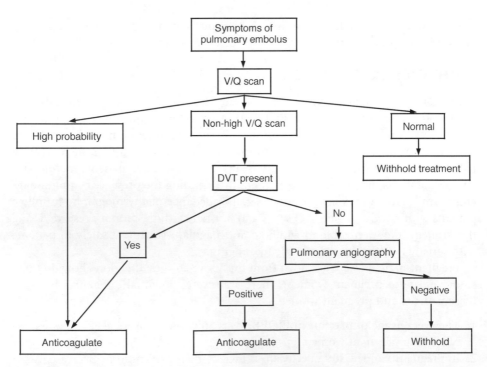

Figure 16.2 *An algorithm for diagnosis of pulmonary embolism. (V/Q = ventilation/perfusion; DVT = deep vein thrombosis.)*

New developments

Recent advances are beginning to offer noninvasive alternatives to pulmonary angiography and venography in nonpregnant patients and may be applicable in the future to pregnant women.

D-DIMER ASSAYS

D-dimer assays have been used for the exclusion of deep vein thrombosis and pulmonary embolism, and in clinical trials the negative predictive value of certain kits is over 95%.[23,24] The sensitivity and specificity of a D-dimer assay for deep vein thrombosis are dependent on the method of testing and, in some cases, on the intrinsic properties of the kit.[24] There have been no prospective clinical trials using D-dimer as a screening investigation in pregnant women, although D-dimers are likely to have high negative predictive value.

SPIRAL COMPUTED TOMOGRAPHY

Spiral computed tomography (CT) is appealing because it is fast and adequate pictures can be obtained on single breath hold at peak opacification. In retrospective small studies of selected patients, the technique has a sensitivity and specificity of over 90% for central emboli. It is, however, insensitive to embolic occlusion of subsegmental vessels and vessels of the lingula and right middle lobe.[25–7] To date, there have been no prospective management studies using spiral CT.

MAGNETIC RESONANCE ANGIOGRAPHY

Preliminary results in a small study with selected patients with symptoms of pulmonary embolism reported a sensitivity of at least 75%, but a specificity of over 95%. As with spiral CT, magnetic resonance angiography is also insensitive for small subsegmental pulmonary vessels. It should be safe in pregnancy as it does not use ionizing radiation and uses a non-nephrotoxic contrast agent.[28,29]

Magnetic resonance angiography is probably as sensitive and specific (96–100%, 92–100%, respectively) for deep vein thrombosis as compression ultrasound.[30] Its utility is limited by its cost, but it may have a role in the diagnosis of isolated iliac vein thrombosis for which, in selected studies of nonpregnant patients, its performance is superior to that of compression ultrasound.[31,32] There is limited experience of its use in pregnancy.[33]

Postpartum ovarian vein thrombosis

Postpartum ovarian vein thrombosis is an uncommon complication, whose exact incidence is not known, but with improved imaging techniques it is being diagnosed more frequently. Current estimates range from 1 in 569 to 1 in 6000 deliveries.[34,35] This syndrome is characterized by fever and right lower quadrant pain, usually occurring 1–2 days postpartum. Typically, the fever fails to respond to antibiotics after 24–48 hours. Vaginal examination often reveals a tender right adnexal mass.

The right ovarian vein is predominantly involved and this predilection for the right side is thought to be secondary to increased antegrade flow into the right side and retrograde flow from the left vein, such that all the pelvic blood flow postpartum is through the right ovarian vein.[36,37] Enlargement of the right ovarian vein is such that it may compress the right ureter, leading to pyuria and infection.

Diagnosis remains difficult unless there is a high index of clinical suspicion, particularly when postpartum pyelonephritis or endometritis fails to resolve with antibiotics. The diagnosis may be made on ultrasound, but CT is more often diagnostic; on CT, an enlarged ovarian vein, often dilated to the size of the inferior vena cava, looks like a sausage-shaped structure in the right paracolic gutter, which disappears at the level of the renal veins.[35,36] Often, thrombus is seen on contrast-enhanced scans and it may extend into the inferior vena cava. The exact incidence of proximal extension and subsequent of pulmonary embolism is not known.

Conventional practice has been to treat affected patients with 1 week of heparin therapy. However, if there is clear extension into the inferior vena cava or beyond, then the women should be treated with long-term anticoagulants, the duration depending on the extent of proximal progression.

MANAGEMENT OF VENOUS THROMBOEMBOLISM

The usual therapy of deep vein thrombosis/pulmonary embolism in nonpregnant patients is initially unfractionated heparin (UFH) or low molecular weight heparin (LMWH), followed by long-term warfarin.

Heparin is a glycosaminoglycan composed of variable-length saccharide units. Its anticoagulant effect is related to its ability to bind to and subsequently cause a conformational change in antithrombin III. The complex of antithrombin III and heparin rapidly increases the inactivation of thrombin, at a rate greater than the inactivation of thrombin by antithrombin III alone. The heparin–antithrombin III complex also inactivates factor Xa.[36] The binding of heparin to antithrombin III is through a critical pentasaccharide sequence. The ability of heparin to bind thrombin is also related to its length, and a minimum of 18 saccharides is required for heparin to bind thrombin and antithrombin III at the same time; in doing so, it acts as a template in hastening the interaction between thrombin and antithrombin III.[37]

Warfarin, a coumarin derivative, is an anticoagulant which inhibits the vitamin K-dependent post-translational carboxylation of prothrombin and factors VII, IX, and X. Post-translational carboxylation allows these proteins to bind calcium and thereby undergo conformational changes essential for binding their cofactors on phospholipid surfaces.[38]

Each of these drugs has been used in pregnant women but, as with any drug in pregnancy, one has to consider the potential for adverse experiences in both the mother and the fetus. For the fetus, the most important potential side-effects are teratogenicity, death, and bleeding, whereas for the mother, relevant issues include efficacy, risks of bleeding, and other side-effects.

Safety for the fetus

UFH and LMWH do not cross the placenta,[39,40] and therefore are unlikely to cause hemorrhage or be teratogenic. Several recent studies support the safety of UFH and LMWH for the fetus.[41–2]

Warfarin is relatively contraindicated in pregnancy, because it is teratogenic and can cause fetal bleeding. Warfarin exposure is associated with embryopathy when used between 6 and 12 weeks of gestation; this clinical syndrome consists of a characteristic facies with nasal hypoplasia, flattening of the nasal bridge, epiphyseal stippling (seen on x-rays), and telecanthus: some infants may have respiratory distress because of nasal hypoplasia.[43]

There are a number of case reports in the literature of central nervous system-related abnormalities and optic atrophy related to warfarin exposure at any time in pregnancy; although the true risk is unknown, it is likely to be small.[44]

Finally, because it crosses the placenta, warfarin can cause hemorrhage in the fetus and is likely to be hazardous at the time of delivery. Neither heparin nor warfarin crosses into breast milk in amounts that cause an anticoagulant effect in the neonate, and it is safe for the baby to breast feed when the mother is taking either or both medications.[44]

Consequently, heparin is the anticoagulant of choice during pregnancy, because it is safe for the fetus. There is no doubt that warfarin should be avoided between 6 and 12 weeks of gestation and close to term, but its use at other times is probably safe.

Safety for the mother

The main side-effects associated with heparin are osteoporosis, thrombocytopenia, bleeding, and skin rash.

OSTEOPOROSIS

Prolonged use of heparin is known to cause osteoporosis. The exact mechanism and etiology are not known; however, there is a preponderance for vertebral bone. Vertebral bone is more metabolically active compared to cortical bone, which may explain its susceptibility.[45]

Bone mass densitometry studies show that UFH can cause a mean bone mass density loss of around 7.1%, which is equivalent to 2 years of postmenopausal bone loss.[46] The heparin-associated bone loss in pregnancy appears to be at least partly reversible.[47] There are no trials which look at interventions to prevent heparin-induced osteoporosis. Dahlman and colleagues reported an incidence of symptomatic fracture of 2.2% of pregnant women treated with UFH;[48] the estimated incidence of symptomatic fracture in pregnant women using LMWH is probably lower.[49–51]

HEPARIN-INDUCED THROMBOCYTOPENIA

The severe life-threatening HIT (type II) is an IgG-mediated immune thrombocytopenia which leads to platelet activation and paradoxical arterial or venous thrombosis.[52] The reported incidence in certain patient populations has been 1–3% for

UFH and lower for LMWH.[53,54] Although there are no accurate estimates of the incidence of type II HIT in pregnancy, it is probably rare in patients treated with UFH and even less common with LMWH.[55]

As there is a high risk of thrombosis in the presence of an HIT antibody, women with HIT should be started on alternative anticoagulant treatment. Danaparoid sodium (Orgaran®) is a heparanoid that has negligible clinical cross-reactivity with the HIT antibody, and has been widely used as an anticoagulant in HIT-positive patients. Orgaran® does not cross the placenta and so it should be safe for the fetus.[56]

BLEEDING

In nonpregnant patients, the incidence of bleeding with UFH is dependent on the dose given, the method of administration, and the clinical context in which it is administered; biologically, there should be no reason why this should be untrue in pregnancy.[57]

The McMaster University experience of bleeding in pregnancy was two major bleeds in 45 women receiving full anticoagulant doses of UFH and no bleeds in a further 55 women receiving UFH 5000 U twice daily.[43] For the prevention and treatment of deep vein thrombosis in nonpregnant patients, LMWHs have generally produced equivalent or less bleeding than UFH[58,59] and are likely to show similar trends in pregnant women.

At McMaster University, an approach to pregnant women receiving full-dose anticoagulants is to discontinue UFH (or LMWH) for at least 24 hours prior to the elective induction of labor, and to monitor the activated partial thromboplastin time (aPTT) (if on UFH) so that hemostasis is normal at the time of delivery. This practice was adopted after a small study showed that women who had received their last subcutaneous injection within 28 hours of delivery were likely to have a prolonged aPTT at the time of delivery. Most patients are started on intravenous heparin within 12–24 hours after delivery.[60]

As intravenous UFH has a short half-life, in many instances stopping therapy will stop blood loss. In patients who have excessive bleeding, a protamine infusion may be required to reverse the effects of subcutaneous heparin. If patients bleed while receiving LMWH, protamine should be considered, because it neutralizes the high molecular weight subfractions thought to contribute most to bleeding.

SKIN REACTIONS

Walker et al.[61] reported a 50% incidence of bruising at the injection site with prolonged use of subcutaneous UFH therapy, with about 4% of patients complaining of severe pain at the injection site. When the injection techniques were checked, 31% required revision of the injection method used. In order to reduce the incidence of pain at injection sites, an indwelling subcutaneous Teflon catheter can be used.[62] Heparin-induced skin necrosis is a rare problem seen with either UFH or LMWH and may be immune mediated.[63,64]

TREATMENT OF ANTEPARTUM ACUTE VENOUS THROMBOEMBOLISM

Conventional treatment for pregnant women with acute venous thromboembolism has been intravenous UFH initially, followed by conversion to subcutaneous treatment. In the nonpregnant population, an appropriate regimen for anticoagulation is to use a 5000-unit bolus of intravenous unfractionated heparin, followed by a starting infusion of at least 30 000 units per day.[65] Table 16.1 outlines an intravenous heparin nomogram that has been validated for dose adjustments in nonpregnant patients and is reasonable in pregnancy. Twice-daily, subcutaneous, full-dose heparin should be continued for the duration of the pregnancy.

Table 16.1 *Full-dose intravenous heparin nomogram*[a]

aPTT (s)	Bolus (U)	Hold (min)	Rate change (mL/min)	Repeat aPTT (hours)
<50[b]	5000	0	+3	6
50–59	0	0	+3	6
60–85	0	0	0	Next morning
86–95	0	0	−2	Next morning
96–120	0	30	−2	6
>120	0	60	−4	6

[a]Indicates activated partial thromboplastin time (aPTT) using Actin FS (Dade).
[b]If the aPTT was subtherapeutic despite a heparin dose of 1440 U/hour (36 mL/hour) or greater at any time during the first 48 hours, the response to an aPTT of less than 50 s was a heparin bolus of 5000 U and a rate increase of 5 mL/hour.
Adapted from Cruickshank MK, Levine MN, Hirsch J, et al. A standard heparin nomogram for the management of heparin therapy. *Arch Intern Med* 1991; **151**: 333–7.

Heparin requirements to meet a target aPTT (or heparin levels) rise around the end of the second trimester.[59] The therapeutic range for heparin adjustment is to achieve an aPTT of 1.5–2.5 times baseline at 6 hours after the last dose. Pregnancy-associated changes in levels of coagulation factors and plasma proteins may change the relationship between the aPTT and plasma heparin level, such that, for a given plasma heparin level, a pregnant woman's aPTT response may be lower than that of a nonpregnant woman. If there are difficulties achieving a therapeutic aPTT, measuring plasma heparin levels (anti-Xa levels) may give an accurate means of adjusting heparin dose, aiming for a 6-hour post-dose anti-Xa level of 0.3–0.7 U/mL.[66]

LMWHs are enzymatically cleaved fractions of unfractionated heparin that have a mean molecular weight of approximately 5000 kD (compared to 15 000 kD for UFH). These agents exert a predominantly anti-Xa effect.[67] LMWHs have more predictable pharmacokinetics because of their reduced binding to endothelium and plasma proteins. This allows for once-daily or twice-daily weight-adjusted dosing.[68–70] LMWHs are at least as efficacious as UFH in the initial treatment of pulmonary embolism and deep vein thrombosis in the nonpregnant population.[58,71]

As with UFH the dose requirement of LMWH is also likely to increase with gestation, even if only because of the usual increase in weight.[50,51,59] The data regarding dose adjustment in pregnancy are limited, and therefore it seems reasonable to adjust the dose according to weight changes; we advise checking plasma anti-Xa levels monthly in the third trimester and to target an anti-Xa level of 0.5–1.0 U/mL.

MANAGEMENT AT THE TIME OF LABOR AND DELIVERY

Delivery of women receiving heparin is likely to be associated with an increased risk of hemorrhage. It is probably prudent to withhold the last dose of subcutaneous UFH for at least 24 hours prior to delivery,[61] to reduce the chance of delivery with an anticoagulant effect; to do this normally requires a planned induction. If a woman delivers within 24 hours of her last injection of UFH, monitoring the aPTT and administering protamine may be necessary.

Heparin should be recommenced as soon as possible postpartum, within 12–24 hours, and therapy is overlapped with coumadin until an International Normalized Ratio (INR) of 2 or greater is reached. Coumadin is continued for a minimum of 4 weeks.

Acute venous thromboembolism occurring within 4 weeks of expected delivery poses a particular problem, as stopping anticoagulant therapy for even a short period (24 hours) may subject the women to a high risk of recurrence.[72] Two management options are:

(a) switch to intravenous heparin therapy (full dose) at the time of labor and stop the infusion around 4–6 hours prior to expected delivery; heparin should be recommenced as soon as possible postpartum (4–6 hours);
(b) insertion of an inferior vena cava filter.

Epidural anesthesia and analgesia

As the true incidence of symptomatic epidural hematoma is likely to be low,[73,74] this issue is unlikely to be addressed by a prospective trial. Recommendations regarding thromboprophylaxis and epidural use are guidelines, based on estimated risk. A decision should be made on a case-by-case basis.

The risk of hematoma formation is thought to be greatest at the time of needle insertion or withdrawal, especially for those patients who are fully anticoagulated at these times.[75] In patients receiving prophylactic UFH or LMWH, we believe that it is reasonable to wait 8 hours after or before the next dose, prior to insertion or withdrawal of the catheter. In the setting of low-dose UFH or LMWH, laboratory monitoring prior to catheter insertion is unlikely to be helpful. The current McMaster practice of planned induction for the majority of patients ensures that most women have sufficient time to stop their heparin and can receive epidural analgesia or anesthesia with minimal risk.

TREATMENT OF POSTPARTUM VENOUS THROMBOEMBOLISM

The treatment of postpartum venous thromboembolism is similar to that of the nonpregnant patient, and should consist of 5 days of UFH or LMWH, followed by long-term warfarin. It is important to advise women that warfarin is teratogenic and that they should take appropriate contraceptive precautions while using it.

PROPHYLAXIS FOR VENOUS THROMBOEMBOLISM

This section is divided into prophylaxis for women with previous venous thromboembolism and no known laboratory abnormality, and prophylaxis for women with a thrombophilic disorder (protein C, protein S, or antithrombin III deficiency, factor V Leiden mutation, anticardiolipin antibodies, and the lupus anticoagulant) with or without previous or recurrent venous thromboembolism. In general, there are three approaches.

1. No antepartum anticoagulation, but careful clinical vigilance. The basis of this approach is reliant on appropriate resources so that symptomatic women can be assessed promptly. Emphasis should be placed on using appropriate objective tests in symptomatic women (see above section on diagnosis of deep vein thrombosis and pulmonary embolism).
2. Antepartum prophylaxis with LMWH or UFH: the guidelines for UFH are shown in Table 16.2 and for LMWH in Table 16.3. It is important to realize that there are no randomized, controlled trials comparing the efficacy of any of the UFH or LMWH regimes.
3. Full-dose UFH or LMWH (see guidelines in preceding section).

All three regimens should be overlapped with postpartum warfarin, and warfarin should be continued for 4–6 weeks.

Table 16.2 *Recommendations for prophylaxis using unfractionated heparin*

American College of Chest Physicians	(1) Surveillance with baseline screening and regular review (2) 5000 U unfractionated heparin starting in the first trimester and continued throughout pregnancy
British Society of Haematology	5000 U twice daily during the first and second trimesters; increase to prolong 6-hour post-dose aPTT to 1.5 times but aim to keep heparin level below 0.3 U/mL
Dahlman et al.[59]	Adjust subcutaneous heparin dose according to a 3-hour post-injection anti-Xa level (aim 0.08–0.15 IU/mL of plasma)

aPTT = activated partial thromboplastin time.

Table 16.3 *Recommendations[a] for low molecular weight heparin prophylaxis[b]*

Formulation	Dosage recommendations
Ardeparin	50 U/kg twice daily
Dalteparin	2500 U twice daily or 5000 U once daily
Nadroparin	60 U/kg once daily
Tinzaparin	75 U/kg once daily
Enoxaparin	3000 U twice daily or 4000 U once daily

[a]Adapted from Weitz.[67]
[b]The doses shown are in anti-Xa factor units and come from recommendations for postoperative prophylaxis for total hip and knee surgery.

Prophylaxis for women with previous venous thromboembolism and no thrombophilia

The true risk of recurrence of venous thromboembolism in such women is not known. Intuitively, the risk of recurrence, as in nonpregnant patients, is unlikely to be uniform. For example, a woman with idiopathic venous thromboembolism is likely to have a greater recurrence risk than a woman who has venous thromboembolism postoperatively or after trauma. A decision to offer prophylaxis should be considered on a case-by-case basis. We believe that either of the first two approaches cited above is reasonable.

Primary prophylaxis for women with thrombophilia and no previous venous thromboembolism

There are no prospective data on the risk of venous thromboembolism in asymptomatic pregnant patients with thrombophilia. Based on retrospective data of the thrombophilic disorders, antithrombin III deficiency may be associated with a relatively high incidence of antepartum venous thromboembolism.[76] However, we believe that either option 1 or 2 is reasonable in these women.

Prophylaxis for thrombophilic women with previous venous thromboembolism

It is important to assess these women properly, with a critical review of the diagnosis of previous venous thromboembolism and a critical review of the diagnosis of thrombophilia. Our recommendation is to offer any of the options listed above, although empirically we favor option 3.

REFERENCES

1   Rutherford S, Montoro M, McGhee W, Strong T. Thromboembolic disease associated with pregnancy: an 11 year review. *Am J Obstet Gynecol* 1991; **164**(Suppl. 1286), abstract.

2   Ginsberg JS, Brill Edwards P, Burrows RF, et al. Venous thrombosis during pregnancy and trimester of presentation. *Thromb Haemost* 1992; **67**: 519–20.

3   Sterling Y, Woolf L, North WRS, Seghatchian, Meade TW. Haemostasis in normal pregnancy. *Thromb Haemost* 1984; **52**: 176–82.

4   Hellgren M, Blomback M. Studies on coagulation and fibrinolysis in pregnancy, during delivery and in the purpureum. *Gynecol Obst Invest* 1981; **12**: 141–54.

5   Faught W, Garner P, Jones GB. Changes to protein C and S levels in normal pregnancy. *Am J Obstet Gynecol* 1995; **172**: 147–50.

6   Bremme K, Ostlund E, Almqvist I, Heinonen K, Blomback M. Enhanced thrombin generation and fibrinolytic activity in normal pregnancy and the puerperium. *Obstet Gynecol* 1992; **80**: 132–7.

7   Halligan A, Bonnar J, Shepard B, Darling M, Walshe J. Haemostatic, fibrinolytic and endothelial variables in normal pregnancies and pre-eclampsia. *Br J Obstet Gynaecol* 1994; **101**: 488–92.

8   Kruithof EKO, Tran-Thang C, Gudicet A, et al. Fibrinolysis in pregnancy. A study of plasminogen activator inhibitors. *Blood* 1987; **69**: 460–6.

9   Goodrich S, Wood JE. Peripheral venous distensibility and velocity of venous blood flow during pregnancy or during oral contraceptive therapy. *Am J Obstet Gynecol* 1964; **90**: 740–4.

10 Ikard RW, Ueland K, Folse R. Lower limb venous dynamics in pregnant women. *Surg Gynecol Obstet* 1971; **132**: 483–8.

11 Meade TW, Chakrabarti R, Haines AP, et al. Haemostatic function and cardiovascular death: early results of a prospective study. *Lancet* 1980; **8177**: 1050–4.

12 Huisman MV, Buller HR, ten Cate JW, et al. Management of clinically suspected acute venous thrombosis in outpatients with serial impedance plethysmography in a community hospital setting. *Arch Intern Med* 1989; **149**: 511–13.

13 Wells P, Hirsh J, Anderson DR, et al. Comparison of the accuracy of impedance plethysmography and compression ultrasound in outpatients with clinically suspected deep venous thrombosis. A two center paired-design prospective trial. *Thromb Haemost* 1995; **74**: 1423–7.

14 Hull RD, Raskob GE, Carter CJ. Serial impedance plethysmography in pregnant patients with clinically suspected deep vein thrombosis. Clinical validity of negative findings. *Ann Intern Med* 1990; **112**: 663–7.

15 Heijboer H, Buller HR, Lensing AWA, et al. Comparison of real time compression ultrasound with impedance plethysmography for the diagnosis of deep venous thrombosis in symptomatic outpatients. *N Engl J Med* 1993; **329**: 1365–9.

16 Ginsberg JS, Hirsh J, Rainbow AJ, Coates G. Risks to the fetus of radiologic procedures used in the diagnosis of maternal venous thromboembolic disease. *Thromb Haemost* 1989; **61**: 189–96.

17 Huisman MV, Buller HR, ten Cate JW, et al. Unexpected high prevalence of silent pulmonary embolism in patients with deep venous thrombosis. *Chest* 1989; **95**: 498–502.

18 Stein PD, Hull RD, Pineo G. Strategy for diagnosis of patients with suspected acute pulmonary embolism. *Chest* 1993; **103**: 1153–9.

19 The PIOPED Investigators. Value of the ventilation/perfusion scan in acute pulmonary embolism. Results of the Prospective Investigation of Pulmonary Embolism Diagnosis. (PIOPED). *JAMA* 1990; **263**: 2753–9.

20 Hull RD, Raskob GE, Ginsberg JS, et al. A noninvasive strategy for the treatment of patients with suspected pulmonary embolism. *Arch Intern Med* 1994; **154**: 289–97.

21 Flick MR. In: Murray and Nadel. *Textbook of respiratory medicine*, 2nd edn. WB Saunders, 1994: 2476–9.

22 Stein PD, Athanasoulis C, Alavi A, et al. Complications and validity of pulmonary angiography in acute pulmonary embolism. *Circulation* 1992; **85**: 462–8.

23 Ginsberg JS, Kearon C, Douketis J, et al. The use of D-dimer testing and impedance plethysmographic examination in patients with clinical indications of deep vein thrombosis. *Arch Intern Med* 1997; **157**: 1077–81.

24 Ginsberg JS, Wells PS, Brill-Edwards P, et al. Application of a novel and rapid whole blood assay for the D-dimer in patients with clinically suspected pulmonary embolism. *Thromb Haemost* 1995; **73**: 35–8.

25 Remy-Jardin M, Remy J, Dechildre F, et al. Diagnosis of pulmonary embolism with spiral CT: comparison with pulmonary angiography and scintigraphy. *Radiology* 1996; **200**: 699–706.

26 van Rossum AB, Pattynama PM, Treurniet FE, Schpers R, Kieft GJ. Spiral CT angiography for detection of pulmonary embolism: validation in 124 patients (abstract). *Radiology* 1995; **197**: 303.

27 Stein PD, Henry JW. Prevalence of acute pulmonary embolism in central and subsegmental pulmonary arteries and relation to probability interpretation of ventilation/perfusion scans. *Chest* 1997; **111**: 1246–8.

28 Gefter WB, Hatabu H, Holland GA, Gupta KB, Henschke CI, Palevsky HI. Pulmonary thromboembolism: recent developments in the diagnosis with CT and MRI imaging. *Radiology* 1995; **197**: 561–74.

29 Meaney JFM, Weg JG, Chnevert TL, Stafford-Johnson D, Hamilton BH, Princer MR. Diagnosis of pulmonary embolism with magnetic resonance angiography. *N Engl J Med* 1997; **336**: 1422–7.

30 Spritzer CE, Norconk JJ, Sostman HD, Coleman RE. Detection of deep venous thrombosis by magnetic resonance imaging. *Chest* 1993; **104**: 54–60.

31 Dupas B, El Kouri D, Curtet C, et al. Angiomagnetic resonance imaging of iliofemorocaval venous thrombosis. *Lancet* 1995; **345**: 17–19.

32 Evans AJ, Sostman HD, Knelson MH, et al. Detection of deep venous thrombosis: prospective comparison of MR imaging with contrast venography. *Am J Roentgenol* 1993; **161**: 131–9.

33 Spritzer CE, Evans AC, Kay HH. Magnetic resonance imaging of deep venous thrombosis in pregnant woman with lower extremity edema. *Obstet Gynecol* 1995; **85**: 603–7.

34 Dunnihoo DR, Gallaspy JW, Wise RB, Otterson WN. Postpartum ovarian vein thrombophlebitis: a review. *Obstet Gynaecol Survey* 1991; **46**: 415–27.

35 Simnos GR, Piwnica-Worms DR, Goldhaber SZ. Ovarian vein thrombosis. *Am Heart J* 1993; **126**: 641–7.

36 Rosenberg RD, Bauer KA. The heparin–antithrombin system: a natural anticoagulant mechanism. In: Colman RW, Hirsh J, Marder VJ, et al. eds *Haemostasis and thrombosis: basic principles and clinical practice*, 3rd edn. Philadelphia: JB Lippincott, 1992: 837–60.

37 Kandrotas RJ. Heparin pharmacokinectics and pharmacodynamics. *Clin Pharmacokinet* 1992; **22**: 359–74.

38 Fiore L, Deykin D. In: E Beutler et al, eds *Williams hematology*, 5th edn. City: New York: McGraw-Hill, 1995: 1567–9.

39 Forestier F, Daffos F, Rainaut M, Toulemonde F. Low molecular weight heparin (CY216) does not cross the placenta during the third trimester of pregnancy. *Thromb Haemost* 1987; **57**: 234.

40 Omri A, Delaloye JF, Andersen H, Bachmann F. Low molecular weight heparin novo (LHN-1) does not cross the placenta during the second trimester of pregnancy. *Thromb Haemost* 1989; **61**: 55–6.

41 Ginsberg JS, Hirsh J, Turner CD, Levine MN, Burrows R. Risks to the fetus of anticoagulant therapy during pregnancy. *Thromb Haemost* 1989; **61**: 197–203.

42 Ginsberg JS, Kowalchuck G, Hirsh J, Brill-Edwards P. Heparin therapy during pregnancy: risks to the fetus and mother. *Arch Intern Med* 1989; **149**: 2233–6.

43 Iturbe-Alessio I, Del Carmen Fonseca M, Mutchinik O, Santo MA, Zajarias A, Salazar E. Risks of anticoagulant therapy in pregnant women with artificial heart valves. *N Engl J Med* 1988; **315**: 1390–3.

44 McKenna R, Cale ER, Vasa U. Is warfarin sodium contraindicated in the lactating mother? *J Paediatr* 1983; **103**: 325–7.

45 Riggs BL, Melton LJ. Involutional osteoporosis. *N Engl J Med* 1986; **314**: 1676–86.

46 Douketis JD, Ginsberg JS, Burrows RF, Duku EK, Webber CE, Brill-Edwards P. The effects of long term heparin therapy during pregnancy on bone density. *Thromb Haemost* 1996; **75**: 254–7.

47 Ginsberg JS, Kowalchuk G, Hirsh J, Brill-Edwards P, Burrows R, Coates G. Heparin effect on bone density. *Thromb Haemost* 1990; **64**: 286–9.

48 Dahlman TC. Osteoporotic fractures and the recurrence of thromboembolism during pregnancy and the puerperium in 184 women undergoing thromboprophylaxis with heparin. *Am J Obstet Gynecol* 1993; **168**: 1265–70.

49 Nelson-Piercy C, Letsky EA, De Swiet M. Low molecular weight heparin for obstetric thromboprophylaxis: experience of sixty nine pregnancies in sixty women at high risk. *Am J Obstet Gynecol* 1997; **176**: 1062–8.

50 Dulitzli M, Pauner R, Langevitz P, Pras M, Many A, Schiff E. Low molecular weight heparin during pregnancy and delivery: preliminary experience with 41 pregnancies. *Obstet Gynecol* 1996; **87**: 380–3.

51 Monreal M, Lafoz E, Olive A, del Rio L, Vedia C. Comparison of subcutaneous unfractionated heparin with a low molecular weight heparin in patients with venous thromboembolism and contraindications to coumarin. *Thromb Haemost* 1994; **71**: 7–11.

52 Amiral J, Bridey F, Dreyfus M, et al. Platelet factor 4 complexed to heparin is the target for antibodies generated in heparin induced thrombocytopenia. *Thromb Haemost* 1992; **68**: 95–6.

53 Warkentin TE, Levine MN, Hirsh J, et al. Heparin-induced thrombocytopenia in patients treated with low molecular weight heparin or unfractionated heparin. *N Engl J Med* 1995; **332**: 1330–5.

54 Chong BH. Heparin-induced thrombocytopenia. *Aust N Z J Med* 1992; **22**: 145–52.

55 Hunt BJ, Doughty HA, Majumdar G, et al. Thromboprophylaxis with low molecular weight heparin in high risk pregnancies. *Thromb Hemost* 1997; **77**: 39–43.

56 Magnani HN. Heparin induced thrombocytopenia (HIT): an overview of 230 patients treated with Orgaran® (Org10172). *Thromb Haemost* 1993; **70**: 554–61.

57 Levine MN, Raskob G, Landefeld S, Hirsh J. Hemorrhagic complications of anticoagulant treatment. *Chest* 1995; **108**: 276S–87S.

58 Koopman MMW, Prandoni P, Piovella F, et al. Treatment of venous thrombosis with intravenous unfractionated heparin administered in the hospital as compared with subcutaneous low molecular weight heparin administered at home. *N Engl J Med* 1996, **334**: 682–7.

59 Dahlman TC, Hellgren MSE, Bloomback M. Thrombosis prophylaxis in pregnancy with the use of subcutaneous heparin adjusted by monitoring heparin concentration in plasma. *Am J Obstet Gynecol* 1989; **161**: 420–5.

60 Anderson DR, Ginsberg JS, Burrows R, Brill-Edwards P. Subcutaneous heparin therapy during pregnancy: a need for concern at the time of delivery. *Thromb Haemost* 1991; **65**: 248–50.

61 Walker MG, Shaw JW, Thomson GJL, Cumming JGR, Thomas ML. Subcutaneous calcium heparin versus intravenous sodium heparin in treatment of established acute deep vein thrombosis of the legs: a multicentre prospective randomised trial. *BMJ* 1987; **294**: 1189–92.

62 Anderson D, Ginsberg JS, Brill-Edwards P, Demers C, Burrows RF, Hirsh J. The use of an indwelling Teflon catheter for subcutaneous heparin administration during pregnancy. A randomised crossover study. *Arch Intern Med* 1993; **153**: 841–4.

63 Sallah S, Thomas DP, Roberts HR. Warfarin and heparin induced skin necrosis and the purple toe syndrome: infrequent complications of anticogulant treatment. *Thromb Haemost* 1997; **78**: 785–90.

64 Ojeda S, Perez MDC, Mataix R, et al. Case reports: skin necrosis with a low molecular weight heparin. *Br J Haemat* 1992; **82**: 620–9.

65 Anand S, Ginsberg JS, Kearon C, Hirsh J. The relationship between the activated partial thromboplastin time response and recurrence in patients with venous thrombosis treated with continuous intravenous heparin. *Arch Intern Med* 1996; **156**: 1677–81.

66 Brill-Edwards P, Ginsberg JS, Johnson M, Hirsh J. Establishing a therapeutic range for heparin therapy. *Ann Intern Med* 1993; **119**: 104–9.

67 Weitz JI. Drug therapy: low molecular weight heparins. *N Engl J Med* 1997; **337**: 688–98.

68 Leizorovicz A, Haugh MC, Chapuis FR, Samama MM, Boissel JP. Low molecular weight heparin in prevention of perioperative thrombosis. *BMJ* 1992; **305**: 913–20.

69 Barzu T, Van Rijn JLMC, Petitou M, et al. Heparin degradation in endothelial cells. *Thromb Res* 1987; **47**: 601–9.

70 Harenburg J. Pharmacology of low molecular weight heparins. *Semin Thromb Hemost* 1990; **16**(Suppl): 12–18.

71 Levine M, Gent M, Hirsh J, et al. A comparison of low molecular weight heparin administered primarily at home with unfractionated heparin administered in the hospital for proximal deep vein thrombosis. *N Engl J Med* 1996; **334**: 677–81.

72 Kearon C, Hirsh J. Management of anticoagulation before and after elective surgery. *N Engl J Med* 1997; **336**: 1506–11.

73 Bergqvist D, Linblad B, Matzch T. Risk of combining low molecular weight heparin for thromboprophylaxis and epidural or spinal anesthesia. *Semin Thromb Hemost* 1993; **19**: 147–51.

74 Tryba M, Wedel DJ. Central neuraxial block and low molecular weight heparin (enoxaparine): lessons learned from different dosage regimes in two continents. *Acta Anaesth Scand* 1997; **111**: 100–4.

75 Wulf H. Epidural anaesthesia and spinal haematoma. *Can J Anaesth* 1996; **43**: 1260–71.

76 McColl M, Ramsay JE, Tait ID, McCall F, Conkie JA, Walker ID. Risk factors for pregnancy associated venous thromboembolism. *Thromb Haemost* 1997; **778**: 1183–8.

17

Upper extremity deep vein thrombosis

INTRODUCTION

The purpose of this chapter is to discuss the incidence, etiology, presentation, and treatment of upper extremity deep vein thrombosis, with an emphasis placed on encouraging prevention of secondary upper extremity deep vein thrombosis. Primary upper extremity deep vein thrombosis is discussed first, and secondary upper extremity deep vein thrombosis is then reviewed distinguishing catheter-related thrombosis from noncatheter-related thrombosis.

Primary deep vein thrombosis of the upper extremity is a phenomenon described by Paget more than 100 years ago and by Von Schroetter a few years later.[1-6] These early investigators described patients who developed spontaneous pain and edema of an upper extremity. Primary upper extremity deep vein thrombosis came to be known early on as Paget–Schroetter syndrome. It has also been termed either effort thrombosis, related to the fact that many patients present after overuse of the involved arm, or primary subclavian–axillary vein thrombosis, as these are the vessels involved. Spontaneous thrombosis is another term used when no history of strenuous activity or trauma is elicited. Patients are usually young and healthy and are often found to have an anatomic abnormality. They present with pain and edema of the involved arm approximately 24 hours after local trauma or strenuous activity. Earlier literature, indeed into the 1980s, generally reflected an attitude that primary upper extremity deep vein thrombosis was a rare entity with no serious acute complications.[5,7–10] There were those who thought differently, but these were in the minority opinion. Some of this earlier literature recognized a moderate but significant amount of chronic complications such as pain and disability, and only a few authors called attention to its serious acute complications [7,9,11,12].

Careful examination of more current literature shows primary upper extremity deep vein thrombosis to be a more serious problem, with not only significant chronic complications, but also acute complications, which occur much more frequently than previously suspected.[8,13]

Secondary upper extremity deep vein thrombosis has been an increasingly recognized entity in the past few decades. Multiple factors have contributed to this, including its increased occurrence, physicians' increasing awareness of the issue, and its frequent serious complications, most notably pulmonary embolism. The literature on this subject does not easily lend itself to analysis for conclusions regarding risk and treatment, let alone a consensus opinion. It is a collection of retrospective analyses, case reports and series, and a few reviews. Many authors have studied upper extremity deep vein thrombosis on an 'all-comers' basis and, once the diagnosis of thrombus has been made, study the patients for risk factors. Although this has provided much useful information, it is often tedious to identify individual risk factors and their relative risks. Much of the literature is comprised of articles in which the lines of etiologic distinction between primary and secondary upper extremity deep vein thrombosis are mingled, and so are the data.

The incidence of upper extremity deep vein thrombosis (primary + secondary) is said to account for 2.1–3.5% of all deep vein thrombosis.[6,10] However, these data were collected at a time when upper extremity deep vein thrombosis was less recognized and the use of venous access devices and central vein cannulation was less frequent.

There has never been a consensus regarding some of the most important and, perhaps, first steps in addressing this issue; what constitutes primary versus secondary upper extremity deep vein thrombosis? The question that directly follows is, once the risk factors are recognized and properly categorized, what are the relative risks of each risk factor? Are they additive? What is their impact on each other? Most importantly, how can we prevent it?

Because this entity is now better recognized, the priorities for the medical community should be to reach agreement regarding the classification of risk factors, prophylaxis, and treatment.

PRIMARY UPPER EXTREMITY DEEP VEIN THROMBOSIS

For the purposes of this discussion, upper extremity deep vein thrombosis associated with an anatomic abnormality, vigorous exercise, and trauma is discussed in the category of primary upper extremity deep vein thrombosis. That associated with congestive heart failure, malignancy, and other thrombophilic states is discussed under secondary upper extremity deep vein thrombosis. Patients with primary upper extremity deep vein thrombosis are usually young, otherwise healthy and active individuals who may take part in exercise or occupations involving strenuous repetitive motions. This type of deep vein thrombosis has been more common in men than women and has had a predeliction for affecting the right side, possibly reflecting the predominantly right-handed population.

Hyperabduction of the arm or overuse ('effort' thrombosis) has been documented in many cases from varying repetitive motions, including, but not limited to: construction work, playing tennis, swimming, throwing a baseball, and weight lifting.[3,14] One report attributed development of a thrombus to a woman who vigorously spanked her child.[5]

The etiology of this entity has not been uniformly identified, but there is often evidence of venous obstruction from an anatomic abnormality. Hyperabduction of the arm, malrotation during sleep, cervical ribs, non-union of clavicular fractures, and sternoclavicular hyperostosis have been described as causative or contributing etiologies. A number of other anatomic abnormalities have been described and the most common is compression of the vein between the first rib and a hypertrophied scalene muscle or subclavius tendon.[3,15] These abnormalities have been found to be bilateral as well, in some series up to 65% of the time.[16] Although this may predispose to thrombosis of the contralateral vessels later, bilateral thrombosis occurs infrequently, at a rate of 2–15%.[17]

Reviewing the anatomy of the costoclavicular space, one can readily see how the subclavian vein is in a position to be easily compromised. The subclavian vein courses through an anatomic tunnel bounded by the first rib, the subclavius muscle, the clavicle, and the anterior scalene muscle. This tunnel is relatively fixed and motions such as those named above directly narrow the channel available for blood-flow, leading to decreased return, stasis, and then thrombosis.

Presentation

Clinically, patients present with acute pain and nonpitting edema of an arm or forearm, usually over a 24-hour period. The pain worsens with use of the affected extremity and abates with rest. Patients may describe or be found to have dilatation of the superficial veins of the anterior chest wall in the region of the shoulder. Several case reports also describe patients presenting with symptoms of pulmonary embolus.[5,7,18]

Complications

As most patients are otherwise young and healthy, minimizing chronic complications should be aggressively pursued as these patients can be left with a considerable degree of disability if vein patency is not restored. Outcome depends on several things: time to diagnosis, mode of treatment, and response to initial therapy.[3,12] Complications leading to disability include chronic venous insufficiency leading to chronic pain and edema. Rarely, these patients develop phlegmasia cerulia dolens, a condition in which deoxygenated hemoglobin in stagnant veins imparts a cyanotic hue to the limb.[9,19] As mentioned above, early investigators believed acute complications to be unusual and chronic complications to be unavoidable. However, we now know from several more recent studies that neither case is true.

Prandoni's group reported chronic complications in only 4 out of 27 patients (15%), but we are not told if these were patients with primary or catheter-related thrombi.[18] Chronic complications of some kind have been noted to occur in up to 68% of patients with this disorder.[12,20] Even patients treated with anticoagulants have been shown to have a significant incidence of chronic problems.[13,20,21] Urschel and Razzuk treated 34 patients with heparin and coumadin shortly before 1980 and found that the majority (25 patients, or 74%) had chronic complications: 21 had chronic intermittent swelling of the arm with use, 2 had constant symptoms, and 2 developed phlegmasia cerulea dolens.[22]

Symptoms are often worsened by exercise, leading to vocational disability and loss of quality of avocational life. Other important complications include pulmonary embolus, venous gangrene, and clot propagation complicated by thoracic duct obstruction or superior vena cava obstruction.[3,15,21]

Whereas it was once believed that pulmonary embolism was a rare complication of upper extremity deep vein thrombosis, more recent investigations have shown a surprisingly high incidence.[5,8,9] In fact, although they did not discern between primary and catheter-related upper extremity thrombi, Prandoni's group reported an incidence of pulmonary embolism in 36% of their patients.[18] Hurlbert's review and others quote an incidence of pulmonary embolism in 12–15% of patients with primary upper extremity deep vein thrombosis.[10,13,17,21,23] Upper extremity deep vein thrombosis is now said to account for 3–6% of all pulmonary emboli and for 1–2% of all fatal pulmonary emboli.[3,17,18,24]

Becker et al. reviewed 71 case reports and 17 case series in 1991 for a total of 329 patients of whom 34% reported post-treatment symptoms, pulmonary embolism in 9.4%, and death in 1.2%, but did not delineate between primary and catheter-related thrombi.[25] It is probably the case that 12% is close to the actual occurrence of pulmonary emboli, based on a review of the literature, but it is clearly difficult to be sure as asymptomatic patients are not evaluated routinely for pulmonary embolus and this may reflect the frequency of only clinically overt emboli.[17,18,21,26–8]

Diagnosis

Many different strategies have been evaluated for confirming the presence of thrombus in the deep venous system of the arm. There are reports in the literature comparing different methods of ultrasound, nuclear imaging techniques, and venography.[29–39] Venography remains the standard, but several authors provide good data for using compression and color-flow Doppler ultrasound (as oppposed to Doppler without color flow) as an initial tool.[18,33,35,36] A reasonable approach after a history and physical examination is to decide what you are going to do with the information. If the patient is not a candidate for thrombolysis, anticoagulation, or surgery, not pursuing a venogram and documenting a thrombus with an initial ultrasound seems reasonable. These patients should be treated conservatively with elevation, pain control, and prophylaxis against propogation, if possible. However, if the patient is otherwise young and healthy and more aggressive therapy is an option, a venogram should be considered as the initial test to evaluate the extent of the thrombus and rule out extrinsic compression of the vein. An initial ultrasound is also a reasonable option, but in a case where there is a high degree of suspicion and aggressive therapy is an option, a venogram should be performed if the screening ultrasound is negative.

Given the significant number of patients with upper extremity deep vein thrombosis found to have a hypercoagulable state,[3,40] an evaluation for a hypercoagulable state is suggested at an appropriate time, especially for patients for whom there is no history of trauma. (See Chapter 2, for more information.)

Treatment

Treatment of this disorder has been said to be 'shrouded in controversy'.[3] Restoring vein patency is the key to minimizing complications. As always, treatment needs to be tailored to the individual patient. The general approaches are: conservative therapy with rest, elevation, and pain control; anticoagulation with heparin and warfarin; thrombolysis; and surgery. Treatment in the past, and mainly still today, usually entails anticoagulation with standard heparin and warfarin for most patients. For patients for whom anticoagulation is contraindicated, a conservative therapy of elevation and immobilization with pain control may be the best approach. Unfortunately, patients treated in this manner have a high incidence of developing postphlebitic syndrome.[11,16] In other patients, several modalities have been employed as well as combinations of approaches. There is much in the literature about thrombolytic therapy for upper extremity deep vein thrombosis. Systemic and local thrombolytic therapies have been utilized, with a significant degree of improvement in a large number of patients, and several trials report no major complications and only some minor complications (such as bleeding at the infusion site).[11,16,17,20,41-4] Surgery may be indicated in patients in whom anatomic obstruction of the vein is revealed by venography; several different procedures to restore proper flow have been utilized (first rib resection, partial resection of the clavicle) depending on the cause of the obstruction.

Machleder has led the way, prospectively studying 50 patients with upper extremity deep vein thrombosis with a staged, multimodal approach. His series showed several important points: thrombolytic therapy with urokinase significantly improved vein patency over heparin (75% compared to 25%); preoperative balloon angioplasty after successful thrombolysis provided no additional benefit and may have had a deleterious effect; and postoperative balloon angioplasty for residual stricture was both helpful (seven of nine patients) and uncomplicated. Complications of therapy in that study were limited and minor: two patients had systemic allergic reactions to streptokinase (and were changed to urokinase), one patient who deviated from protocol had an axillary hematoma; one patient had transient gastrointestinal and urinary tract bleeding while on warfarin; and, importantly, two patients who were subtherapeutic on their warfarin regimens rethrombosed at the site which had been successfully recannulized.[40]

Urschel and Razzuk studied two groups of patients, the first treated with heparin and warfarin. This first group had a high incidence of recurrent symptoms necessitating rib resection or thrombectomy. The second group of patients comprised 33 patients who were treated with thrombolysis and early decompressive surgery. These patients had no major complications, and 32 out of 36 extremities treated had good results, which were defined as the ability to return to work without symptoms. Two patients experienced intermittent swelling and two had chronic swelling.[22]

In another study, Molina showed the efficacy and safety of thrombolytic therapy among 18 patients.[45] Although the sample sizes of the studies are small, the literature shows a trend toward using lytic therapy for young patients and that it can be done safely.

This author's preference, based on the review of the current literature, is for local urokinase infusion by a catheter embedded directly into the clot, followed by anticoagulation with heparin. Surgery should then be undertaken to repair an obstruction, if present, and postsurgical balloon angioplasty for any residual stricture. Finally, the patient should be treated with 3 months of warfarin therapy. Surgical resection of persistent obstruction should be strongly considered.

Primary upper extremity deep vein thrombosis is an under-recognized and often under-treated entity, which is often misdiagnosed because of many physicians' unfamiliarity with it. Although this is a rare syndrome, its early diagnosis is paramount as we have a safe and effective method of treating it and the results are best if therapy is initiated quickly.

SECONDARY UPPER EXTREMITY DEEP VEIN THROMBOSIS

Noncatheter related

Noncatheter-related upper extremity deep vein thrombosis has been associated with multiple etiologies, including heart failure, malignancies, other thrombophilic states, trauma, and the administration of various medications through peripheral catheters.[13,46,47] Another etiology of upper extremity deep vein thrombosis is that associated with oral contraceptives and/or smoking cigarettes. The largest group of patients with noncatheter-related upper extremity deep vein thrombosis today is patients with malignancies. Upper extremity deep vein thrombosis has been associated with many different malignancies unrelated to central venous cannulation.[25,28,47–55] Some cases of thrombosis were felt to be related to venous compression by the tumor itself or to the induction of a hypercoagulable state. Another mechanism involving a tumor in the chest is diffuse adenopathy (particularly in the axillary/subclavian region) leading to decreased venous return.

Haire notes personal experience with protein C and antithrombin III deficiencies in patients with this syndrome, and Prandoni found 6/14 patients to have a thrombophilic state associated with spontaneous or effort-related thrombi.[3,18] Prandoni's investigation also found an association with a history of prior lower extremity deep vein thrombosis. There are also reports of primary upper extremity deep vein thrombosis associated with the use of oral contraceptives (we have recently seen such a case at our institution), and it is also a well-recognized complication of congestive heart failure.[7,10,12,19,46,56]

Loring reasoned that the cause of thrombosis originated in the pooling of blood in the capillary network in patients with congestive heart failure and the prolonged circulation time associated with myocardial failure.[46] He correlated this with the most common site of origin of the thrombi being the junction of large veins where blood that is already low in oxygen content tends to eddy. Prescott and Tickoff further reasoned that noncatheter-related upper extremity deep vein thrombosis occurred so much less frequently than the lower extremity for several reasons: there is no analog to the soleal network in the upper extremities; there are fewer valves in the upper extremities (because thrombi often originate at the valves); and, even in bedridden patients, there is less likely to be cessation of arm movement (and so less stagnation).[13] They also discussed literature reflecting less hydrostatic pressure in the arms and the increased fibrinolytic activity of the vascular epithelium in the upper extremity as opposed to that in the lower extremity.

Symptoms are similar to those of primary upper extremity deep vein thrombosis. Patients may experience pulmonary emboli in approximately 10% of cases and chronic sequelae in approximately 34%, even when treated with anticoagulation.[5,8,9,13,25] An effort should be made to distinguish whether an anatomic abnormality (Paget–Schroetter syndrome) is present, as this clearly alters therapeutic considerations. For patients who are candidates for surgical correction, a venogram should be performed to evaluate the presence of an anatomic abnormality. Once an anatomic abnormality is ruled out, the patient should be evaluated for the presence of a thrombophilic state, especially if no other obvious risk factor is present. In one study of risk factors in 27 patients with upper extremity deep vein thrombosis, eight were felt to be related to catheters, seven had a thrombophilic state, six had a malignancy, and five had a prior lower extremity deep vein thrombosis.[18]

Diagnosis depends on a high index of suspicion. Compression and Duplex ultrasound have been shown to be good screening tests.[18,29,35,36,39] Patients with the above risk factors and symptoms who have a negative ultrasound should undergo venography.

Treatment should be similar to the treatment of lower extremity deep vein thrombosis (see Chapter 5).

Catheter related (see chapters 5 and 10)

Catheter-related upper extremity deep vein thrombosis has become a much more important issue in the last 2–3 decades, mainly as a result of the increased use of large vein cannulation. This procedure is usually performed to place central venous catheters. In studies of all upper extremity deep vein thrombosis, catheters are felt to be the inciting cause in 33–65% of cases.[15,49,57] Patients most commonly seen with catheters, and hence catheter-related thromboses, include those with varying types of malignancies and those who require venous access for long-term antibiotic therapy or for nutritional support. This classification should also include patients with transvenous pacemakers.

However, most patients with central venous catheters do not develop thrombi. There are many risk factors, including a history of or concomitant lower extremity deep vein thrombosis, the circumference of the catheter, presence of malignancy, and those risk factors also associated with noncatheter-related upper extremity deep vein thrombosis such as a thrombophilic state, sepsis, and an intensive care unit (ICU) setting, among others.[3,18,21,51,57,58] Active inflammatory bowel disease, known to be associated with increased risk of thrombus development, has anecdotally been associated with upper extremity deep vein thrombosis.

Most of the literature on catheter-related thrombosis is comprised of retrospective analyses and case reports or case series on specific populations. Therefore, the reported incidence of catheter-related thrombosis ranges widely, from 3.2% to 41%.[12,21,28,49,50,52-5] This is a result of several issues, not limited to: the particular at-risk population studied; the total number of patients studied; the length of the study; and comorbid conditions. Also, unless these studies were designed to look prospectively for upper extremity deep vein thrombosis, the true incidence may well be underestimated as a result of the vague signs and symptoms associated with upper extremity deep vein thrombosis, particularly catheter-related upper extremity deep vein thrombosis. Screening venography has been used for this purpose and has demonstrated thrombus in 33–60% of patients with catheters.[25] Fortunately, not all of these patients become symptomatic and the number of patients who develop clinically evident upper extremity deep vein thrombosis is probably closer to 3%.[25,28,52,53] If one stops to consider the number of central venous catheters placed in a single 500-bed hospital in a given year (outpatient plus inpatient), 3% is actually a quite significant number.

The signs and symptoms include pain or a 'tightness' in the shoulder area, ipsilateral upper extremity edema and/or cyanosis, and anterior chest wall superficial vein dilatation. Patients can also present with catheter malfunction, phlegmasia cerulea dolens and symptoms of pulmonary embolism.

Patients with catheter-related upper extremity deep vein thrombosis have been shown to have pulmonary embolism in up to 25% of cases. The controversy over the rate of pulmonary embolism is that not all of these patients are symptomatic. However, in one small series, four of the five known pulmonary emboli were symptomatic and one was felt to be contributory to the patient's death. Other authors have shown symptomatic pulmonary emboli occurring in approximately 4% of patients with catheter-related upper extremity deep vein thrombosis.[28,32,49,59]

The chronic complications of catheter-related upper extremity deep vein thrombosis are similar to those of primary upper extremity deep vein thrombosis and include chronic pain, edema, and loss of use of the affected extremity. However, most authors have found that these chronic complications occur much less frequently in this population as compared to those with primary upper extremity deep vein thrombosis.[1,3,25,49]

Diagnosis depends on a clinical suspicion – the practitioner needs to be vigilant as the symptoms are often vague. Duplex (as opposed to Doppler) ultrasound has been shown to be reliable in several studies, but venography remains the gold standard. Patients who have a negative ultrasound but have signs/symptoms should undergo a venogram.

Treatment of catheter-related upper extremity deep vein thrombosis is another gray area. Patients have been treated with thrombolytic therapy, heparin, superior vena cava filters, and conservative therapy consisting of elevation and pain control.[15,20,28,42,59] Currently, it is suggested that the catheter be removed and, if there are no contraindications, heparin (or low molecular weight heparin) should be started at therapeutic doses. The patient should then be placed on warfarin for at least 3 months. Patients with additional risk factors for thrombosis should be considered for longer treatment with anticoagulants. There is a great need for further trials of locally delivered, low-dose thrombolytic therapy, which has been shown to be safe and effective in primary upper extremity deep vein thrombosis.

Prophylaxis of patients with central venous catheters is the best opportunity to decrease its incidence. The question is who to prophylaxis, at what dose, and which agent to use. At this point, all patients with indwelling central catheters used for chemotherapy should be given prophylaxis with very low doses of warfarin and monitored closely. Bern and colleagues, as well as others, have shown this to be safe and effective.[47,50] When patients with malignancies and central access devices were given 1 mg of warfarin daily, the incidence of upper extremity deep vein thrombosis was reduced from 37.5% to 9.5%.[50] It is important to note that nearly 10% of these patients still developed a thrombus, and that some patients may require higher doses or other anticoagulants.

With the aging population, the ability to detect more cancers at an early stage, and the continuing advancements in chemotherapy, it is possible that the number of patients receiving long-term intravenous access will continue to increase. Therefore, it is imperative that these patients be educated as to the signs and symptoms of upper extremity deep vein thrombosis and receive adequate prophylaxis. Ongoing research into less thrombogenic catheters is an area they may decrease the incidence of secondary upper extremity deep vein thrombosis in the future, but currently prophylaxis is the greatest single area in which an impact can be made at this time.

ASYMPTOMATIC UPPER EXTREMITY DEEP VEIN THROMBOSIS

The literature on asymptomatic upper extremity deep vein thrombosis is severely limited by its inherent nature. Patients with asymptomatic upper extremity deep vein thrombosis are those usually found serendipitously on an imaging study performed for follow-up of their underlying diagnosis or for another unrelated reason. Obviously, the question is then what to do with this information. Several factors need to be evaluated, including whether the patient is a candidate for anticoagulation, whether there is a significant benefit to anticoagulation in this patient, and whether the patient has been receiving prophylaxis. Other questions include whether the catheter's function has been impaired, and whether the vessel's lumen is completely or partially obstructed. If a patient not receiving prophylaxis is found to have an asymptomatic upper extremity deep vein thrombosis that is not completely obstructing the lumen or interfering with catheter function, the patient should be started on 1 mg daily of warfarin. The patient could also be started on prophylactic doses of heparin or low molecular weight heparin. Of course, thought must be given first to whether the patient can be treated with peripheral access and, if so, the catheter should be removed.

If the patient has an asymptomatic upper extremity clot related to either an implanted venous access device (passport) or other permanent central venous catheter and the catheter's function has been compromised, streptokinase/urokinase or tissue plasminogen factor can be instilled through the catheter (if the patient has no major contraindications) and the patient subsequently begun on prophylaxis, if not already on it.[41,51–5,60] This may be effective in restoring catheter function and lysing the clot. If the patient has already been on prophylaxis, thought should be given to either increasing the dose of the same anticoagulant to a therapeutic range or changing to a different anticoagulant.

Currently, it is difficult to suggest therapeutic levels of anticoagulation for asymptomatic upper extremity deep vein thrombosis that are associated with catheters. Of course, once it is known that a patient has an asymptomatic clot, he or she should be placed on prophylaxis and educated about the signs and symptoms of upper extremity deep vein thrombosis and clot propagation. An asymptomatic upper extremity deep vein thrombosis should be followed clinically; the decision to obtain serial imaging studies to rule out propagation is difficult to suggest on the basis of a cost–benefit ratio, but is left to the clin individual practitioner. If the patient becomes symptomatic or if there is evidence of clot propagation despite catheter removal, the patient should be treated with therapeutic levels of anticoagulation.

SUMMARY

Primary upper extremity deep vein thrombosis is an under-recognized and potentially treatable disease that is associated with a significant degree of morbidity. It is often associated with exertion, and an anatomic abnormality is often present. Patients are usually young and present with pain, edema, and limitation of motion. The diagnosis is made with venography, which should be performed on most patients; ultrasonography is an adequate screening test. Aggressive therapy including thrombolytics, anticoagulation, and surgery should be instituted quickly.

Secondary upper extremity deep vein thrombosis is a phenomenon occurring increasingly, mainly as a result of central vein cannulation. It may occur as a complication of tumors, other thrombophilic states, catheters of all types, congestive heart failure, and, commonly, from a combination of factors. There is a significant degree of morbidity associated with catheter-related upper extremity deep vein thrombosis as a result of venous insufficiency and pulmonary embolism. Therapy is directed at removing the inciting agent (catheter), if present, and using anticoagulation in symptomatic patients. The most important impact that can be made today is with prevention. With the increasing age of the population and the ability to treat patients with chronic disease processes longer, it is likely that the incidence will continue to rise. Further trials are needed to better define the relative risks predisposing toward upper extremity deep vein thrombosis and the best methods for prevention.

REFERENCES

1 Paget J. *Clinical lectures and essays*. Longmans Green, 1875.
2 Von Schroetter L. Enkrankungen der Gefasse. In: *Nathnagel handbuch der pathologie und therapie*. Wein: Holder, 1884.
3 Haire WD. Arm vein thrombosis. *Clin Chest Med* 1995; **16**: 341–51.
4 Demeter SL, Pritchard JS, Piedad OH, et al. Upper extremity thrombosis: etiology and prognosis. *Angiology* 1982; November: 743–55.

5 Barnett T, Levitt LM. 'Effort' thrombosis of the axillary vein with pulmonary embolism. *JAMA* 1951; **146**.

6 Featherstone T, Bayliss AP. Deppe venous thrombosis of the upper extremity – a case report. *Angiology* 1987; October: 793–6.

7 Tomlin CE. Pulmonary infarction complicating thrombophlebitis of the upper extremity. *Am J Med* 1952; April.

8 Coon WW, Willis PW. Thrombosis of axillary and subclavian veins. *Arch Surg* 1967: **94**.

9 Tilney NL, Griffiths HJ, Edwards EA. Natural history of major venous thrombosis of the upper extremity. *Arch Surg* 1970; **101**.

10 Lindblad B, Tengborn L, Bergvist D. Deep vein thrombosis of the axillary-subclavian veins: epidemiologic data, effects of different types of treatment and late sequele. *Eur J Vasc Surg* 1988; **2**: 161–5.

11 Swinton NW, Edgett JW, Hall RJ. Primary subclavian–axillary vein thrombosis. *Circulation* 1968; **XXXVIII**.

12 AbuRahma AF, Sadler DL, Robinson PA. Axillary–subclavian vein thrombosis. *Am Surg* 1991; **57**.

13 Prescott SM, Tikoff G. Deep venous thrombosis of the upper extremity: a reappraisal. *Circulation* 1979; **59**.

14 Vogel CM, Jensen JE. 'Effort' thrombosis of the subclavian vein in a competitive swimmer. *Am J Sports Med* 1985; **13**.

15 Hill SL, Berry RE. Subclavian vein thrombosis: a continuing challenge. *Surgery* 1990; **108**.

16 Machleder H. The role of thrombolytic agents for acute subclavian vein thrombosis. *Semin Vasc Surg* 1992; **5**.

17 Hurlbert SN, Rutherford RB. Primary subclavian–axillary vein thrombosis. *Ann Vasc Surg* 1995; **9**.

18 Prandoni et al. Upper extremity deep venous thrombosis. *Arch Int Med* 1997; **57**.

19 Kammen BF and Soulen MC. Phlegmasia cerulea dolens of the upper extremity. *J Vasc Intervent Radiol* 1995; **6**.

20 Becker GJ, Holden RW, Rabe FE, et al. Local thrombolytic therapy for subclavian and axillary vein thrombosis. *Radiol* 1983; **149**.

21 Horattas MC, Wright DJ, Fenton AH, et al. Changing concepts of deep venous thrombosis of the upper extremity – Report of a series and review of the literature. *Surg* 1988; **104**.

22 Urscel HC, Razzuk MA. Improved management of the Paget–Schroetter syndrome secondary to thoracic outlet compression. *Ann Thor Surg* 1991; **52**.

23 Harley DP, White RA, Nelson RJ, Mehringer CM. Pulmonary embolism secondary to venous thrombosis of the arm. *Am J Surg* 1984; **147**.

24 Stephens MB. Deep venous thrombosis of the upper extremity. *Am Fam Phys* 1997; **55**.

25 Becker DM, Philbrick JT, Walker FB IV. Axillary and subclavian venous thrombosis – prognosis and treatment. *Arch Int Med* 1991; **151**.

26 Moser KM, Fedullo PF, LittleJohn, JK. Frequent asymptomatic pulmonary embolism in patients with deep venous thrombosis. *JAMA* 1994; **271**.

27 Monreal M, Ruiz J, Olazabal A, et al. Deep venous thrombosis and the risk of pulmonary embolism. *Chest* 1992; **102**.

28 Monreal M, Lafoz E, Ruiz J, et al. Upper-extremity deep venous thrombosis and pulmonary embolism. *Chest* 1991; **99**.

29 Sottiuri VS, Towner K, McDonnell AE, et al. Diagnosis of upper extremity deep venous thrombosis using noninvasive technique. *Surg* 1982; **91**: 582–5.

30 Patwardhan NA, Anderson FA, Cutler BS, Wheeler HB. Noninvasive detection of axillary and subclavian venous thrombosis by impedence plethysmography. *J Cardiovasc Surg* 1983; **24**: 250–5.

31 Silverstein AM, Turbiner EH. Technetium-99m red blood cell venography in upper extremity deep venous thrombosis. *Clin Nucl Med* 1987; **2**: 421–3.

32 Monreal M, Montserrat E, Salvador R, et al. Real-time ultrasound for diagnosis of symptomatic venous thrombosis and for screening of patients at risk: correlation with ascending conventional venography. *Angiology* 1989.

33 Grassi CJ and Polak JF. Axillary and subclavian vein thrombosis: follow-up evaluation with color doppler flow US and Vvenography. *Radiology* 1990; **175**: 651–4.

34 Erdman WA, Jayson HT, Redman HC, et al. Deep venous thrombosis of extremities: role of MR imaging in the diagnosis. *Radiology* 1990; **174**: 425–31.

35 Baxter GM, Kincaid W, Jeffrey RF, et al. Comparison of colour Doppler ultrasound with venography in the diagnosis of axillary and subclavian vein thrombosis. *Brit J Radiol* 1991; **64.**

36 Cronan JJ. Venous thromboembolic disease: the role of US. *Radiology* 1993; **186**: 619–30.

37 Fielding JR, Nagel S, Pomeroy O. Upper extremity DVT-correlation of MR and nuclear medicine flow imaging. *Clin Imag* 1997; **21**: 260–3.

38 Chang Y-C, et al. 2–D Time-of-Flight (TOF) MRA of thrombophlebitis of upper extremity and subclavian veins. *Angiology* 1996; **47**.

39 Longley DG, Finlay DE, Letourneau JG. Sonography of the upper extremity and jugular veins. *Am J Radiol* 1993; **160**.

40 Machleder HI. Evaluation of a new treatment strategy for Paget–Schroetter syndrome: Spontaneous thrombosis of the axillary-subclavian vein. *J Vasc Surg* 1993; **17**.

41 AbuRahma AF, Sadler D, Stuart P, et al. Conventional versus thrombolytic therapy in spontaneous (effort) axillary-subclavian vein thrombosis. *Am J Surg* 1991; **161**.

42 Appleby DH, Heller MS. Low-dose streptokinase therapy for subclavian vein thrombosis. *South Med J* 1984; **77**.

43 Pires LA, Jay G. Upper-extremity deep-vein thrombosis: thrombolytic therapy with antistrepalase. *Ann Emerg Med* 1993; **2**.

44 Chang, et al. Pulse-spray treatment of subclavuian and jugular venous thrombi with recombinant TPA. *J Vasc Intervent Radiol* 1996.

45 Molina JE. Surgery for effort thrombosis of the subclavian vein. *J Thor Cardiovasc Surg* 1992; **103**.

46 Loring WE. Venous thrombosis in the upper extremities as a complication of myocardial failure. *Am J Med* 1952.

47 Borakas P, Seale J, Price J, et al. Prevention of central venous catheter associated thrombus using minidose warfarin in patients with haematological malignancies. *Br J Haemat* 1998; **101**: 483–6.

48 Monreal M, et al. Upper extremity deep venous thrombosis in cancer patients with venous access devices – prophylaxis with a low-molecular weight heparin (Fragmin). *Thromb Hemost* 1996; **75**: 251–3.

49 Burihan E, de Figueiredo LF, Francisco J Jr, Miranda F Jr. Upper extremity deep venous thrombosis: analysis of 52 cases. *Cardiovasc Surg* 1993; **1**.

50 Bern MM, Lokich JJ, Wallach SR, et al. Very low doses of warfarin can prevent thrombosis in central venous catheters. *Ann Intern Medic* 1990; **112**: 423–8.

51 Haire WD, Lieberman RP, Edney J, et al. Hickman catheter-induced thoracic vein thrombosis. Frequency and long-term sequellae in patients receiving high-dose chemotherpay and marrow transplantation. *Cancer* 1990; **66**.

52 Oakley GJ, Downey GO, King LA, et al. Symptomatic central venous thrombosis and long-term right atrial catheters. *Gynecologic Oncology* 1990; **36**: 405–8.

53 Anderson AJ, Krasnow SH, Boyer MW et al. Thrombosis: the major Hickman catheter complication in patients with solid tumor. *Chest* 1989; **95**.

54 Huisman MV, Buller HR, ten Cate JW, et al. Unexpected high prevalence of silent pulmonary embolism in patients with deep venous thrombosis. *Chest* 1989; **95**.

55 Hung SS. Deep vein thrombosis of the arm associated with malignancy. *Cancer* 1989.

56 Stricker SJ, Sowers DK, Sowers JR, et al. 'Effort thrombosis' of the subclavian associated with oral contraceptives. *Ann Emerg Med* 1981; **10**: 11.

57 Hingorani AH, et al. Upper extremity versus lower extremity deep venous thrombosis. *Am J Surg* 1997; **174**.

58 Hirsch DR, Ingenito EP, Goldhaber SZ. Prevalence of deep venous thrombosis among patients in medical intensive care. *JAMA* 1995; **274**.

59 Monreal M, Raventos A, Lerma R, et al. Pulmonary embolism in patients with upper extremity DVT associated to venous central lines – a prospective study. *Thromb Hemost* 1994; **72**.

60 Leiby JM, Purcell H, DeMaria JJ, et al. Pulmonary embolism as a result of Hickman catheter-related thrombosis. *Am J Med* 1989; **86**.

18

Antithrombotic therapy in atrial fibrillation

BRIAN F GAGE, TAMMY L LIN

THE RELATIONSHIP BETWEEN ATRIAL FIBRILLATION AND STROKE

Over 2 million North Americans have atrial fibrillation and they suffer approximately 75 000 strokes annually.[1] The morbidity and mortality caused by these strokes catalyzed the inception of 10 randomized trials of antithrombotic therapy (Table 18.1)[2–11] and exploration of various techniques to cardiovert these patients to sinus rhythm. However, even in patients who are cardioverted to sinus rhythm initially, atrial fibrillation usually becomes chronic or intermittent (paroxysmal), with an associated fivefold increase in the risk of stroke.[12,13] Thus, the important challenge in caring for patients who have atrial fibrillation is to prevent them from suffering a stroke.

ETIOLOGY AND PATHOPHYSIOLOGY OF ATRIAL FIBRILLATION

The most common causes of atrial fibrillation are hypertension, ischemic heart disease, congestive heart failure, and rheumatic valvular disease.[14,15] Advanced age is

Table 18.1 *Randomized trials of antithrombotic therapy in atrial fibrillation*

Trials	Mean age (years)	Mean duration (years)	Number of participants	No Rx	ASA	Warf	Dual Rx
AFASAK I	74	1.2	1007	X	X	X	
AFASAK II	73	2.2	677		X	X	X
BAATAF	68	2.2	420	X		X	
CAFA	67	1.3	383	X		X	
EAFT	72	2.3	1007	X	X	X	
MWNAF	74	1.2	303			X	
SIFA	72	1.0	916		X	X	
SPAF I	66	1.3	1330	X	X	X	
SPAF II, younger	64	3.1	715		X	X	
SPAF II, older	80	2.0	385		X	X	
SPAF III, high-risk	72	1.1	1044			X	X
SPAF III, low-risk	67	2.0	892		X		
SPINAF	67	1.8	525	X		X	

AFASAK I and II are the Atrial Fibrillation, Aspirin, and Anticoagulation Studies.[2,3]
BAATAF is the Boston Area Anticoagulation Trial for Atrial Fibrillation.[4] About half of the patients in the No Rx arm of this trial took aspirin.
CAFA is the Canadian Atrial Fibrillation Anticoagulation Study.[5]
EAFT is the European Atrial Fibrillation Trial.[6]
MWNAF is the minidose warfarin in Nonrheumatic Atrial Fibrillation Study.[59]
SIFA is the Studio Italiano Fibrillazione Atriale.[7] The antiplatelet agent used in the trial was indobufen rather than aspirin.
SPAF I, II, and III are the Stroke Prevention in Atrial Fibrillation Studies.[8–10, 36] Some patients participated in more than one SPAF study.
SPINAF is the Stroke Prevention in Nonrheumatic Atrial Fibrillation Study.[11]
(No Rx = neither warfarin nor ASA therapy; ASA = aspirin therapy; Warf = warfarin therapy; Dual Rx = both aspirin and warfarin therapy.)

also associated with atrial fibrillation: 70% of North Americans with atrial fibrillation are between the ages of 65 and 85.[1] Other causes of atrial fibrillation include myocardial infarction, alcohol intoxication, stroke, pulmonary embolism, and genetic predisposition.[14,16]

Atrial fibrillation is characterized by the loss of coordinated electrical and mechanical atrial activity.[17] The loss of mechanical contraction results in impaired ventricular filling, thereby favoring the formation of atrial thrombi.[14,18]

DIAGNOSIS OF ATRIAL FIBRILLATION

Atrial fibrillation can be diagnosed from the bedside. Symptoms include palpitations, chest discomfort, fatigue, and breathlessness.[14] Signs include rapid ventricular response, an irregular cardiac rhythm, pulmonary edema, and dyspnea. Once suspected, the diagnosis of atrial fibrillation should be confirmed by electrocardiogram.

ANTITHROMBOTIC THERAPY FOR ACUTE ATRIAL FIBRILLATION

Cardioversion of acute atrial fibrillation to normal sinus rhythm is often attempted to improve cardiac function, to relieve symptoms, and to decrease the potential risk for thromboembolism. The hypothesis that cardioversion of atrial fibrillation will decrease the risk for thromboembolism is being tested by a National Institutes of Health (NIH) trial (the AFFIRM trial).

For new-onset atrial fibrillation (i.e., atrial fibrillation that began in the preceding 48 hours), cardioversion can be attempted without prescribing antecedent warfarin therapy (Fig. 18.1). Intravenous heparin is usually prescribed at the time of hospital admission for cardioversion and then is continued for at least 24 hours after the cardioversion.[19] Warfarin therapy (International Normalized Ratio, INR, of 2–3)

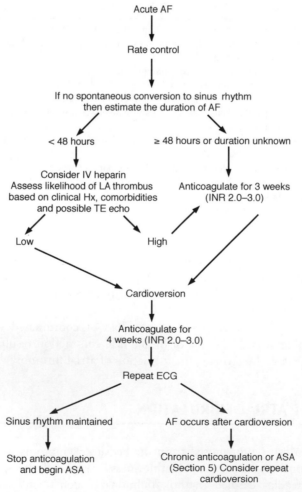

Figure 18.1 *Acute atrial fibrillation (AF) algorithm. (INR = International Normalized Ratio; IV = intravenous; TE = transesophageal; Hx = History; ECG = electrocardiogram; ASA = aspirin.)*

should be initiated prior to hospital discharge and continued for 4 weeks after the cardioversion. Assuming that the patient remains in normal sinus rhythm throughout these 4 weeks, the warfarin therapy can then be stopped in most patients.

Warfarin should be prescribed for approximately 4 weeks after successful cardioversion because there is usually a delay between the time of cardioversion and the return of mechanical atrial contractions. Echocardiographs performed after cardioversion to electrical normal sinus rhythm sometimes demonstrate the complete absence of mechanical atrial contractions.[20] In fact, the atria may require 3 weeks to recover their normal mechanical function.[18] If anticoagulation is withheld during this 3-week postcardioversion period, a thromboembolism may occur.[21]

Patients with atrial fibrillation lasting 48 hours or longer should receive 3 weeks of anticoagulation prior to any elective cardioversion. Cardioversion of these patients without antecedent anticoagulation causes thromboembolism from 1% to 6% of the time.[19,22-4] Prescribing approximately 3 weeks of antecedent anticoagulation therapy lowers this probability to approximately 1%.[19,23-5]

Although prescribing 3 weeks of warfarin prior to cardioversion is safe, this strategy has certain disadvantages. First, delaying cardioversion can lead to clinical instability, especially if the rate of ventricular response is not well controlled. Second, delaying cardioversion may decrease the likelihood of maintenance of normal sinus rhythm.[26] Third, prescribing antecedent warfarin increases the potential risk of hemorrhage.

To overcome these problems, patients who have atrial fibrillation can be cardioverted immediately if they have a high-quality transesophageal echocardiogram (TEE) that documents the absence of left atrial thrombi.[17,27] The risk of thromboembolism in these patients is no more than 1%, as long as they do not also have a very high-risk clinical condition such as mitral stenosis or a prior thromboembolism.[28-30] A multicentered, randomized clinical trial comparing TEE-guided cardioversion with traditional cardioversion (the ACUTE study) is underway.[17]

After any successful cardioversion, 4 weeks of warfarin is usually sufficient to prevent thromboembolism in the short term. However, in some atrial fibrillation patients – patients with mitral stenosis, cardiomyopathy, or prior cerebral ischemia – warfarin should be continued long term, even if normal sinus rhythm is maintained after cardioversion.[15] Most patients who do not need long-term warfarin therapy should switch to aspirin therapy to help prevent a myocardial infarction or stroke (see Efficacy of antiplatelet therapy, below).

In summary, how one should treat a patient with acute atrial fibrillation depends on the duration of the atrial fibrillation, the availability of an accurate TEE, and the risks of hemorrhage. If atrial fibrillation has been present for less than 48 hours, then begin intravenous heparin and assess the likelihood of left atrial thrombus based on the clinical history (Fig. 18.1). If there is high suspicion of thrombus or if the patient is not a good candidate for TEE, then prescribe 3 weeks of oral anticoagulant prior to cardioversion and at least 4 weeks of warfarin after the cardioversion. If suspicion of thrombus is low and no thrombus is detected by TEE, one can cardiovert immediately. Regardless of the duration of atrial fibrillation, prescribing 4 weeks of warfarin after cardioversion will limit the risk of stroke.

ANTITHROMBOTIC THERAPY FOR CHRONIC ATRIAL FIBRILLATION

In the past 10 years, knowledge about atrial fibrillation and the role of antithrombotic therapy in chronic atrial fibrillation has mushroomed. An individual's risk of stroke can now be estimated from his or her comorbid conditions and from findings on an echocardiogram. If this risk is high, the patient can take warfarin to decrease his or her relative risk of stroke by two-thirds. If the risk is low, or if the patient has a contraindication to warfarin therapy, he or she can take aspirin, thereby decreasing the risk of stroke by one-fifth. Appropriate prescription of stroke prophylaxis prolongs life, improves quality of life, and reduces medical expenditure.[31]

Risk of an ischemic event

Without antithrombotic therapy, the annual rate of ischemic stroke among patients with chronic atrial fibrillation varies from less than 1% to over 10%. The lowest rate occurs in patients younger than 60 years who have atrial fibrillation but no other risk factor for stroke – i.e., no history of cerebral ischemia, hypertension, diabetes, or heart disease (mitral stenosis, heart failure, left ventricular dysfunction, or coronary artery disease). These patients, who have *lone atrial fibrillation,* have an annual stroke rate of 0.35%[32] or less.[33] However, older patients who have atrial fibrillation but no other stroke risk factors have annual rates of stroke between 1% and 3%.[34–6] In contrast to these low-risk populations, patients who have already suffered a prior stroke or transient ischemic attack have an annual stroke rate of approximately 12% without antithrombotic therapy.[6,10]

By estimating each patient's risk of stroke, healthcare providers can assess the risks and benefits of antithrombotic therapy for their atrial fibrillation patients. For example, healthcare providers have little to gain by prescribing warfarin to a young man who has lone atrial fibrillation: his annual risk of stroke without warfarin therapy is too low to justify the risk of hemorrhage from warfarin therapy. In contrast, a patient with a high-risk of stroke can prolong his or her quality-adjusted life expectancy by taking warfarin, even if the risk of hemorrhage from warfarin therapy is relatively high.[31] Thus, the healthcare provider should take into account each patient's risk of stroke, as well as other factors, before choosing antithrombotic therapy.

CLINICAL RISK FACTORS FOR STROKE

Recent clinical trials have defined the relationship between clinical risk factors and risk of stroke. Not surprisingly, a history of neurological ischemia is a key risk factor for stroke – a prior stroke or transient ischemic attack triples the risk of a subsequent stroke.[7,10,33,37–40]

A history of hypertension or diabetes probably increases the risk of stroke in the atrial fibrillation population. Hypertension approximately doubles the risk of stroke.[33,35,36,39–41] Diabetes may increase the risk of stroke by a factor of 1.7,[33] but the relationship between diabetes and stroke has not been corroborated in the atrial fibrillation population.[35,42]

Certain types of heart disease are also risk factors for stroke. Mitral stenosis doubles or triples the risk of stroke in patients who have atrial fibrillation.[12,43] A history of heart failure – especially recent heart failure[35,42] – increases the risk of stroke by a factor of approximately 1.4.[33] A prior myocardial infarction also increases the risk of stroke.[3,7,39,44,45] The significance of any type of heart disease is most apparent in patients who have no other risk factors for stroke: it raises their annual risk of stroke sufficiently high (to 3%) that they generally should receive warfarin therapy.[3,33,35,46]

Several characteristics do not appear to affect the rate of stroke significantly. In contrast to earlier studies that found lower rates of stroke in patients whose atrial fibrillation was intermittent rather than chronic,[43,47] a recent pooled analysis found equivalent rates of stroke for these two populations.[33] Likewise, initial findings that the risk of stroke was higher in patients whose atrial fibrillation was of recent onset[43,48] have not been confirmed.[33,35,39] Findings that females have a higher rate of stroke than males[7,35,46] have not been corroborated in recent analyses that controlled for age and for comorbid conditions.[10,33]

ECHOCARDIOGRAPHIC RISK FACTORS FOR STROKE

Knowing that mitral stenosis[12] or a thrombus in the left atrium or left ventricle[49,50] increases the risk of stroke in patients who have atrial fibrillation, researchers have searched for relationships between stroke and other findings seen on transthoracic echocardiogram. The Stroke Prevention in Atrial Fibrillation I (SPAF I) investigators identified two echocardiographic findings that predicted stroke – left atrial enlargement and left ventricular dysfunction. Although retrospective studies also had found that left atrial enlargement was associated with stroke,[41,44,46] several recent prospective studies have not corroborated this association.[4,51] In contrast, recent trials have confirmed the association between left ventricular dysfunction and stroke:[51] patients with moderate to severe left ventricular dysfunction were 2.5 times as likely to suffer a stroke as were patients without this dysfunction. Finally, although controversial, mitral annular calcification may also be a stroke risk factor.[4,41,44] In summary, findings on transthoracic echocardiogram that predict stroke are mitral stenosis, thrombus, left ventricular dysfunction, and possibly left atrial enlargement and mitral annual calcification.

Because TEE provides greater resolution of the left atrium than does transthoracic echocardiography, TEE can detect otherwise-invisible harbingers of stroke: dense spontaneous echocardiographic contrast, small thrombi of the left atrium or left atrial appendage, enlargement of the left atrial appendage, and complex aortic plaque. Although all these factors have been associated with stroke in at least one study, the findings of these studies vary.[40,52–4] Thus, the role of TEE in estimating long-term stroke risk in the atrial fibrillation population remains controversial.

Efficacy of antithrombotic therapy

In the last decade, 10 randomized, controlled trials documented the effectiveness of antithrombotic therapy in preventing stroke in patients who have atrial fibrillation. When taken together, the trials provide overwhelming evidence that warfarin therapy can prevent about two-thirds of strokes in the atrial fibrillation population. The effectiveness of antiplatelet therapy is not as great as that of warfarin therapy: administration of aspirin prevents about one-fifth of strokes in the atrial fibrillation population.

EFFICACY OF ANTICOAGULANT THERAPY

Six randomized trials compared warfarin to no antithrombotic therapy in atrial fibrillation patients: the Copenhagen Atrial Fibrillation, Aspirin, Anticoagulation Study (AFASAK I),[2] the Boston Area Anticoagulation Trial for Atrial Fibrillation (BAATAF),[4] the Canadian Atrial Fibrillation Anticoagulation Study (CAFA),[5] the European Atrial Fibrillation Trial (EAFT),[6] the Stroke Prevention in Nonrheumatic Atrial Fibrillation Study (SPINAF),[11] and the SPAF I[8] (Table 18.1). The results of these trials so favored adjusted-dose warfarin therapy (over no antithrombotic therapy) that subsequent randomized trials have compared adjusted-dose warfarin to other regimens of antithrombotic therapy.

Five trials showed statistically significant reductions in the rate of ischemic stroke; the sixth (CAFA) was stopped prematurely based on the results of the others. Pooling the raw data of these trials (Fig. 18.2), the Atrial Fibrillation Investigators (i.e., investigators from AFASAK, BATAAF, CAFA, EAFT, SPAF, and SPINAF) demonstrated that warfarin had a relative risk reduction of 68%, with a narrow 95% confidence interval (50–79%). The absolute risk reduction was 3.1% per year of warfarin therapy: the annual ischemic stroke rate was 4.5% in patients randomized to no antithrombotic therapy, and 1.4% in patients randomized to warfarin therapy. Thus, for every 100 patient-years of warfarin therapy, 3.1 strokes were prevented.[33,55]

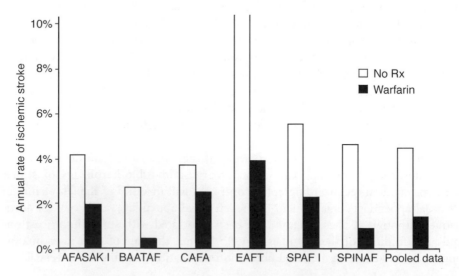

Figure 18.2 *Stroke rate with warfarin versus no antithrombotic therapy. Bars represent the annual rate of stroke in atrial fibrillation patients randomized to no antithrombotic therapy (white) or adjusted-dose warfarin (black). The annual rate of stroke in EAFT participants randomized to no antithrombotic therapy (12.3%) was truncated at 10%. Because EAFT was a trial of secondary prophylaxis, it was not included in the pooled data. (For explanations of acronyms, see Table 18.1.)*

Participants in these trials differed from the atrial fibrillation population at large. Potential participants who were very elderly or who had contraindications to antithrombotic therapy were excluded, with exclusion rates of 60% or greater in the trials. Because of these exclusions, the average age of trial participants was approximately 5 years younger than the median age (75 years) of the North American atrial fibrillation population.[1,56] The prevalences of stroke risk factors in the trial participants were typical of the general atrial fibrillation population: hypertension was present in 45% of participants, diabetes in 14%, congestive heart failure in 19%, angina in 22%, and history of myocardial infarction in 13%. Although most trials excluded patients who had a history of neurological ischemia, all the EAFT participants had suffered such an event. Despite their history of stroke and their frequent use of acenocoumarol rather than warfarin, EAFT participants taking an anticoagulant enjoyed the same 68% relative risk reduction as participants in other trials who took warfarin.[6]

EFFICACY OF ANTIPLATELET THERAPY

The benefit of aspirin therapy is less clear than that of anticoagulation. AFASAK I, SPAF I, and EAFT all compared aspirin to no antithrombotic therapy. In SPAF I, aspirin therapy had a relative risk reduction of 42% compared to no antithrombotic therapy;[8] in the other two trials, the benefit of aspirin therapy was not statistically significant (18% in AFASAK I; 15% in EAFT).[57] Analyses of pooled data from these trials found that aspirin prevented 21–22% of ischemic strokes, but the 95% confidence interval of this relative risk reduction was large (0% to 38%).[55,57,58]

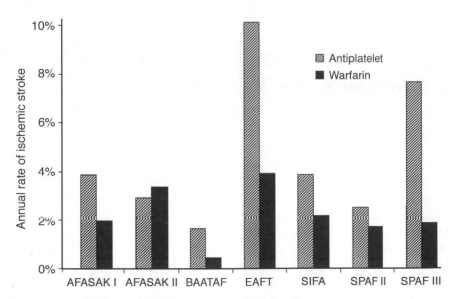

Figure 18.3 *Stroke rate with warfarin versus antiplatelet therapy. Bars represent the annual rate of stroke in atrial fibrillation patients randomized to antiplatelet therapy (hatched) or adjusted-dose warfarin (black). In all of the trials except SIFA, the antiplatelet therapy was aspirin (75–325 mg). SIFA participants were randomized to either indobufen or warfarin. In half of the AFASAK II participants and all of the SPAF III participants, aspirin was prescribed in combination with minidose warfarin. (For explanations of acronyms, see Table 18.1.)*

Although the seven randomized trials that compared adjusted-dose warfarin to antiplatelet therapy had different protocols, all trials reported results consistent with a 46% relative risk reduction in the rate of ischemic stroke with warfarin rather than antiplatelet therapy (Fig. 18.3).[55] The AFASAK I investigators found that warfarin (INR 2.8–4.2) halved the rate of stroke, compared to daily aspirin (75 mg).[2] The AFASAK II (Atrial Fibrillation, Aspirin, Anticoagulation Study II)[3] investigators randomized patients to one of four regimens: adjusted-dose warfarin (INR 2.0–3.0), minidose warfarin (1.25 mg), aspirin (300 mg), or both minidose warfarin and aspirin. The rate of stroke was insignificantly higher in patients randomized to adjusted-dose warfarin than in those randomized to one of the aspirin arms. Although the BAATAF investigators randomized participants to warfarin versus no warfarin, enough participants in the no-warfarin cohort took aspirin and later suffered a stroke that the benefits of warfarin over aspirin therapy were apparent.[4] The EAFT investigators found a significant 62% reduction in the rate of stroke in patients randomized to warfarin (INR 2.5–4.0) rather than aspirin (300 mg).[6] The Studio Italiano Fibrillazione Atriale (SIFA)[7] investigators randomized patients who had atrial fibrillation and recent cerebral ischemia to either warfarin (INR 2.0–3.5) or the antiplatelet agent indobufen; they found a 44% relative risk reduction with warfarin therapy. The SPAF II investigators[9] randomized patients to aspirin (325 mg) or adjusted-dose warfarin (prothrombin time ratio 1.3–1.8). They found a 31% relative risk reduction with warfarin therapy, but an absolute reduction in the stroke rate that was less than 1% – about the same magnitude as the rate of intracranial events in patients assigned warfarin. The SPAF III investigators randomized participants to either adjusted-dose warfarin (INR 2.0–3.0) or combined therapy with aspirin (325 mg) and minidose warfarin (INR 1.2–1.5). Participants taking adjusted-dose warfarin had a significant 75% relative risk reduction in the rate of stroke.[10] Averaging the stroke rates from all of these atrial fibrillation trials, Hart and colleagues calculated that warfarin has a relative risk reduction of about 46% as compared to aspirin therapy.[55]

EFFICACY OF MINIDOSE WARFARIN THERAPY

SPAF III demonstrated that minidose warfarin was less effective than adjusted-dose warfarin. In SPAF III, the annual rate of stroke was 1.9% with adjusted-dose warfarin (INR 2.0–3.0) and 7.7% with minidose warfarin (INR 1.2–1.5) plus aspirin (325 mg). The Minidose Warfarin in Nonrheumatic Atrial Fibrillation Study (MWNAF) also found a lower stroke rate in participants randomized to adjusted-dose warfarin (INR 2.0–3.0) rather than to min-dose warfarin (1.25 mg/day).[59] Because of these results, a third trial (AFASAK II) that was comparing minidose warfarin to adjusted-dose warfarin was halted early. At the time of cessation of AFASAK II, there was no significant difference between any of the arms of the trial.[3] Because SPAF III had more patient-years of therapy and results that strongly favored adjusted-dose therapy, most experts have accepted their findings and concluded that mini-dose warfarin is a relatively ineffective regimen for patients who have atrial fibrillation.

Safety of antithrombotic therapy

In the clinical trials, adjusted-dose warfarin caused fewer major hemorrhages than the number of ischemic strokes it prevented. Trial participants randomized to adjusted-dose warfarin therapy had annual rates of major hemorrhage (typically defined as bleeding requiring hospitalization or the transfusion of at least 2 U of blood) that averaged 1.9%,[3,6,10,33,60] approximately 1% higher than the hemorrhage rate in participants taking aspirin or no antithrombotic therapy.[33,36,57] Thus, for every 100 participant-years of warfarin therapy, rather than no antithrombotic therapy, 3.1 ischemic strokes were prevented and one major hemorrhage was caused. Thus, in the clinical trials, the benefit of adjusted-dose warfarin therapy outweighed its risk.

Because trial participants were selected carefully and received their medical care in carefully controlled settings, they may have benefited more from antithrombotic therapy than would typical patients. As mentioned, prospective participants were often excluded from the trials because of advanced age or a contraindication to antithrombotic therapy. As a result of these and other exclusions, only from 7%[11,61] to 40%[2] of screened patients ultimately enrolled in the trials. Thus, participants were younger and healthier than typical atrial fibrillation patients. Furthermore, most trial participants were cared for in carefully controlled settings. Typical care may be associate with a higher hemorrhage rate: in their review of anticoagulant-related bleeding, Landefeld and Beyth concluded that the risk of hemorrhage is approximately twofold higher in patients prescribed anticoagulants outside of experimental trials.[62] Thus, prescribing warfarin to typical patients may have an annual rate of major hemorrhage of 3–4% – an absolute increase in hemorrhage of 2–3% as compared with aspirin therapy. Likewise, because of the careful participant selection and the excellent medical care in the trials, the 68% efficacy of warfarin therapy observed in the trials may be difficult to emulate in clinical practice.[63]

Selection of antithrombotic therapy

The optimal antithrombotic therapy for atrial fibrillation patients depends on their risk of stroke, risk of hemorrhage, and personal preferences.[64] Circumstances that favor warfarin therapy include higher risk of stroke, lower risk of hemorrhage, and individual preference endorsing that therapy.

RISK OF ISCHEMIC EVENT

Because the relative risk reductions of antithrombotic therapy (68% for warfarin, 21% for aspirin) are consistent across subgroups of patients who have atrial fibrillation, the absolute benefit of antithrombotic therapy depends on an individual's risk of stroke. For example, consider a high-risk patient – a man who has atrial fibrillation and at least two of the following stroke risk factors: a history of cerebral ischemia, hypertension, diabetes, or heart disease. If his risk factors include a prior stroke, for example, then his risk of a recurrent stroke is about 12% per year without antithrombotic therapy.[6] Warfarin will reduce this annual stroke risk by approximately 8% per year; aspirin will reduce it by just over 2% per year. Because of its 6% per year incremental absolute reduction in stroke rate, warfarin is the first-line therapy for this high-risk patient (Table 18.2).

The benefit of antithrombotic therapy is more modest in a woman* who has atrial fibrillation and a single stroke risk factor. She is a medium-risk patient, with a

---

*The patient's gender does not affect the choice of therapy: antithrombotic therapy is as effective[33] and as safe[60] in women as it is in men.

Table 18.2 *Recommended antithrombotic therapy for atrial fibrillation*

Stroke risk factors[a]	1st-line therapy	Alternate therapy
Absent	ASA	Warf
Present	Warf	ASA

[a]Stroke risk factors: history of an ischemic neurological event, hypertension, diabetes, or heart disease (mitral stenosis, coronary artery disease, or heart failure).
ASA = Aspirin (e.g., 325 mg daily); Warf = warfarin (e.g., target INR 2.5).

stroke risk of approximately 3–4% per year.[33,36] Her absolute risk reduction from antithrombotic therapy would be about 2.4% per year with warfarin and 0.7% per year with aspirin therapy. Warfarin's incremental reduction in the rate of ischemic stroke (1.7% per year) would be worth its risk of major hemorrhage (approximately 2% per year) because, on average, strokes are more severe than major hemorrhages. Thus, warfarin is the first-line therapy for patients who have atrial fibrillation and at least one additional risk factor for stroke (Table 18.2).[65,66]

In contrast to higher risk patients, low-risk atrial fibrillation patients gain little by taking warfarin instead of aspirin. Without antithrombotic therapy, these low-risk patients have an annual stroke rate of 3% or less.[33,35] With either aspirin or warfarin therapy, this rate is reduced to 1% or 2%, depending on patient age.[9,33,36] Although warfarin may decrease the rate of ischemic stroke more than aspirin therapy does, the two agents have equivalent effectiveness at reducing the combined endpoint of ischemic stroke plus intracranial hemorrhage in low-risk patients.[3,9] Thus, for patients who have atrial fibrillation and no (additional) risk factors for stroke, aspirin is the first-line therapy. Although young patients with lone atrial fibrillation have a risk of stroke of 0.35% or less, even without antithrombotic therapy, prescribing aspirin therapy in this subpopulation is recommended to lower cardiovascular mortality.[67–9]

QUALITY-OF-LIFE CONSIDERATIONS

Decision analyses have demonstrated that prescription of antithrombotic therapy for patients who have atrial fibrillation prolongs quality-adjusted survival.[31,70–8] *Decision analysis* is a technique that combines uncertain, heterogeneous outcomes – strokes, hemorrhages, and antithrombotic therapy, in this case – into a common currency, such as quality-adjusted life years (QALYs).[79] These recent decision analyses have demonstrated that the benefits of antithrombotic therapy depend on a patient's risk of stroke. In high-risk patients, prescribing warfarin (rather than no antithrombotic therapy) improved quality-adjusted survival by 0.50 QALY. For medium-risk patients, warfarin improved survival by 0.37 QALY as compared with no antithrombotic therapy. Finally, for low-risk patients, either warfarin or aspirin prolonged quality-adjusted survival by about 0.20 QALY. Thus, on average, there is little to be gained by prescribing warfarin instead of aspirin in a typical low-risk patient, especially if one takes into account the lower cost of aspirin therapy.[31]

On the other hand, whether warfarin or aspirin should be prescribed to an individual low-risk patient depends on that individual's preferences (and risk of hemorrhage). Surveys of patients who have atrial fibrillation have shown great variability in preferences regarding stroke and antithrombotic therapy.[80] This variability affects the quality-adjusted survival. For example, in a 75-year-old, low-risk patient whose quality of life would not be adversely affected by taking warfarin, warfarin therapy has a slightly greater projected quality-adjusted survival than does aspirin.[64] Likewise, medium-risk patients (of any age) who would have a very low quality of life from daily warfarin therapy would have a greater quality-adjusted survival with aspirin therapy. Thus, one should prescribe antithrombotic therapy tailored to a patient's risks of adverse events and personal preferences.[64,65,77,81] The best way to accommodate a patient's preference is unknown, but techniques to engage a patient in the selection of antithrombotic therapy are being developed.[73,82,83]

Although incorporation of patient preferences into the choice of therapy for atrial fibrillation may be an unfamiliar proposition for many clinicians, promotion of patient involvement has improved the outcomes of patients who have other chronic diseases. A physician's participatory decision-making style can help to reduce pain in arthritic patients,[84] blood pressure in hypertensive patients,[85] and glycosylated hemoglobin in diabetics.[86,87] Patient participation probably improves outcomes in these populations by enhancing patient knowledge[82] and compliance.[88,89] If so, a participatory decision-making style may be especially important for clinicians whose patients take warfarin therapy – a regimen that requires high levels of patient knowledge and compliance.

IN SPECIAL POPULATIONS

The recommendations – to prescribe aspirin to low-risk patients and warfarin to others – apply to almost all atrial fibrillation populations. An exception is that one may prescribe aspirin (or even no antithrombotic therapy) to patients whose risk of hemorrhage is exceptionally high. Patients who are very elderly or who have coronary artery disease also require special consideration.

Patients older than 75 years
Although there are exceptions,[90–4] most investigators have found that older patients who take warfarin have significantly higher rates of major hemorrhage than do younger patients on the same regimens.[60,90,95–100] For example, in the elderly cohort (mean age 80 years) of SPAF II, the lower rate of ischemic stroke in participants prescribed warfarin instead of aspirin was offset by their higher rate of intracranial hemorrhage: the annual rate of all intracranial events combined was 4.6% in elderly patients randomized to warfarin versus 4.3% in similar participants randomized to aspirin.[9] Although other atrial fibrillation trials did not find a significantly increased risk of hemorrhage in the elderly,[6,101] they included fewer octogenarians.

In contrast to the results of SPAF II, other data strongly support the use of warfarin in the very elderly. First, coincidentally, the risk of ischemic stroke and the risk of major hemorrhage both increase by a factor of approximately 1.4 per decade of life.[33,95,96] Thus, the increased risk of prescribing warfarin in the elderly is offset by a commensurate increased benefit. Second, atrial fibrillation trials have shown no significant benefit of aspirin in patients older than age 75.[57,102] Because trials of aspirin in other elderly populations have found reductions in stroke and myocardial infarction,[67] aspirin's lack of efficacy in elderly atrial fibrillation patients may be spurious. Finally, in an atrial fibrillation cohort of frail Medicare beneficiaries who had a median age of 80 years, warfarin was associated with a lower incidence of the composite endpoint of stroke or death, whereas aspirin had no significant benefit.[63]

Our guidelines for prescribing antithrombotic therapy (Table 18.2) are not age linked: warfarin is the first-line therapy for patients who have atrial fibrillation with additional stroke risk factors, whereas aspirin is the first-line therapy for patients who have atrial fibrillation alone (and for patients who have contraindications to warfarin). Other published guidelines are similar to ours, except that some of them have advocated the prescription of warfarin in the entire elderly atrial fibrillation population, including those patients whose only stroke risk factor is atrial fibrillation.[65,66]

Patients who have coronary artery disease

Because warfarin is as effective as aspirin in preventing myocardial infarction,[69, 103–6] aspirin does not need to be added to warfarin therapy in patients who have atrial fibrillation and stable coronary artery disease. The two atrial fibrillation trials that randomized participants to either adjusted-dose warfarin or to the combination of minidose warfarin plus aspirin found no advantage of the combination therapy.[3,10] Other trials of combination therapy have found increased rates of hemorrhage,[69,107,108] sometimes without greater effectiveness.[108] Thus, given its increased risk of hemorrhage and its uncertain added benefit in this population, combination therapy should not be used routinely in patients who have atrial fibrillation and stable coronary artery disease. However, in patients who have atrial fibrillation and acute coronary-artery syndromes, the benefits of combination therapy are likely to outweigh the risks. When combination therapy is necessary, prescribing aspirin at low doses (e.g., enteric-coated aspirin 81 mg per day) can minimize aspirin's risk of causing gastric hemorrhage.[109]

Selection of the target INR atrial fibrillation

Recent guidelines recommend a target INR of 2.5.[65] Some of the larger trials targeted INRs that were higher than this recommendation, but the INRs achieved in these trials averaged no higher than 2.9 (Fig. 18.4). In contrast to these trials, BAATAF and SPINAF targeted prothrombin time ratios of only 1.2–1.5, equivalent to INRs of approximately 1.4–2.8. The remaining studies targeted INRs of 2.0–3.0[3,5,10] or 2.0–3.5.[7] Because adjusted-dose warfarin appeared to be equally effective in all of these trials (see Fig. 18.2) experts have advocated an intermediate level of anticoagulation: typically a target INR of 2.5,[65,66] although a target INR of 3.0 has sometimes been recommended.[110] An INR range of 2.0–3.5 approximates the target INRs used in the clinical trials.

Other studies also support the use of INRs greater than 2.0. The SPAF III investigators demonstrated that minidose warfarin (INR 1.5 or less) was ineffective, even when combined with aspirin, and that rates of ischemic events were lowest in patients whose INR was greater than 2.0.[10] Likewise, in a case-controlled study, Hylek and colleagues found that the odds of an ischemic stroke were lowest in patients who had an INR above 2.0.[111] In a similar study, Brass and colleagues found that the odds of an ischemic stroke decreased with increasing INRs. For example, they found that the odds of stroke were halved by an INR of 3.0 or greater, compared with an INR of 2.0–2.9.[112] The EAFT Study Group found the lowest rate of stroke in patients who had an INR of 2.0–3.9.[113] Finally, Azar and colleagues found that higher INRs also decreased the risk of myocardial infarction.[114]

Because the risk of hemorrhage rises with increasing INR,[60,95,96,114–16] an INR of 2.5 may minimize the risk of all (hemorrhagic and ischemic) adverse events in typical

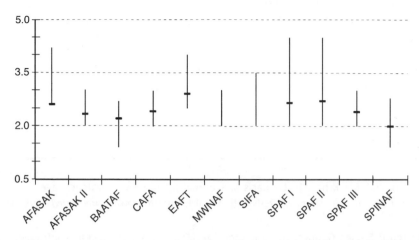

Figure 18.4 *Target and mean International Normalized Ratios (INRs) in atrial fibrillation trials of adjusted-dose warfarin. Lines represent the targeted INR ranges and tick marks denote the average INR reported in each of the trials. (NB: the average INR was not reported from all trials.)*

patients who have atrial fibrillation. However, for patients who have already suffered cerebral ischemia, a target INR of 3.0 (range 2.5–3.5) may confer more overall benefit.[110,113,117,118] Recommended INRs should be interpreted with caution: they represent an ideal level of anticoagulation, rather than a standard of practice, and a given patient's dose of warfarin need not be changed just because a single INR is slightly above or below the ideal INR range. Furthermore, for patients at high risk of hemorrhage, lower INRs may confer a more favorable risk–benefit ratio.

Current use of antithrombotic therapy in atrial fibrillation

In light of the evidence supporting the prescription of antithrombotic therapy in patients who have atrial fibrillation,[2–9,11,33,36] the use of antithrombotic therapy is surprisingly low. Chart reviews have documented that only one-half of the atrial fibrillation population is receiving therapy with warfarin (or other vitamin K antagonist).[119–23] Furthermore, the use of warfarin is even lower in the elderly[112,119–21,123–8] – the population at highest risk of stroke. To reverse this underuse of antithrombotic therapy, clinicians should increase awareness about the benefits of antithrombotic therapy, and should adopt systems, such as anticoagulation services,[129] that decrease the burden of anticoagulation.

THE FUTURE OF ANTITHROMBOTIC THERAPY FOR PATIENTS WITH ATRIAL FIBRILLATION

Current research promises to help clinicians refine the choice of antithrombotic therapy, to use cardioversion more judiciously, and to improve anticoagulation monitoring. To refine their choice of antithrombotic therapy, clinicians will consider their patients' comorbid conditions, personal preferences, and echocardiographic findings to select the regimen that will maximize quality-adjusted survival. To use cardioversion more judiciously, clinicians will be guided by the results of a multi-centered, randomized trial (AFFIRM) that is comparing rate control versus rhythm control. To improve anticoagulation monitoring, clinicians will have greater access to anticoagulation clinics and to newer hematological assays.[130-3]

REFERENCES

1 Feinberg WM, Blackshear JL, Laupacis A, Kronmal R, Hart RG. Prevalence, age distribution, and gender of patients with atrial fibrillation. *Arch Intern Med* 1995; **155**: 469–73.

2 Petersen P, Boysen G, Godtfredsen J, Andersen ED, Andersen B. Placebo-controlled, randomised trial of warfarin and aspirin for prevention of thromboembolic complications in chronic atrial fibrillation: the Copenhagen AFASAK Study. *Lancet* 1989; **1**: 175–9.

3 Gulløv AL, Koefoed BG, Petersen P, et al. Fixed minidose warfarin and aspirin alone and in combination vs adjusted-dose warfarin for stroke prevention in atrial fibrillation: Second Copenhagen Atrial Fibrillation, Aspirin, and Anticoagulation Study. *Arch Intern Med* 1998; **158**: 1513–21.

4 The Boston Area Anticoagulation Trial for Atrial Fibrillation Investigators. The effect of low-dose warfarin on the risk of stroke in patients with nonrheumatic atrial fibrillation. *N Engl J Med* 1990; **323**: 1505–11.

5 Connolly SJ. Canadian Atrial Fibrillation Anticoagulation (CAFA) Study. *J Am Coll Cardiol* 1991; **18**: 349–55.

6 The European Atrial Fibrillation Trial Study Group. Secondary prevention in non-rheumatic atrial fibrillation after transient ischaemic attack or minor stroke. *Lancet* 1993; **342**: 1255–62.

7 Morocutti C, Amabile G, Fattapposta F, et al. Indobufen versus warfarin in the secondary prevention of major vascular events in nonrheumatic atrial fibrillation. *Stroke* 1997; **28**: 1015–21.

8 Stroke Prevention in Atrial Fibrillation Investigators. Stroke Prevention in Atrial Fibrillation (SPAF) Study. Final results. *Circulation* 1991; **84**: 527–39.

9 Stroke Prevention in Atrial Fibrillation Investigators. Warfarin versus aspirin for prevention of thromboembolism in atrial fibrillation: Stroke Prevention in Atrial Fibrillation II Study. *Lancet* 1994; **343**: 687–91.

10 Stroke Prevention in Atrial Fibrillation Investigators. Adjusted-dose warfarin versus low-intensity, fixed-dose warfarin plus aspirin for high-risk patients with atrial fibrillation: Stroke Prevention in Atrial Fibrillation III randomised clinical trial. *Lancet* 1996; **348**: 633–38.

11 Ezekowitz MD, Bridgers SL, James KE, et al. Warfarin in the prevention of stroke associated with nonrheumatic atrial fibrillation. *N Engl J Med* 1992; **327**: 1406–12.

12 Wolf PA, Dawber TR, Thomas HE Jr, Kannel WB. Epidemiologic assessment of chronic atrial fibrillation and risk of stroke: the Framingham Study. *Neurology* 1978; **28**: 973–7.

13 Flegel KM, Shipley MJ, Rose G. Risk of stroke in non-rheumatic atrial fibrillation. *Lancet* 1987; **1**: 526–9.

14 Alpert JS, Petersen P, Godtfredsen J. Atrial fibrillation: natural history, complications, and management. *Annu Rev Med* 1988; **39**: 41–52.

15 Laupacis A, Albers GW, Dalen JE, Dunn MI, Feinberg W, Jacobson AK. Antithrombotic therapy in atrial fibrillation. *Chest* 1995; **108**(Suppl.): 352–9.

16 Brugada R, Tapscott T, Czernuszewicz GZ, et al. Identification of a genetic locus of familial atrial fibrillaiton. *N Engl J Med* 1997; **336**: 905–11.

17 Klein AL, Grimm RA, Black IW, et al. Cardioversion guided by transesophageal echocardiography: the ACUTE pilot study. *Ann Intern Med* 1997; **126**: 200–9.

18 Manning WJ, Leeman DE, Gotch PJ, Come PC. Pulsed Doppler evaluation of atrial mechanical function after electrical cardioversion of atrial fibrillation. *J Am Coll Cardiol* 1989; **13**: 617–23.

19 Weigner MJ, Caulfield TA, Danias PG, Silverman DI, Manning WJ. Risk for clinical thromboembolism associated with conversion to sinus rhythm in patients with atrial fibrillation lasting less than 48 hours. *Ann Intern Med* 1997; **126**: 615–20.

20 O'Neill PG, Puleo PR, Bolli R, Rokey R. Return of atrial mechanical function following electrical conversion of atrial dysrhythmias. *Am Heart J* 1990; **120**: 353–9.

21 Navab A, La Due JS. Postconversion systemic arterial embolism. *Am J Cardiol* 1965; **16**: 452–3.

22 Iglehart JK. The American health care system – Medicare. *N Engl J Med* 1992; **327**: 1467–72.

23 Bjerkelund CJ, Orning OM. The efficacy of anticoagulant therapy in preventing embolism related to D.C. electrical conversion of atrial fibrillation. *Am J Cardiol* 1969; **23**: 208–16.

24 Mancini GB, Goldberger AL. Cardioversion of atrial fibrillation: consideration of embolization, anticoagulation, prophylactic pacemaker, and long-term success. *Am Heart J* 1982; **104**: 617–21.

25 Freeman I, Wexler J, Howard F. Anticoagulants for treatment of atrial fibrillation. *JAMA* 1963; **184**: 1007–10.

26 Van Gelder IC, Crijns HJGM, Tieleman RG, et al. Chronic atrial fibrillation: success of serial cardioversion therapy and safety of oral anticoagulation. *Arch Intern Med* 1996; **156**: 2585–92.

27 Manning WJ, Weintraub RM, Waksmonski CA, et al. Accuracy of transesophageal echocardiography for identifying left atrial thrombi: a prospective, intraoperative study. *Ann Intern Med* 1995; **12**: 817–22.

28 Salka S, Saeian K, Sagar KB. Cerebral thromboembolization after cardioversion of atrial fibrillation in patients without transesophageal echocardiographic findings of left atrial thrombus. *Am Heart J* 1993; **126**: 722–4.

29 Black IW, Hopkins AP, Lee LC, Walsh WF. Evaluation of transesophageal echocardiography before cardioversion of atrial fibrillation and flutter in nonanticoagulated patients. *Am Heart J* 1993; **126**: 375–81.

30 Black IW, Fatkin D, Sagar KB, et al. Exclusion of atrial thrombus by transesophageal echocardiography does not preclude embolism after cardioversion of atrial fibrillation. *Circulation* 1994; **89**: 2509–13.

31 Gage BF, Cardinalli AB, Albers GW, Owens DK. Cost-effectiveness of warfarin and aspirin for prophylaxis of stroke in patients with nonvalvular atrial fibrillation. *JAMA* 1995; **274**: 1839–45.

32 Kopecky SL, Gersh BJ, McGoon MD, et al. The natural history of lone atrial fibrillation: a population-based study over three decades. *N Engl J Med* 1987; **317**: 669–74.

33 Atrial Fibrillation Investigators. Risk factors for stroke and efficacy of antithrombotic therapy in atrial fibrillation. *Arch Intern Med* 1994; **154**: 1449–57.

34 Brand FN, Abbott RD, Kannel WB, Wolf PA. Characteristics and prognosis of lone atrial fibrillation: 30-year follow-up in the Framingham Study. *JAMA* 1985; **254**: 3449–53.

35 Stroke Prevention in Atrial Fibrillation Investigators. Risk factors for thromboembolism during aspirin therapy in patients with atrial fibrillation: the Stroke Prevention in Atrial Fibrillation study. *J Stroke Cerebrovasc Dis* 1995; **5**: 147–57.

36 Stroke Prevention Atrial Fibrillation III Writing Committee. Patients with nonvalvular atrial fibrillation at low risk of stroke during treatment with aspirin: Stroke Prevention in Atrial Fibrillation III Study. *JAMA* 1998; **279**: 1273–7.

37 Bogousslavsky J, Adnet-Bonte C, Regli F, Van Melle G, Kappenberger L. Lone atrial fibrillation and stroke. *Acta Neurol Scand* 1990; **82**: 143–6.

38 Flegel KM, Hanley J. Risk factors for stroke and other embolic events in patients with non-rheumatic atrial fibrillation. *Stroke* 1989; **20**: 1000–4.

39 van Latum JC, Koudstaal PJ, Venables GS, van Gijn J, Kappelle LJ, Algra A. Predictors of major vascular events in patients with a transient ischemic attack or minor ischemic stroke and with nonrheumatic atrial fibrillation. European Atrial Fibrillation Trial (EAFT) Study Group. *Stroke* 1995; **26**: 801–6.

40 Stollberger C, Chnupa P, Kronik G, et al. Transesophageal echocardiography to assess embolic risk in patients with atrial fibrillation. *Ann Intern Med* 1998; **128**: 630–8.

41 Moulton AW, Singer DE, Hass JS. Risk factors for stroke in patients with nonrheumatic atrial fibrillation: a case-control study. *Am J Med* 1991; **91**: 156–61.

42 Stroke Prevention in Atrial Fibrillation Investigators. Predictors of thromboembolism in atrial fibrillation: I. Clinical features of patients at risk. *Ann Intern Med* 1992; **116**: 1–5.

43 Petersen P, Godtfredsen J. Embolic complications in paroxysmal atrial fibrillation. *Stroke* 1986; **17**: 622–6.

44 Aronow WS, Gutstein H, Hsieh FY. Risk factors for thromboembolic stroke in elderly patients with chronic atrial fibrillation. *Am J Cardiol* 1989; **63**: 366–7.

45 Petersen P, Kastrup J, Helweg-Larsen S, Boysen G, Godtfredsen J. Risk factors for thromboembolic complications in chronic atrial fibrillation. The Copenhagen AFASAK Study. *Arch Intern Med* 1990; **150**: 819–21.

46 Cabin HS, Clubb KS, Hall C, Perlmutter RA, Feinstein AR. Risk for systemic embolization of atrial fibrillation without mitral stenosis. *Am J Cardiol* 1990; **65**: 1112–6.

47 Aboaf AP, Wolf PS. Paroxysmal atrial fibrillation: a common but neglected entity. *Arch Int Med* 1996; **156**: 362–7.

48 Wolf PA, Kannel WB, McGee DL, et al. Duration of atrial fibrillation and imminence of stroke: The Framingham Study. *Stroke* 1983; **14**: 664–7.

49 Manning WJ, Silverman DI, Keighley CS, Oettgen P, Douglas PS. Transesophageal echocardiographically facilitated early cardioversion from atrial fibrillation using short-term anticoagulation: final results of a prospective 4.5 year study. *J Am Coll Cardiol* 1995; **25**: 1254–61.

50 Chiang C, Lo S, Ko Y, Cheng N, Lin PJ, Chang C. Predictors of systemic embolism in patients with mitral stenosis. *Ann Intern Med* 1998; **128**: 885–9.

51 Atrial Fibrillation Investigators. Echocardiographic predictors of stroke in patients with

atrial fibrillation: a prospective study of 1066 patients from 3 clinical trials. *Arch Intern Med* 1998; **158**: 1316–20.

52 Stroke Prevention in Atrial Fibrillation Investigators Committee on Echocardiography. Transesophageal echocardiographic correlates of thromboembolism in high-risk patients with nonvalvular atrial fibrillation. *Ann Intern Med* 1998; **128**: 639–47.

53 Manning WJ, Douglas PS. Transesophageal echocardiography and atrial fibrillation: Added value or expensive toy? *Ann Intern Med* 1998; **128**: 685–7.

54 Fatkin D, Kelly RP, Feneley MP. Relations between left atrial appendage blood flow velocity, spontaneous echocardiographic contrast and thromboembolic risk in vivo. *J Am Coll Cardiol* 1994; **23**: 961–9.

55 Hart RG, Benavente O, McBride R, Pearce LA. Antithrombotic therapy to prevent stroke in patients with atrial fibrillation: a meta-analysis. *Ann Intern Med* 1999; **131**: 492–501.

56 Domanski MJ. The epidemiology of atrial fibrillation. *Coron Artery Dis* 1995; **6**: 95–100.

57 Laupacis A, Boysen G, Connolly S, et al. The efficacy of aspirin in patients with atrial fibrillation: analysis of pooled data from 3 randomized trials. *Arch Intern Med* 1997; **157**: 1237–40.

58 Barnett HJM, Eliasziw M, Meldrum HE. Drugs and surgery in the prevention of ischemic stroke. *N Engl J Med* 1995; **332**: 238–48.

59 Pengo V, Zasso A, Barbero F, et al. Effectiveness of fixed minidose warfarin in the prevention of thromboembolism and vascular death in nonrheumatic atrial fibrillation. *Am J Cardiol* 1998; **82**: 433–7.

60 Stroke Prevention in Atrial Fibrillation Investigators. Bleeding during antithrombotic therapy in patients with atrial fibrillation. *Arch Intern Med* 1996; **156**: 409–16.

61 Stroke Prevention in Atrial Fibrillation Investigators. Preliminary report of the Stroke Prevention in Atrial Fibrillation Study. *New Engl J Med* 1990; **322**: 863–8.

62 Landefeld CS, Beyth RJ. Anticoagulant-related bleeding: clinical epidemiology, prediction and prevention. *Am J Med* 1993; **95**: 315–28.

63 Gage BF, Boechler M, Doggette AL, et al. Adverse outcomes and predictors of underuse of antithrombotic therapy in Medicare beneficiaries with chronic atrial fibrillation. *Stroke* 2000; **31**: 822–7.

64 Gage BF, Cardinalli AB, Owens DK. Cost-effectiveness of preference-based antithrombotic therapy for patients with nonvalvular atrial fibrillation. *Stroke* 1998; **29**: 1083–91.

65 Laupacis A, Albers G, Dalen J, Dunn MI, Jacobson AK, Singer DE. Antithrombotic therapy in atrial fibrillation. *Chest* 1998; **114**: 579S-89S.

66 Matchar DB, McCrory DC, Barnett HJM, Feussner JR. Guidelines for medical treatment for stroke prevention. *Ann Intern Med* 1994; **121**: 54–5.

67 Steering Committee of the Physicians' Health Study Research Group. Final report on the aspirin component of the ongoing physicians' health study. *N Engl J Med* 1989; **321**: 129–35.

68 Hansson L, Zanchetti A, Carruthers SG, et al. Effects of intensive blood-pressure lowering and low-dose aspirin in patients with hypertension: principal results of the Hypertension Optimal Treatment (HOT) randomised trial. HOT Study Group. *Lancet* 1998; **351**: 1755–62.

69 The Medical Research Council's General Practice Research Framework. Thrombosis prevention trial: randomised trial of low-intensity oral anticoagulation with warfarin

and low-dose aspirin in the primary prevention of ischaemic heart disease in men at increased risk. The Medical Research Council's General Practice Research Framework. *Lancet* 1998; **351**: 233–41.

70 Eckman MH, Levine HJ, Pauker SG. Making decisions about antithrombotic therapy in heart disease: decision analytic and cost-effectiveness issues. *Chest* 1995; **108**(Suppl): 457–70.

71 Eckman MH, Falk RH, Pauker SG. Cost-effectiveness of therapies for patients with nonvalvular atrial fibrillation. *Arch Intern Med* 1998; **159**: 1669–77.

72 Naglie G, Detsky AS. Treatment of chronic nonvalvular atrial fibrillation in the elderly: a decision analysis. *Med Decis Making* 1992; **12**: 239–49.

73 Nadeau SE. The use of expected value as an aid to decisions regarding anticoagulation in patients with atrial fibrillation. *Stroke* 1993; **24**: 2128–34.

74 Disch DL, Greenberg ML, Holzberger PT, Malenka DJ, Birkmeyer JD. Managing chronic atrial fibrillation: a Markov decision analysis comparing warfarin, quinidine, and low-dose amiodarone. *Ann Intern Med* 1994; **120**: 449–57.

75 Caro JJ, Groome PA, Flegel KM. Atrial fibrillation and anticoagulation: from randomised trials to practice. *Lancet* 1993; **341**: 1381–84.

76 Beck JR, Pauker SG. Anticoagulation and atrial fibrillation in the bradycardia–tachycardia syndrome. *Med Decis Making* 1981; **1**: 284–301.

77 Flegel KM, Hutchinson TA, Groome PA, Tousignant P. Factors relevant to preventing embolic stroke in patients with non-rheumatic atrial fibrillation. *J Clin Epidemiol* 1991; **44**: 551–60.

78 Gustafsson C, Asplund K, Britton M, Norrving B, Olsson B, Marke LA. Cost effectiveness of primary stroke prevention in atrial fibrillation: Swedish national perspective. *BMJ* 1992; **305**: 1457–60.

79 Pauker SG, Kassirer JP. Decision analysis. *N Engl J Med* 1987; **316**: 250–8.

80 Gage BF, Cardinalli AB, Owens DK. The effect of stroke and stroke prophylaxis with aspirin or warfarin on quality of life. *Arch Intern Med* 1996; **156**: 1829–36.

81 Matchar DB, McCrory DC, Barnett HJM, Feussner JR. Medical treatment for stroke prevention. *Ann Intern Med* 1994; **121**: 41–53.

82 Man-Son-Hing M, Laupacis A, O'Connor A, et al. Warfarin for atrial fibrillation: the patient's perspective. *Arch Intern Med* 1996; **156**: 1841–8.

83 Sumner W, Nease R, Littenberg B. U-Titer: a utility assessment tool. *Proceedings of the Fifteenth Annual Symposium on Computer Applications in Medical Care, Washington, DC.* 1991: 701–5.

84 Kaplan SH, Greenfield S, Dukes K. The effects of a joint physician–patient intervention program on health outcomes and interpersonal care (abstract). *Clin Res* 1993; **41**: 541A.

85 Kaplan SH, Greenfield S, Ware JE, Jr. Assessing the effects of physician–patient interactions on the outcomes of chronic disease. *Med Care* 1989; **27**(Suppl. 3): S110–27.

86 Greenfield S, Kaplan SH, Ware JE Jr, Yano EM, Frank HJL. Patients' participation in medical care: effects on blood sugar control and quality of life in diabetes. *J Gen Intern Med* 1988; **3**: 448–57.

87 Rost KM, Flavin KS, Cole K, McGill JB. Change in metabolic control and functional status after hospitalization: impact of patient activation intervention in diabetic patients. *Diabetes Care* 1991; **14**: 881–9.

88 Thompson CE, Wankel LM. The effects of perceived activity choice upon frequency of exercise behaviour. *J Appl Soc Psychol* 1980; **10**: 436–43.

89 Janis I, Mann L. *Decision making: a psychological analysis of conflict, choice, and commitment*. New York: Free Press; 1977.

90 Fihn SD, Callahan CM, Martin DC, et al. The risk for and severity of bleeding complications in elderly patients treated with warfarin. *Ann Intern Med* 1996; **124**: 970–9.

91 Forfar J. A 7-year analysis of haemorrhage in patients on long-term anticoagulant treatment. *Br Heart J* 1979; **42**: 128–32.

92 Gurwitz JH, Goldberg RJ, Holden A, Knapic N, Ansell J. Age-related risks of long-term oral anticoagulant therapy. *Arch Intern Med* 1988; **148**: 1733–6.

93 Gitter MJ, Jaeger TM, Petterson TM, Gersh BJ, Silverstein MD. Bleeding and thromboembolism during anticoagulant therapy: a population-based study in Rochester, Minnesota. *Mayo Clin Proc* 1995; **70**: 725–33.

94 Petty GW, Lennihan L, Mohr JP, et al. Complications of long-term anticoagulation. *Ann Neurol* 1988; **23**: 570–4.

95 Hylek EM, Singer DE. Risk factors for intracranial hemorrhage in outpatients taking warfarin. *Ann Intern Med* 1994; **120**: 897–902.

96 van der Meer FJM, Rosendaal FR, Vandenbroucke JP, Briet E. Bleeding complications in oral anticoagulant therapy: an analysis of risk factors. *Arch Intern Med* 1993; **153**: 1557–62.

97 Landefeld CS, Goldman L. Major bleeding in outpatients with warfarin: incidence and prediction by factors known at the start of outpatient therapy. *Am J Med* 1989; **87**: 144–52.

98 Coon W, Willis P III. Hemorrhagic complications of anticoagulant therapy. *Arch Intern Med* 1974; **133**: 386–92.

99 Launbjerg J, Egeblad H, Heaf J, Nielsen NH, Fugleholm AM, Ladefoged K. Bleeding complications to oral anticoagulant therapy: multivariate analysis of 1010 treatment years in 551 outpatients. *J Int Med* 1991; **229**: 351–5.

100 Landefeld CS, Cook EF, Flatley M, Weisberg M, Goldman L. Identification and preliminary validation of predictors of major bleeding in hospitalized patients starting anticoagulant therapy. *Am J Med* 1987; **82**: 703–13.

101 Connolly S. Stroke Prevention in Atrial Fibrillation II Study (letter). *Lancet* 1994; **343**: 1509.

102 Stroke Prevention in Atrial Fibrillation Investigators. A differential effect of aspirin on prevention of stroke in atrial fibrillation. *J Stroke Cerebrovasc Dis* 1993; **3**: 181–8.

103 Smith P, Arnesen H, Holme I. The effect of warfarin on mortality and reinfarction after myocardial infarction. *N Engl J Med* 1990; **323**: 147–52.

104 ASPECT Research Group. Effect of long-term anticoagulant treatment on mortality and cardiovascular morbidity after myocardial infarction: antcoagulants in the Secondary Prevention of Events in Coronary Thrombosis (ASPECT) Research Group. *Lancet* 1994; **343**: 499–503.

105 The E.P.S.I.M. Research Group. A controlled comparison of aspirin and oral anticoagulants in prevention of death after myocardial infarction. *N Engl J Med* 1982; **307**: 701–8.

106 van Bergen PFMM, Jonker JJC, van Hout BA, et al. Costs and effects of long-term oral anticoagulant treatment after myocardial infarction. *J Am Med Assoc* 1995; **273**: 925–8.

107 Turpie AG, Gent M, Laupacis A, et al. A comparison of aspirin with placebo in patients treated with warfarin after heart-valve replacement. *N Engl J Med* 1993; **329**: 524–9.

108 Coumadin Aspirin Reinfarction Study (CARS) Investigators. Randomised double-blind trial of fixed low-dose warfarin with aspirin after myocardial infarction. *Lancet* 1997; **350**: 389–96.

109 Hirsh J, E Dalen JE, Fuster V, Harker LB, Patrono C, Roth G. Aspirin and other platelet-active drugs: the relationship among dose, effectiveness, and side-effects. *Chest* 1995; **108**(Suppl.): 247S–57S.

110 Rosendaal FR. The Scylla and Charybdis of oral anticoagulant treatment. *N Engl J Med* 1996; **335**: 587–9.

111 Hylek EM, Skates SJ, Sheehan MA, Singer DE. An analysis of the lowest effective intensity of prophylactic anticoagulation for patients with nonrheumatic atrial fibrillation. *N Engl J Med* 1996; **335**: 540–6.

112 Brass L, Krumholz H, Scinto J, Radford M. Warfarin use among patients with atrial fibrillation. *Stroke* 1997; **28**: 2382–9.

113 The European Atrial Fibrillation Trial Study Group. Optimal oral anticoagulant therapy in patients with nonrheumatic atrial fibrillation and recent cerebral ischemia. *N Engl J Med* 1995; **333**: 5–10.

114 Azar AJ, Cannegieter SC, Deckers JW, et al. Optimal intensity of oral anticoagulant therapy after myocardial infarction. *J Am Coll Cardiol* 1996; **27**: 1349–55.

115 Cannegieter SC, Rosendaal FR, Wintzen AR, van der Meer FJM, Vandenbroucke JP, Briet E. Optimal oral anticoagulant therapy in patients with mechanical heart valves. *N Engl J Med* 1995; **333**: 11–17.

116 Palareti G, Leali N, Coccheri S, et al. Bleeding complications of oral anticoagulant treatment: an inception-cohort, prospective collaborative study (ISCOAT). *Lancet* 1996; **348**: 423–8.

117 McCrory DC, Matchar DB. Stroke prevention: the emerging strategies. *Hosp Practice* 1996; **31**: 123–34.

118 Gage B, Cardinalli AB, Wyrwich KW, Albers GW, Rich MW, Owens DK. Meta-analysis of the optimal INR in nonvalvular atrial fibrillation (abstract). *J Gen Intern Med* 1998; **13**(Suppl.): 25.

119 Flaker GC, McGowan DJ, Boechler M, Fortune G, Gage B. Underutilization of antithrombotic therapy in elderly rural patients with atrial fibrillation. *Am Heart J* 1999; **137**: 307–12.

120 Albers GW, Yim JM, Belew KM, et al. Status of antithrombotic therapy for patients with atrial fibrillation in university hospitals. *Arch Intern Med* 1996; **156**: 2311–16.

121 Stafford RS, Singer DE. National patterns of warfarin use in atrial fibrillation. *Arch Intern Med* 1996; **156**: 2537–41.

122 Bath PMW, Prasad A, Brown MM, MacGregor GA. Survey of use of anticoagulation in patients with atrial fibrillation. *Br Med J* 1993; **307**: 1045.

123 Antani MR, Beyth RJ, Covinsky KE, et al. Failure to prescribe warfarin to patients with nonrheumatic atrial fibrillation. *J Gen Intern Med* 1996; **11**: 713–20.

124 Monette J, Gurwitz JH, Rochon PA, Avorn J. Physician attitudes concerning warfarin for stroke prevention in atrial fibrillation: results of a survey of long-term care practitioners. *J Am Geriatr Soc* 1997; **45**: 1060–5.

125 Gurwitz JH, Monette J, Rochon P, Eckler MA, Avorn J. Atrial fibrillation and stroke

prevention with warfarin in the long-term care setting. *Arch Intern Med* 1997; **157**: 978–84.

126 Lackner TE, Battis GN. Use of warfarin for nonvalvular atrial fibrillation in nursing home patients. *Arch Fam Med* 1995; **4**: 1017–26.

127 Munschauer FE, Priore RL, Hens M, Castilone A. Thromboembolism prophylaxis in chronic atrial fibrillation. *Stroke* 1997; **28**: 72–6.

128 Whittle J, Wickenheiser L, Venditti LN. Is warfarin underused in the treatment of elderly persons with atrial fibrillation? *Arch Intern Med* 1997; **157**: 441–5.

129 Matchar DB, Samsa GP, Cohen SJ. Should we just let the anticoagulation service do it? The conundrum of anticoagulation for atrial fibrillation. *J Gen Intern Med* 1996; **11**: 768–70.

130 Kornberg A, Francis CW, Pellegrini VD Jr, Gabriel KR, Marder VJ. Comparison of native prothrombin antigen with the prothrombin time for monitoring oral anticoagulant prophylaxis. *Circulation* 1993; **88**: 454–60.

131 Millenson MM, Bauer KA, Kistler JP, Barzegar S, Tulin L, Rosenberg RD. Monitoring 'mini-intensity' anticoagulation with warfarin: comparison of the prothrombin time using a sensitive thromboplastin with prothrombin fragment F1+2 levels. *Blood* 1992; **79**: 2034–8.

132 Takahashi H, Kashima T, Nomizo Y, et al. Metabolism of warfarin enantiomers in Japanese patients with heart disease having different CYP2C9 and CYP2C19 genotypes. *Clin Pharmacol Ther* 1998; **63**: 519–28.

133 Furuya H, Fernandez-Salguero P, Gregory W, et al. Genetic polymorphism of CYP2C9 and its effect on warfarin maintenance dose requirement in patients undergoing anticoagulation therapy. *Pharmacogenetics* 1995; **5**: 389–92.

19

Anticoagulation in patients with mechanical and biological prosthetic heart valves

NICOLAS L DEPACE, GENO J MERLI, CHERYL COSTELLO

INTRODUCTION

Whereas the availability of prosthetic heart valves extends the lives of patients by many years, thromboembolism and bleeding during therapeutic anticoagulation are still a major cause of morbidity and mortality. The American College of Physician Consensus Conference on antithrombotic therapy recently recommended that lifelong anticoagulation offered the most consistent protection against thromboembolic events in patients with mechanical prosthetic valves.[1] These optimal anticoagulation guidelines for different prosthetic valves in various subsets of patients represent an evidence-based approach combined with expert consensus opinion. In this chapter, the recommendations for anticoagulation options in patients with mechanical and bioprosthetic heart valves are reviewed.

PROSTHETIC HEART VALVES

The incidence of thromboembolic events depends in part on the type of material from which the prosthetic valve is made, the number of valves inserted, and their

Table 19.1 *Types of mechanical prosthetic heart valves*

1. First-generation
   a. Starr–Edwards (caged ball type)
   b. Smeloff–Cutler (caged ball type)
   c. Bjork–Shiley standard (caged disc)
2. Second-generation
   a. Medtronic Hall (disc)
   b. St Jude Medical (bileaflet)
   c. Bjork–Shiley monostrut (tilting disc)

location. There are two major types of prosthetic heart valves, bioprosthetic valves (made of tissue components) and mechanical valves (Table 19.1). Mechanical heart valves are more durable but also more thrombogenic than bioprostheses.[2–6] Table 19.1 lists the first-generation and second-generation mechanical heart valves. The first-generation prosthetic valves are more thrombogenic than the newer, second-generation of valves.

First-generation valves

It is impossible to attribute to each type of prosthesis an unqualified embolic rate. Patient-related risk factors (see below) and the level of anticoagulation are important with respect to embolic events. Caged ball valves have a higher incidence of major embolism than bileaflet and tilting disc valves. At an International Normalized Ratio (INR) of 2.0–2.9, the frequency of thromboemboli was 0.5% per year with bileaflet valves, 0.7% per year with tilting disk valves, and 2.5% per year with caged ball and caged disc valves.[7] This high incidence of embolic events in this latter group was reduced with an INR of 4.0–4.9. However, others have shown a high rate of major hemorrhage with an INR between 3.0 and 4.5.[8] Stein et al. recommend that the level of 4.0–4.9 for the INR be recommended for patients with caged ball or caged disc valves, but randomized trials are required to clarify this issue.[1,7]

Second-generation valves

The frequency of thromboembolic events is lower with the second-generation mechanical valves than with the first-generation valves. Among patients with St Jude valves in the aortic position, thromboembolic events were not statistically more prevalent at an INR of 2.0–3.0 than at higher INR ranges, provided the patient was in sinus rhythm and the left atrium was not enlarged.[9,10] Horstkotte et al. analyzed a subset of patients with St Jude aortic valves, normal sinus rhythm, and normal left atrial diameters.[10] An INR of 1.8–2.7 was compared to an INR of 2.5–3.2. There was no statistically significant reduction in the frequency of thromboembolic events and the incidence of major bleeding in the 1.8–2.7 group. In a retrospective case series of 670 patients aged 70 years or older with St Jude aortic valves, Arom et al. showed a frequency of thromboemboli of 0.7% per year at an INR of 1.8–2.5.[2] The prevalence of atrial fibrillation was not reported in this study. In patients with St Jude aortic valves and comorbidities such as atrial fibrillation and a left atrium of >30 mm/m^2, an INR of 2.5–3.2 was optimal.[10] A low ejection fraction also increased the risk of thromboemboli.[3]

In patients with St Jude valves in the mitral position, normal sinus rhythm, and a left atrial diameter of < 26 mm/m^2, an INR of 2.4–3.4 was optimal to prevent embolic events.[10] For those patients with atrial fibrillation and a left atrial diameter of > 30 mm/m^2, an INR of 2.7–3.6 was ideal.[10]

The use of antiplatelet therapy in combination with warfarin has demonstrated good results in case series and nonrandomized trials (Table 19.2). Skudicky et al. evaluated warfarin at an INR of 2.0–2.5 in combination with dipyridamole in a case series of patients with St Jude valves in the aortic, mitral, and double valve positions.[4] The thromboembolic frequency was 0.6% per year and the frequency of major bleeding was 1.1% per year. The use of aspirin and dipyridamole with warfarin in fixed dose with no adjustment of the INR also showed good results in patients with St Jude aortic and mitral valves.[5] Antiplatelet therapy alone in patients in sinus rhythm with St Jude aortic valves has also shown a reduction of embolic events, although not as much as warfarin alone.[6,11]

Table 19.2 *Anticoagulation recommendations: mechanical prosthetic valves*

1. Bileaflet aortic valve, normal left atrium, NSR, normal ejection fraction	Warfarin (INR 2–3)
2. Bileaflet aortic valve and atrial fibrillation	Warfarin (INR 2.5–3.5)
3. Tilting disc or bileaflet mitral valve	Warfarin (INR 2.5–3.5)
4. Caged ball or caged disc valves	Warfarin (INR 2.5–3.5) and aspirin (80–100 mg/day)
5. Additional risk factors	Warfarin (INR 2.5–3.5) and aspirin (81 mg/day)
6. Systemic embolism, despite adequate therapy with warfarin	Warfarin (INR 2.5–3.5) and aspirin (81 mg/day)

(NSR = Normal sinus rhthym.)

BIOPROSTHETIC HEART VALVES

The frequency of thromboembolic events in patients receiving bioprosthetic valve replacement is high during the first 3 months following surgery. Bioprosthetic mitral valves have been shown to have a higher frequency of events compared to similar aortic valves.

A case series study by Heras et al. reported a thromboembolic rate extrapolated to 1 year of 41% per year for aortic and 55% per year for bioprosthetic mitral valves. These extrapolated rates were observational during the first 10 days following surgery as the warfarin anticoagulation was being adjusted.[7] Another case series of bioprosthetic mitral valves not anticoagulated during the first 3 months postsurgery demonstrated a 17.6% per year rate.[12] Horstkotte et al. published a case series of patients with bioprosthetic aortic valves and on full anticoagulation with warfarin (INR 3–4.5). Nineteen of 298 patients developed thromboemboli during the first 3 months following surgery. Extrapolated to 1 year, the rate of thromboembolic events was 25.6% per year.[3] Another approach to anticoagulation in a similar group of bioprosthetic aortic valves was the use of subcutaneous heparin (22 500 IU/day) and aspirin (100 mg/day) for the first 14–22 days after surgery.[7] The extrapolated frequency of thromboemboli during the first 6 months was 3.5% per year.

Looking long-term at patients in normal sinus rhythm with bioprosthetic aortic valves and not on warfarin therapy, the frequency of thromboembolic events was between 0.2% and 2.9% per year. This frequency is closer to that in patients with St Jude aortic valves on anticoagulation at an INR of 2.5–3.5, which was reported to be 1.6–2.6% per year. For patients with bioprosthetic mitral valves in normal sinus rhythm and not anticoagulated, the frequency of thromboembolic events was reported to be 0.4–1.9% per year. The thromboembolic incidence in patients with fully anticoagulated mitral St Jude valves is 2.2–2.9% per year.

Whereas the above describes bioprosthetic valves with normal sinus rhythm, risk factors such as atrial fibrillation, the presence of a pacemaker, and dilated left atrium all contribute to a higher risk scenerio for this patient group. Louagie et al. documented an 8.3% per year frequency of thrombotic events in patients with bioprosthetic valves and pacemakers.[13] The presence of atrial fibrillation with a bioprosthetic valve has been shown to be associated with a thrombotic event frequency as high as 16% in the first 3 years following placement of the valve. The data from these different clinical situations do not support management either with or without anticoagulation.

RISK FACTORS FOR THROMBUS FORMATION

Prosthesis-related risk factors are identified by their type and location. It is important to identify the prosthesis at high risk of cardiac emboli because one can titrate the anticoagulant treatment to modify the risk. Therefore, tracking the influence of anticoagulation, the risks of valve thrombosis, and/or systemic embolism in an individual patient is a combination of the patient's inherent risk factors and type and location of prosthesis implanted.

Patient risk factors

There are various patient risk factors that may increase the probability of embolism in an individual patient. Patients with the highest risk for thromboembolism are those with large mitral gradients especially if they are in atrial fibrillation. Atrial fibrillation without heart disease carries an 0.5% thromboembolic risk per year, but if associated with other cardiac conditions such as hypertension (risk stroke 4–6% per year) or mitral stenosis (risk up to 20% per year), the increase in risk of embolic stroke is evident. Decreased left ventricular function and left atrial enlargement are risks easily identified with the echocardiogram. Prior emboli may lead to a 20% recurrence rate within the first year.

Prosthesis-related risk factors

Cardioembolic risk, as mentioned previously, depends on the type, location, and number of prosthetic heart valves. In general, first-generation prostheses (see Table

19.1) have higher thromboembolic risks than second-generation valves. Most prostheses of the second generation with warfarin have a thromboembolic risk of 0.5–2.2% per year in the aortic position, and of 2–3% per year in the mitral position.[14] During the first 90 days, the risk is also highest until the postoperative coagulable state improves and the endothelialization process of the implanted valve occurs. Bioprosthetic valves should be anticoagulated during this 90-day interval but no longer, unless atrial fibrillation or other complicated risk factors are present (Table 19.3).

Table 19.3 *Anticoagulation recommendations: bioprosthetic heart valves*

1. Mitral or aortic valves, NSR	Warfarin (INR 2–3) for first 3 months following placement
2. Mitral or aortic valves, atrial fibrillation	Long-term warfarin (INR 2–3)
3. Mitral or aortic valves with left atrial enlargement	Long-term warfarin (INR 2–3)
4. Mitral or aortic valves with permanent pacemaker	Optional anticoagulation (INR 2–3)
5. Mitral or aortic valves with history of systemic embolization	Warfarin 3–12 months (INR 2–3)
6. After first 3 months, mitral or aortic valves, NSR	Aspirin 162 mg/day

(NSR = normal sinus rhythm.)

Tables 19.2 and 19.3 detail how to intensify the target level of anticoagulation when various risk factors are present. Some experts even advocate using low-dose aspirin in addition to warfarin in high-risk patients. First-generation valves in individuals with recurrent emboli are at highest risk and the addition of aspirin is recommended.

COMBINING ANTIPLATELET AGENTS WITH ANTICOAGULANTS

Aspirin has been used with anticoagulants in treating heart valve replacement patients. Up to 1200 mg of aspirin was used, with a significant reduction of thromboemboli but an increased risk of bleeding, particularly gastrointestinal,[15,16] because the antithrombotic risk of aspirin is similar for 100–1000 mg/per day,[17] but the gastrointestinal hemorrhage rate increases.[18] Turpie and coworkers[19] combined 100 mg of aspirin with warfarin therapy in patients with prosthetic valves. They showed that the addition of aspirin in the treatment of patients with prosthetic mechanical valves and high-risk tissue valves reduced mortality, especially cerebrovascular. It also reduces systemic embolism with a negligible increase in bleeding. Their mean INR was 3.1 (although their target was 3.0–4.5). These investigators raise the issue of whether a lower target INR (2.0) would also be effective and have a lower bleeding incidence. Trials are currently underway.

Patients with concomittant ischemic heart disease would benefit from aspirin therapy because they have higher rates of adverse outcome. Tables 19.2 and 19.3 highlight where the combination of low-dose aspirin and warfarin may be beneficial but, again, further research is warranted.

NATIVE VALVULAR HEART DISEASE

As with prosthetic heart valves, treatment with anticoagulant in patients with native valvular heart disease balances benefit with risk. The following guidelines are based mostly on empirical and clinical observations and not on controlled trials.

Mitral valve disease

The highest systemic emboli rates occur in rheumatic mitral valve disease. A prevalance of 9–14% has been noted for systemic emboli in several large series of mitral stenosis patients, and embolism rates increased sevenfold with the onset of atrial fibrillation.[20] The risk of emboli is greater in older patients, those with low cardiac output, and those with increased left atrial diameter. Mitral valvuloplasty does not decrease the risk of thromboembolism.[21]

All patients with sustained or paroxysmal atrial fibrillation and mitral stenosis should be anticoagulated. In patients in normal sinus rhythm,[21] older age of the patient, increased size of the left atrium (greater than 50 mm cutoff), severity of the stenosis, presence of left atrial thrombi, spontaneous echo contrast (indicative of slow blood flow in the left atrium), and a history of prior emboli are important indicators of need for anticoagulation.

In patients with predominant mitral regurgitation, anticoagulation is indicated in the presence of atrial fibrillation. If the patient is in normal sinus rhythm, anticoagulation is indicated in the presence of congestive heart failure, extreme cardiac enlargement with a low cardiac output, a large left atrium (> 50 mm), or a history of prior emboli. In patients with mitral valve prolapse and transient ischemic attacks, aspirin is the first-line drug, followed by warfarin only in the case of recurrence.

In mitral valve repair with sinus rhythm, the type of ring used is important when determining if anticoagulation is necessary. No anticoagulation is necessary with the Coagrove Ring. With the Carpentier Ring, 3 months of anticoagulation is usually required, longer if the patient remains in congestive heart failure.[22]

Cardiac emboli in patients with mitral annular calcification have been described.[23] According to the Framingham Heart Study,[24] those with mitral annular calcification have a 2.1 times relative risk of stroke compared to those without it. Anticoagulation is definitely indicated if a prior embolic event occurs, if atrial fibrillation is present, or if severe acquired mitral stenosis from mitral annular calcification occurs.[25] Otherwise, aspirin may be a reasonable compromise as prophylaxis, because the incidence of cardiac emboli is unknown and many of these patients are elderly and at risk for bleeding.

Nonmitral valvular heart disease

Anticoagulation treatment is not indicated in patients with normal sinus rhythm with aortic valve disease or tricuspid valve disease unless other indications for coagulation are present.

The incidence of a paradoxical embolism with patent foramen ovale and atrial septal aneurysm is unknown. This is because 27–29% of normal hearts at autopsy have patent foramen ovale.[26,27] The association of patent foramen ovale and stroke is higher among younger patients. Atrial septal aneurysms have been found in 1% of autopsies and 3% of nonstroke patients examined by transesophageal echocardiography.[28] Anticoagulants should only be used in these patients if the data supporting an embolus in a given patient are strong. A low-dose aspirin is a possible prophylactic measure in asymptomatic patients.

In treating infective endocarditis of both native and prosthetic valves, antibiotic therapy is more important than anticoagulant therapy in preventing neurological complications. Therefore, when a patient is in normal sinus rhythm with native valves or bioprosthetic valves, anticoagulants in the setting of endocarditis are not indicated. For patients with mechanical valve endocarditis, anticoagulation is indicated, as it is in mechanical valves that are not infected.

REFERENCES

1 Stein P, Alpert J, Dalen J, et al. Antithrombotic therapy in patients with mechanical and biological prosthetic heart valves. *Chest* 1998; **114**: 602S–10S.

2 Arom K, Emery R, Nicoloff D, et al. Anticoagulant related complications in elderly patients with St Jude mechanical valve prosthesis. *J Heart Valve Dis* 1996; **5**: 505–10.

3 Horstkotte D, Scharf R, Schultheiss H. Intracardiac thrombosis: patient-related factors. *J Heart Valve Dis* 1995; **4**: 114–20.

4 Skudicky D, Essop M, Wisenbaugh T, et al. Frequency of prosthetic valve complications with very low level warfarin anticoagulation combined with dipyridamole after valve replacement using St Jude medical prosthesis. *Am J Cardiol* 1994; **74**: 1137–41.

5 Yamak B, Karagoz H, Zorlutuna Y, et al. Low dose anticoagulant management of patients with St Jude medical mechanical valve prosthesis. *Thorac Cardiovasc Surg* 1993; **41**: 38–42.

6 Hartz H, LoCicero J, Kucich V, et al. Comparative study of warfarin versus antiplatelet therapy in patients with a St Jude medical valve: the aortic position. *J Thorac Cardiovasc Surg* 1986; **92**: 684–90.

7 Heras M, Chesebro J, Fuster V, et al. High risk of early thromboemboli after bioprosthetic cardiac valve replacement. *J Am Coll Cardiol* 1995; **25**: 1111–19.

8 Cannegieter S, Rosendaal F, Wintzen A, et al. Optimal oral anticoagulant therapy with mechanical heart valves. *N Engl J Med* 1995; **333**: 11–17.

9 Acar J, Iung B, Boissel J, et al. AREVA: multicenter randomized comparison of low dose versus standard dose anticoagulation in patients with mechanical prosthetic heart valves. *Circulation* 1996; **94**: 2107–12.

10 Horstkotte D, Schulte H, Bircks W, et al. Unexpected findings concerning

thromboembolic complications and anticoagulation after complete 10 year follow-up of patients with St Jude medical prosthesis. *J Heart Valve Dis* 1993; **2**: 291–301.

11 Ribeiro P, Al Zaibag M, Idris M, et al. Antiplatelet drugs and the incidence of thromboembolic complications of the St Jude medical aortic prosthesis in patients with rheumatic heart disease. *J Thorac Cardiovasc Surg* 1986; **91**: 92–8.

12 Babin-Ebell J, Schmidt W, Eigel P, et al. Aortic bioprosthesis without early anticoagulations: risk of thromboembolism. *Thorac Cardiovasc Surg* 1995; **43**: 212–14.

13 Louagie Y, Jamart J, Eucher P, et al. Mitral valve Carpentier–Edwards bioprosthetic replacement, thromboembolism, and anticoagulants. *Ann Thorac Surg* 1993; **56**: 931–7.

14 Barwolf G, Kremer R. Prevention of thromboembolic events in valvular heart disease. *Acta Cardiol* 1996; 129–42.

15 Dale J, Mybre E, Storstein O, Stormorken H, Efskind L. Prevention of arterial thromboembolism with acetylsalicylic acid: a controlled clinical study in patients with aortic ball valves. *Am Heart J* 1977; **94**: 101–11.

16 Altman R, Boullon F, Bouvier J, et al. Aspirin and prophylaxis of thromboembolic complications in patients with substitute heart valves. *J Thorac Cardiovasc Surg* 1976; **72**: 127–9.

17 Hirsh J, Salzman EW, Harker L, et al. Aspirin and other platelet active drugs: relationship among dose, effectiveness and side-effects. *Chest* 1989; **95**(Suppl.): 125–85.

18 Hawthorne AB, Mahida YR, Cole AT, Hawkey CJ. Aspirin-induced gastric mucosal damage: prevention by enteric-coating and relation to prostaglandin synthesis. *Br J Clin Pharmacol* 1991; **32**: 77–83.

19 Turpie AG, Gest M, Laupacis A, et al. A comparison of aspirin with placebo in patients treated with warfarin after heart valve replacement. *N Engl J Med* 1993; **329**: 524–9.

20 Szekely P. Systemic emboli and anticoagulant prophylaxis in rheumatic heart disease. *BMJ* 1964; **1**: 209–12.

21 Coulshed N, Epstein EJ, McKendrick CS, et al. Systemic embolism in mitral valve disease. *Br Heart J* 1990; **32**: 26–34.

22 Bolooki H, Kaiser G, Mallon S, et al. Comparison of long-term results of Carpentier–Edwards and Hancock bioprosthetic valves. *Ann Thorac Surg* 1986; **42**: 494–9.

23 Kallman, DePace NL, Kotler MN, et al. Unusual presentation of patients with mitral annular calcification. *J Cardiovasc Ultrason* 1982; **1**: 155–60.

24 Benjamin EJ, Plehn JF, D'Agostino RB, et al. Mitral annular calcification and the risk of stroke in the elderly cohort. *N Engl J Med* 1992; **327**: 374–9.

25 DePace NL, Nestico PF, Morganroth J. Acute severe mitral regurgitation pathophysiology, clinical recognition and management. *Am J Med* 1985; February 28, (2): 293–306.

26 Thompson T, Evans W. Paradoxical embolism. *Am J Med* 1930; **23**: 135–50.

27 Hagen PJ, Schultz DG, Edwards WD. Incidence and size of the patent foramen ovale during the first 10 years of life, an autopsy study of 965 normal hearts. *Mayo Clin Proc* 1984; **59**: 17–20.

28 Pearson AC, Nagelhout D, Castello R, et al. Atrial septal aneurysm and stroke: a transesophageal echocardiographic study. *J Am Coll Cardiol* 1991; **18**: 1223–9.

20

Antithrombotic therapy in left ventricular dysfunction and coronary artery disease

JAMES T FITZPATRICK, NEAL F SKOP, EDGAR J MASSABNI

INTRODUCTION

Gaining an understanding of thrombosis is fundamental to understanding the pathophysiology of many cardiovascular diseases. Many of the recent advances in treating heart disease consist of methods to influence clot formation and degradation. This chapter addresses disorders in which pathologic thrombus formation in coronary arteries and in the left ventricle leads to the array of manifestations of coronary artery disease and cardioembolic disease.

The management of acute coronary syndromes constitutes a major challenge for the practicing clinician. Acute coronary syndromes is a term used to describe the spectrum of conditions that include unstable angina, non-Q-wave myocardial infarction, and Q-wave myocardial infarction. These terms describe a heterogeneous group of patients, both in presentation and prognosis. More recently, acute coronary syndromes have been classified according to the presence or absence of ST segment elevation. Although for many years non-ST elevation myocardial infarction was considered prognostically similar to unstable angina, recent longitudinal studies indicate that long-term prognosis more closely follows that in ST elevation myocardial infarction.[1]

The syndrome of unstable angina alone encompasses a wide spectrum of clinical manifestations. The diagnosis is made for more than 1 million hospitalized patients annually,[2] and between 6% and 8% of patients with this condition suffer a nonfatal myocardial infarction within a year of the sentinel event.[3] The diagnosis itself implies recognition of symptoms of myocardial ischemia, either of new onset or an aggravation of symptoms departing from the usual pattern of chest pain. In 1994, the Agency for Health Care Policy and Research and the National Heart, Lung, and Blood Institute published, as part of clinical practice guidelines, a working definition of unstable angina.[4] This syndrome is described as having four possible presentations: symptoms of angina at rest (usually prolonged > 20 minutes), new-onset (< 2 months), exertional angina of at least Canadian Cardiovascular Society Classification (CCSC) class III in severity, or recent (< 2 months) acceleration of angina as reflected by an increase in the severity of at least one CCSC class to at least CCSC class III. Variant (Prinzmetals) angina, non-ST elevation myocardial infarction, and post-ST elevation infarction chest pains are also included in the syndrome.[5] Whereas the use of clinical guidelines can help the clinician in appropriately managing patients with acute coronary syndromes the diagnosis itself can often be elusive and ultimately only confirmed hours or days from onset, after diagnostic blood tests become available.

The following section focuses on the pathophysiology of acute coronary syndromes, specifically on the evolution of the unstable or 'vulnerable' atherosclerotic plaque and the mechanism of plaque disruption. It examines the essential role of coagulation and platelet aggregation in acute coronary syndromes and discusses the use of antithrombotic therapies for the management of patients presenting with acute coronary syndromes, both acutely (in the first 48 hours of presentation) and long term.

PATHOPHYSIOLOGY OF ACUTE CORONARY SYNDROMES

Central to the development of acute coronary syndromes is the disruption of a mature atherosclerotic plaque in the coronary vessel. Disruption of a plaque ultimately leads to thrombosis, mediated by a cascade of platelet aggregation and fibrin deposition, resulting in a reduction of myocardial blood supply to areas distal to the ruptured plaque. The process is complex and highly unpredictable. It has been well documented via angiographic studies that sudden total or near-total arterial occlusion frequently develops in arteries that previously appeared to have minimal stenosis.[6,7] Two-thirds of arteries with plaques that ruptured and in which a totally occlusive thrombus subsequently develops have stenoses of 50% or less before plaque rupture, and in 97% of patients with plaque rupture, these stenotic lesions were noted to occupy less than 70% of the vessel lumen angiographically.[6] Furthermore, pathologic studies of patients dying of noncardiac causes have documented evidence for plaque disruption even without clinical symptoms of myocardial ischemia or acute myocardial infarction, thus suggesting that not all disruptions of plaques lead to clinically apparent or symptomatic events.[8] Thus, severe stenoses in the coronary artery angiographically (> 70%), may only serve as a marker for more modest plaques which are more prone to rupture.

Over the past decade, coronary pathology and bench research devoted to the molecular basis of acute coronary syndromes have contributed greatly to the understanding of the evolution and composition of the atherosclerotic plaque. Atherosclerosis itself is, simply stated, the response of the arterial intima to the deposition of oxidized lipoprotein and cholesterol. These plaques are deposited along the vessel wall in a non-uniform manner, with focal areas of plaque deposition interspersed with relatively 'normal' areas of vascular endothelium. The development of the atherosclerotic plaque is characterized by a latent phase that may last many years or even decades. This process, which has been termed vascular remodeling, refers to the phase in the development of the plaque in which growth occurs by outward, abluminal expansion, without encroaching on the lumen of the vessel.[9,10] Only after the plaque burden approaches half the luminal area does the plaque usually protrude into the lumen of the vessel, becoming angiographically visible.

The atherosclerotic plaque typically consists of a central, lipid-rich core, surrounded by a thin, fibrous cap (Fig. 20.1). The core is comprised of many lipid-laden macrophages (foam cells), derived from blood monocytes. These cells produce a large quantity of tissue factor (peptide initiating the intrinsic component of the coagulation cascade), which is one of the most potent stimuli of thrombus formation when in contact with blood (see Chapter 1). A dense, fibrous matrix principally composed of interstitial collagen and elastin surrounds the central lipid-rich core of the plaque. Smooth muscle cells recruited from the vascular media by local inflammatory mediators (neutrophils, T cells, macrophages, and growth-promoting cytokines) synthesize this cap, as the plaque develops over time.

Central to the understanding of acute coronary syndromes is the concept of the 'vulnerable plaque' – a plaque that is vulnerable or prone to rupture and has certain characteristic features. Plaque rupture occurs most frequently where the fibrous cap tends to be the thinnest, most heavily infiltrated by foam cells, and thus the weakest structurally. This tends to occur at the shoulder of the plaque, near the adjacent vessel wall. Factors that influence plaque rupture include location, size, and consistency of the lipid core, hemorheology of blood flow, and circumferential wall stress or cap 'fatigue'.[11] Furthermore, an active process of degradation of the fibrous cap has been described in which macrophages play a central role by secreting proteolytic enzymes such as plasminogen activators and a family of matrix metalloproteinases (collagenases, gelatinases, and stromelysins) which predispose the cap to rupture.[12,13] In addition, systemic factors have been described which exert an influence on plaque stability and may contribute to plaque rupture. These include physical exertion, mechanical stress due to increase in cardiac contractility, and vasoconstriction. There is increasing evidence of the role of chronic inflammation as a progenitor of plaque instability.[14]

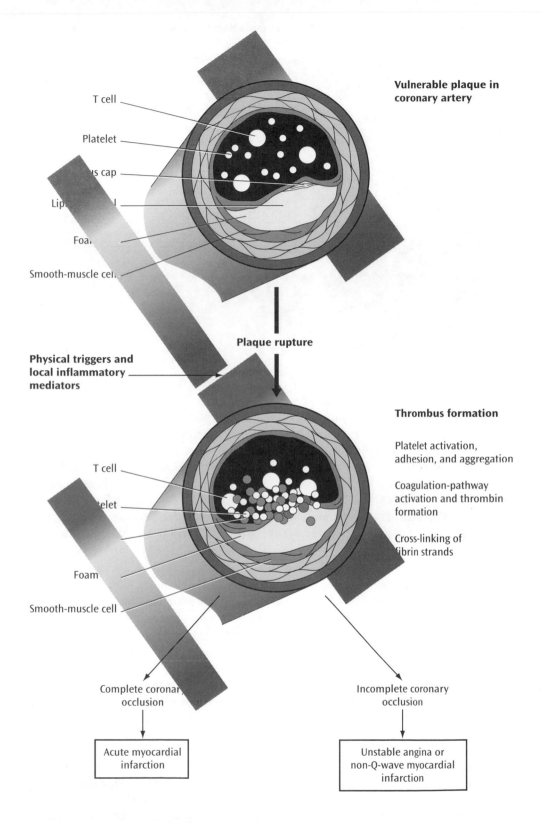

Figure 20.1 *Pathophysiologic events leading to the syndrome of unstable angina.*

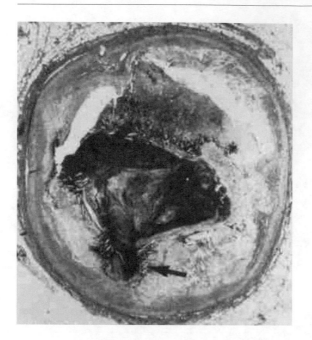

Figure 20.2 *Atherosclerotic plaque in a coronary artery.*

Rupture of an unstable or vulnerable atherosclrotic plaque acts as the inciting event in acute coronary syndromes, primarily by exposing the thrombogenic, lipid-rich core of the plaque to blood-borne elements. The result of this interaction is the formation of thrombus within the vessel (Fig. 20.2). The principal mediators of this event are thrombin, necessary for the formation, growth, maintenance, and consolidation of a thrombus, and activated platelets, which adhere to intimal collagen via specific platelet receptors (Fig. 20.3). These principal factors and their regulation become important in our discussion of the pharmacotherapy and management of acute coronary syndromes.

In normal coronary arteries, the underlying connective tissue of the vessel wall is prevented from contact with platelets by the intact endothelium. Normal arteries rarely undergo thrombosis, by virtue of the protective effect of the normally functioning endothelial monolayer. During the early stages of atherogenesis, endothelial cells may become dysfunctional, manifested by overexpression of certain adhesion molecules and impaired nitric oxide synthesis. At this stage, however, there is no exposure of the underlying collagen and thus minimal platelet deposition is noted. In plaque rupture, the fibrous cap tears to expose the thrombogenic core of the atherosclerotic plaque. The exposure of the blood pool to the lipid core expressing large amounts of tissue factor sets off a complex cascade leading to thrombus formation. Initially, the thrombus is rich in platelets and red blood cells, lending the name 'white clot' to this early thrombus. Subsequently, the thrombus becomes richer in fibrin via activation of the coagulation cascade and thrombin formation. For this stage, the term 'red clot' has been used to describe the thrombus. This process of platelet deposition and fibrin formation may wax and wane for hours or days, depending on the relative balance of factors which promote thrombus growth with those which inhibit thrombus growth (i.e., natural lysis). Other factors, such as

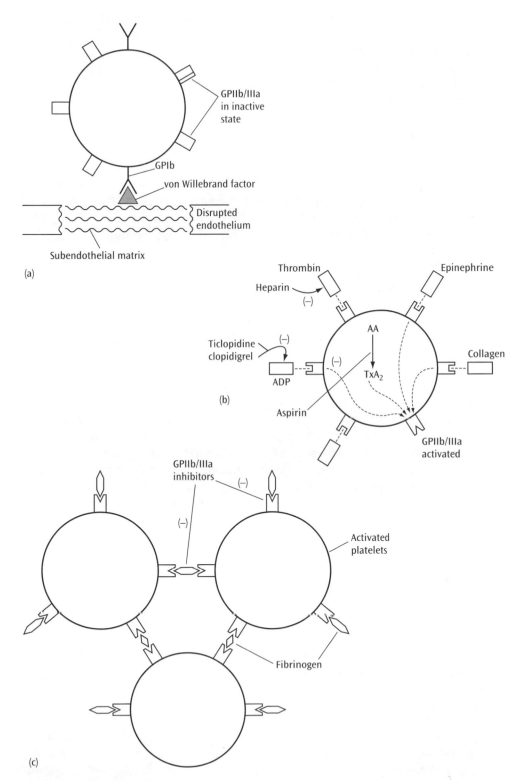

(a)

(b)

(c)

Figure 20.3 *Platelet activation.*

coronary vasospasm and distal embolization of thrombus, may contribute to the clinical syndrome of chest pain and myocardial ischemia classically described in acute coronary syndromes.

Platelets possess multiple surface receptors, which allow them to adhere to sub-endothelial von Willebrand Factor collagen and fibrogen (IIb/IIIa) to form a platelet plug. This is a normal response to tissue injury and functions to prevent bleeding from damage to the vessel following trauma. The evolution of this hemostatic plug requires platelet adherence to the site of injury, platelet aggregation, and platelet activation, which are mediated by release of adenosine diphosphate (ADP) and thromboxane A2, both potent platelet recruiters (Fig. 20.3). The concept of antiplatelet therapy in acute coronary syndromes is to inhibit platelet aggregation. Similarly, the concept of antithrombotic therapy in acute coronary syndromes is aimed at the inhibition of thrombin generation or of thrombin activity, with the goal of dissolution of the thrombus and restoration of coronary blood flow.

ANTIPLATELET THERAPY

The effect of antiplatelet therapy in reducing recurrent vascular-related events in acute coronary syndromes is well substantiated in clinical trials. Aspirin traditionally has been viewed as the gold standard in antiplatelet therapy. The mechanism accounting for the beneficial effect of aspirin in unstable coronary syndromes is mediated via irreversible inhibition of the platelet cyclo-oxygenase pathway, blocking formation of thromboxane A2 and ultimately platelet aggregation as is discussed further in Chapter 6. Aspirin has no effect on platelet aggregation induced by other agonists and thus is a relatively weak platelet inhibitor. Nonetheless, numerous clinical trials have shown a benefit favoring aspirin use in acute coronary syndromes.

In 1988, the Second International Study of Infarct Survival (ISIS-2) investigators studied approximately 17 000 patients presenting to the hospital up to 24 hours (median 5 hours) after the onset of suspected acute myocardial infarction. The patients were randomized to one of four therapeutic arms: (1) a 1-hour intravenous infusion of 1.5 MU streptokinase; (2) 1 month of 160 mg/day enteric-coated aspirin; (3) both active treatments; or (4) neither. Both streptokinase alone and aspirin alone produced a highly significant reduction in 5-week vascular mortality when compared with the placebo group (Fig. 20.4). An odds reduction in 5-week vascular mortality of 23% compared with placebo was seen when using aspirin alone during acute myocardial infarction. A similar reduction was seen with thrombolytic therapy. The reduction in both vascular and all-cause mortality persisted after a median 15-month follow-up. The trial showed that 1 month of low-dose aspirin started immediately in 1000 patients with suspected acute myocardial infarction would typically avoid about 25 deaths and 10–15 nonfatal reinfarctions or strokes, with benefit persisting well beyond the treatment period.[15] This study also differed from previous trials using aspirin after myocardial infarction in that a lower dose was chosen (160 mg/day as compared to 300–1500 mg/day). This avoided the gastro-intestinal toxicity commonly seen when using higher doses of aspirin, without loss of efficacy.[16]

It should be noted that aspirin therapy was initiated immediately on suspicion of acute myocardial infarction in the ISIS-2 trial. This is important in that platelet activation and aggregation occur in the acute phase of myocardial infarction and are further increased by fibrinolytic therapy, increasing the risk of early coronary artery reocclusion and reinfarction.[17,18] Based on these data, patients presenting with acute myocardial infarction should be given a dose of at least 160 mg of aspirin. This dose has been shown to produce virtually complete inhibition of cyclo-oxygenase in less than 1 hour.[19] Complete inhibition can be maintained at doses of 75 mg daily. There is no clinical evidence of therapeutic benefit with doses higher than 325 mg daily.[20]

In 1994, the Antiplatelet Trialists' Collaboration updated their meta-analysis to include 145 randomized trials of prolonged antiplatelet therapy. Approximately 70 000 patients with acute coronary syndromes were studied, the majority of whom were high-risk patients with occlusive vascular disease. The analysis revealed a significant reduction in the risk of death, myocardial infarction, and stroke by prolonged antiplatelet therapy. The most widely used antiplatelet agent was aspirin, with similar effectiveness demonstrated with doses of 500–1500 mg daily, 160–325 mg daily, and 75–100 mg daily.[20]

The data supporting the use of aspirin in treating unstable angina are equally as convincing as in acute myocardial infarction. The Research on Instability in Coronary Artery Disease (RISC) group studied 796 men admitted to the coronary care unit with the diagnosis of unstable angina or non-Q-wave myocardial infarction. They were randomized in a double-blind manner to treatment with oral aspirin

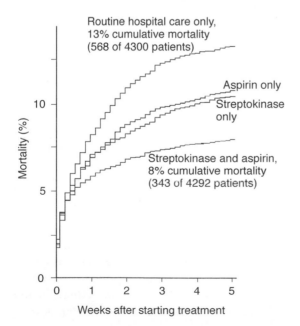

Figure 20.4 *Effects of aspirin and streptokinase on mortality in acute myocardial infarction.*

75 mg daily or placebo. This study showed a reduction of almost 50% in the risk of subsequent myocardial infarction at 3 months after the index event. Treatment with aspirin was shown to be equally as effective after a non-Q-wave myocardial infarction in unstable angina.[21] Other trials using aspirin in variable doses similarly demonstrated a significant risk reduction in mortality and subsequent nonfatal myocardial infarction in patients presenting with unstable angina or non-Q-wave myocardial infarction. There trials are summarized in Table 20.1. Overall, these studies showed a 52% reduction in the risk of fatal or nonfatal myocardial infarction at 2 years.

Table 20.1 *Aspirin in unstable angina*

Study	Design	Entry window/ follow-up	All-cause mortality (RRR %)	Cardiac death or nonfatal myocardial infarction (RRR %)
Lewis et al.[22]	ASA (325 mg/day) versus placebo	51 hours/3 months	51[a]	51[a]
Cairns et al.[23]	ASA (1300 mg/day) versus placebo	8 days/24 months	71[a]	51[a]
Theroux et al.[24]	ASA (650 mg/day) versus placebo	24 hours/6 days	0	72[a]
RISC[21]	ASA (75 mg/day) versus placebo	5 hours/5 days	0	57[a]

[a]$p < 0.05$
(RRR = relative risk reduction; ASA = aspirin.)

There is controversy, however, concerning whether aspirin should be used in the primary prevention of coronary artery disease. Two large studies in the late 1980s looked at this question. The first was the British Doctors Study. This was an open-label, randomized trial of aspirin, 500 mg daily, versus no aspirin. The population included British male physicians without a clinical history of vascular disease. They were followed for up to 6 years. The study revealed a trend, though not statistically significant, toward a reduction in vascular death rates, total mortality, and myocardial infarction. There was a significant reduction in confirmed transient ischemic attacks and, surprisingly, an increase in the risk of disabling stroke in the aspirin group.[25]

Similarly, the Physicians Health Study looked at 22 071 US male physicians aged 40–80 years who were in good health at the time of entry into the study. They were randomly allocated to receive aspirin 325 mg every other day or placebo plus beta-carotene (50 mg every other day) in a 2 × 2 factorial design. The study was stopped early by the Data and Safety Monitoring Board because of a clear reduction of myocardial infarction, a low likelihood of detecting a beneficial effect of aspirin on cardiovascular mortality before the year 2000, and the high prevalence of aspirin use among participants following a nonfatal vascular event. Subgroup analysis only found the protective effect against myocardial infarction in those over 50 years old. Overall, the study showed a significant reduction in the combined incidence of nonfatal myocardial infarction, nonfatal stroke, and death from any cardiovascular cause. Again, there was a trend toward an increase in the rate of hemorrhagic stroke in the aspirin group that was not statistically significant.[26]

Taken together, these studies show that aspirin consistently reduces ischemic cardiac events. There was a consistent failure in these trials to show a mortality benefit in this group. The absolute benefit of aspirin in primary prevention was greatest among older men, those with diabetes mellitus, those with systolic or diastolic hypertension, cigarette smokers, and patients who did not exercise. There are no large trials looking at the use of aspirin in the primary prevention of coronary artery disease in women. Consensus recommendations for the use of aspirin in primary prevention do not support its routine use in individuals free of a history of acute myocardial infarction, stroke, or transient ischemic attacks, and who are under 50 years old. It is recommended that aspirin (80–325 mg/day) be considered for individuals over 50 years of age who have at least one major risk factor for coronary artery disease and have no contraindications to aspirin.[27,28]

GLYCOPROTEIN IIb/IIIa INHIBITORS

Platelet activation follows adhesion to the subendothelial matrix, and is mediated by multiple mechanical and chemical stimuli involving complex intracellular pathways (as discussed in Chapter 6). These potent agonists include thromboxane A2, thrombin, norepinephrine, collagen and ADP. This activation results in conformational and metabolic changes, leading ultimately to activation of the fibrinogen receptor glycoprotein IIb/IIIa on the platelet surface and recruitment of additional platelets to form the hemostatic plug (Fig. 20.3).

Aspirin and heparin each inhibits only one of many pathways leading to platelet aggregation (thromboxane A2 and thrombin, respectively) and have generally weak antiplatelet effects at therapeutic doses. Recognition of these limitations provided the impetus for targeting the final common pathway through the development of specific inhibitors of glycoprotein IIa/IIIa.

Most of the clinical experience with glycoprotein IIb/IIIa inhibitors consists of the use of three intravenous agents: the chimeric human–murine antibody fragment abciximab, the peptide eptifibatide, and the nonpeptide tirofiban. More than 30 000 patients have been enrolled in clinical trials involving glycoprotein IIb/IIIa antagonists. Most of these trials used the combination incidence of major adverse cardiac events as the primary endpoint. The first area of investigation was in conjunction with percutaneous coronary interventions, an obligatory endothelial injury model. Significant reductions in adverse events were seen in a broad range of patients, especially those presenting with unstable angina.[28]

Over the past few years, nine large clinical trials evaluated abciximab, tirofiban, and eptifibatide in the setting of unstable coronary syndromes with and without high-risk angioplasty. The data consistently showed a reduction in the risk of death or nonfatal myocardial infarction at 30 days when a IIb/IIIa inhibitor was added to aspirin and heparin.[29-32] The initial benefit appears to translate into a sustained and incremental long-term benefit. In a 3-year follow-up of the Evaluation of C7E3 Fab in the Prevention of Ischemic Complications (EPIC) trial, patients who presented with acute coronary syndromes had a 60% reduction in mortality if they were assigned to abciximab bolus and infusion at the time of original enrollment.[33]

The elevation of serum levels of troponin T identified patients most likely to benefit from glycoprotein IIb/IIIa inhibition in a post-hoc analysis of the Chimeric 7E3 Antiplatelet Therapy in Unstable Angina Refractory to Standard Treatment (CAPTURE) trial. At 6-month follow-up, patients with troponin T levels of 2.0 ng/ml or greater had fewer clinical endpoints (i.e., myocardial infarction or death) if they received abciximab in conjunction with conventional therapy versus conventional therapy alone (9.5% versus 2.5%; $p = 0.004$). Patients with a low troponin T level had no discernible benefit from abciximab over placebo (8.2% versus 9.5%; $p = 0.52$). These findings help to identify those most likely to benefit from the early institution of glycoprotein IIb/IIIa antagonists.[33]

In patients undergoing coronary interventions, the bleeding rate was higher when abciximab was added to heparin in the EPIC trial. Further studies found no increased risk when weight-based heparin dosage was used (70 units/kg per hour). Furthermore, a meta-analysis of the abciximab trials EPIC, Evaluation in PTCA to Improve Long-term Outcome with abciximab glycoprotein IIb/IIIa Blockade (EPILOG), and CAPTURE showed no clinically significant increase in the risk of stroke with abciximab compared to herparin alone (0.13% versus 0.19% for hemorrhagic stroke).[31]

Another potential complication is thrombocytopenia, more commonly seen with abciximab but possible with all parenteral IIb/IIIa inhibitors. In clinical trials, reversible thrombocytopenia has been observed at a low rate (ranging from 1.1% to 5.6%). However, profound thrombocytopenia ($< 20\,000/\mu L$) within 24 hours has been observed with abciximab in 0.3–0.8% of patients, which requires immediate discontinuation of the drug. Complete resolution occurs in 5–7 days and no major sequelae have been reported. To monitor for thrombocytopenia, a platelet count should be performed 2–4 hours and 24 hours after initiation of therapy with all intravenous IIb/IIIa inhibitors.

Trials are presently underway to examine the role of glycoprotein IIb/IIIa inhibitors in conjunction with thrombolytic agents in ST-segment elevation acute coronary syndromes. Initial pilot studies showed significant improvement in the reperfusion rate, accelerated thrombolysis, and more sustained vascular patency with combination therapy versus thrombolytics alone. Ongoing trials will seek to validate these promising results and define the optimal dosage of each agent.

Potent long-term antiplatelet therapy with oral IIb/IIIa antagonists for the secondary prevention of coronary events is also being studied. Initial enthusiasm was tempered by disappointing results of a large multicenter trial using sibrafiban, an oral IIb/IIIa inhibitor. In patients with recent myocardial infarction, long-term therapy with sibrafiban resulted in recurrent event rates similar to those of aspirin, with a higher incidence of bleeding complications.[32]

THIENOPYRIDINE ANTIPLATELET AGENTS

Ticlopidine and clopidogrel are two thienopyridine derivatives that decrease platelet aggregation by inhibiting the binding of adenosine 5'-diphosphate (ADP) to its receptor on glycoprotein IIb/IIIa (see Chapter 6 for more information). These agents do not affect the cyclo-oxygenase–thromboxane A2 pathway and can potentiate aspirin's antiplatelet effect when given with aspirin. Aggressive antiplatelet therapy is an important element of the medical management after interventional procedures. Ticlopidine or clopidogrel added to aspirin for 4 weeks after intracoronary stent placement lowered the risk of stent thrombosis, while reducing bleeding complications and length of hospital stay compared to anticoagulant therapy.[34–7]

Only one randomized trial examined ticlopidine for the treatment of unstable angina. The Studio della Ticlopidine nell'Angina Instabile trial enrolled 652 patients with unstable angina within 48 hours of admission. They were randomly assigned to ticlopidine 250 mg twice daily plus conventional therapy or conventional therapy alone. Aspirin was not a standard treatment at the time of study design. Overall, there was a 46% reduction at 6-months follow-up in the combined endpoint of vascular death and nonfatal myocardial infarction in the ticlopidine arm (7.3% compared with 13.6%; $p = 0.009$).[38] Clinical practice guidelines for the management of unstable angina and acute myocardial infarction only recommend using ticlopidine in substitution for aspirin in patients with gastrointestinal intolerance and hypersensitivity to aspirin.[45]

The usefulness of ticlopidine is limited by its potential side-effects. Although the risk of minor bleeding is increased, data from the stroke prevention trials reveal a low incidence of major bleeding and intracranial hemorrhage. An uncommon, but more serious, consequence is neutropenia. This potentially fatal complication has been reported with an incidence of 0.9–2.4% in clinical trials. It is reversible in most, but not all, cases. Neutropenia usually develops within the first few months of treatment. It is therefore recommended to monitor serial blood counts at the initiation of drug use.[39] Thrombotic thrombocytopenia purpura is another rare complication, with fewer than 100 cases reported worldwide. It is associated with a devastating 33% mortality rate.[44]

These hematologic complications are almost never encountered in the first 2–3 weeks of therapy, allowing for relatively safe short-term use of ticlopidine following intracoronary stent placement.

Clopidogrel is a thienopyridine derivative structurally related to ticlopidine that has a more favorable safety profile. It was initially compared with aspirin for the secondary prevention of ischemic vascular events in the large multicenter Clopidogrel versus Aspirin in Patients at Risk of Ischemic Events (CAPRIE) study.[41] In this trial, 19 185 patients with atherosclerotic vascular disease, including prior myocardial infarction, ischemic stroke, or symptomatic peripheral arterial disease, were randomized to receive either clopidogrel or aspirin and were followed for a mean of 1.9 years. Clopidogrel 75 mg/day reduced the incidence of the combined endpoint of ischemic stroke, myocardial infarction, or death from peripheral vascular disease (5.3% versus 5.8%; $p = 0.04$). However, no significant benefit was seen in the subgroup of patients with a history of myocardial infarction (5.0% versus 4.8%; $p = 0.66$).

An excellent long-term safety profile was seen with clopidogrel use, with neutropenia and bleeding complications similar to those with aspirin over the study period. The 1999 revised American College of Cardiology/American Heart Association (ACC/AHA) guidelines for the management of acute myocardial infarction recognize clopidogrel as an acceptable alternative antiplatelet agent for patients unable to receive aspirin. Ongoing randomized trials will help to define the role of clopidogrel as an adjunct to aspirin in the setting of unstable coronary syndromes and as a substitute to ticlopidine to prevent intracoronary stent thrombosis.

ANTITHROMBIN THERAPY

Unfractionated heparin is a glycosaminoglycan made up of polysaccharide chains ranging in molecular weight from 3000 to 30 000 kD.[42] These polysaccharide chains bind to antithrombin II and cause a conformational change in the molecule that accelerates the inhibition of thrombin and factor X. There have been several trials examining the efficacy of unfractionated heparin in acute coronary syndromes. Most of the evidence regarding the addition of unfractionated heparin to aspirin in patients suspected of having an acute myocardial infarction comes from the work done in the Second Gruppo Italiano per lo Studio della Sopravvivenza nell'Infarto Miocardico (GISSI-2) trial, and the Third International Study of Infarct Survival (ISIS-3) study.[43,44] These studies looked at a total of 62 067 patients with suspected acute Q-wave myocardial infarction who received fibrinolytic therapy. Beyond the effect of aspirin alone, the reduction in the incidence of death or other major vascular events with the addition of heparin was small. This was at the expense of a small increase in the incidence of major bleeding in the heparin plus aspirin group. Furthermore, the benefit diminished over time. Any early mortality benefit gained by the addition of heparin in these studies was lost at 35 days and at 6 months. In both studies, however, heparin was begun with a significant delay (12 hours in GISSI-2 and 4 hours in ISIS-3) and the dose was given subcutaneously, which may have caused a further delay in achieving therapeutic levels of anticoagulation.

The Global Utilization of Streptokinase and Tissue Plasminogen Activator for Occluded Coronary Arteries Trial (GUSTO-1) studied more than 20 000 patients with suspected acute myocardial infarction who were assigned to therapy with streptokinase. An intravenous dose of unfractionated heparin (5000 IU bolus followed by an intravenous infusion of 1000 IU per hour) plus aspirin was compared to the treatment regimen used in the ISIS-3 trial. Therapy was adjusted to achieve an activated partial thromboplastin time of 60–85 seconds. In this trial, intravenous heparin therapy was not associated with any reduction in mortality or in stroke, and there was also a trend toward increased rates of major or severe bleeding in the intravenous heparin group (see Table 20.2).[45] More intensive intravenous heparin

Table 20.2 *Results of the GUSTO-1 trial*[a]

Event	ASA plus intravenous heparin (n = 10 410)	ASA plus high-dose subcutaneous heparin (n = 9841)	Effect/1000 patients assigned intravenous instead of subcutaneous heparin	p value
Death	763 (7.3)	712 (7.2)	0.9 ± 3.8	0.8
Reinfarction	438 (4.2)	343 (3.5)	7.2 ± 2.7	< 0.01
Any stroke	144 (1.4)	117 (1.2)	2.0 ± 1.6	0.2
Hemorrhagic stroke	59 (0.6)	45 (0.5)	1.1 ± 1.0	0.3
Major or severe bleeding	151 (1.5)	117 (1.2)	2.6 ± 1.6	0.1

[a]Results are only for patients randomly assigned to receive streptokinase therapy.
( ) = numbers in parenthesis are percentages; ASA = aspirin.

regimens have been studied, and although these regimens have improved early coronary artery patency, the trials had to be stopped due to an unacceptable rate of intracerebral hemorrhage and other major bleeding.[46]

Currently, in patients with ST segment elevation acute coronary syndromes who will not be given thrombolytic therapy, there is little evidence supporting the benefit of intravenous heparin. Subcutaneous heparin (7500 IU twice daily) is recommended in all patients with acute myocardial infarction not treated with thrombolytic therapy. Results of clinical trials such as the GUSTO trial do favor heparin administration intravenously in patients receiving thrombolytic therapy with alteplase (TPA). For patients with acute myocardial infarction treated with nonselective thrombolytics (streptokinase, anistreplase), intravenous therapy should be reserved for those at high risk for systemic emboli (large or anterior myocardial infarction, atrial fibrillation, previous embolus, or known left ventricular thrombus).

The benefit of unfractionated heparin in unstable angina has been well documented. Oler et al. published a meta-analysis in 1996 in which they looked at six randomized studies which enrolled patients with unstable angina or non-Q-wave myocardial infarction to aspirin plus heparin versus aspirin alone, and reported the incidence of myocrdial infarction or death.[47] The combined data from these clinical trials suggested a 33% reduction in the risk of myocardial infarction of death during heparin therapy in patients treated with heparin plus aspirin compared with aspirin alone. Although these results did not reach statistical significance, there was clearly a trend favoring the reduction of acute ischemic events in patients receiving heparin plus aspirin. In individual trials the small risk of bleeding on heparin was offset in these studies by the low number needed to treat to prevent an event (29–34 individuals treated to prevent one death or myocardial infarction).

Although unfractionated heparin continues to be used by many physicians as antithrombotic therapy for acute coronary syndromes, it has a few notable disadvantages. First, anticoagulation with unfractionated heparin is associated with a significant failure to achieve therapeutic dosing in a timely manner due to its unpredictable anticoagulant response, secondary to competitive binding to plasma proteins other than antithrombin.[48] Second, neutralization of the drug via activated platelets can further reduce the antithrombotic efficacy of unfractionated heparin. Finlly, unfractionated heparin has been associated with rebound clinical events following discontinuation as well as a small but significant incidence of heparin-induced thrombocytopenia.[49,50]

More recently there has been a growing body of evidence favoring the use of low molecular weight heparins (LMWHs) in the treatment of acute coronary syndromes (see Chapter 5). The efficacy of LMWHs for unstable coronary artery disease has been examined in several controlled clinical trials (Table 20.3). In the Efficacy and

Table 20.3 *Trials using low molecular weight heparin in unstable coronary syndromes*

Study	Drug	Group	Dose	Outcome
FRIC[52]	Dalteparin versus UFH acutely (first 6 days) then dalteparin versus placebo continued to day 45[a]	1482 patients with unstable angina or non-Q wave MI	Weight-adjusted, subcutaneous	No significant difference in combined endpoints (death, MI, recurrent angina) at 6 days and 45 days
FRISC[53]	Dalteparin + ASA compared with ASA alone[a]	1506 patients with unstable angina	120 IU subcutaneously every 12 hours up to 6 days followed by 7500 IU for 50 days	Relative risk reduction of 48% in death or MI at 40 days No significant difference at 150-day follow-up
FRISC II[54]	Dalteparin twice daily versus placebo	2267 patients with acute coronary syndromes	120 IU/kg subcutaneously every 12 hours	Significant decrease in combined endpoint death, MI or revascularization at 3 months. Benefits were not sustained at 6-month follow-up
ESSENCE[51]	Enoxaparin versus UFH[a]	3171 patients with unstable angina/non-Q wave MI	1 mg/kg given 2–8 days after hospitalization	Significant reduction in combined endpoint (death, MI, recurrent angina) in enoxaparin group both at 14-day and 30-day follow-up
TIMI-11B[55]	Enoxaparin versus UFH[a]	4020 patients with unstable angina/non-Q-wave MI	Weight adjusted, subcutaneously	Relative risk reduction of 15% in the combined endpoint of death, MI, and urgent revascularization, which continued at day 43

[a]All patients received standard-dose aspirin.
(ASA = aspirin; UFH = unfractionated heparin; MI = myocardial infarction.)

Safety of Subcutaneous Enoxaparin in Non-Q-wave Coronary Events Study Group (ESSENCE) trial, enoxaparin (1 mg/kg body weight) administered subcutaneously twice daily was compared with continuous intravenous unfractionated heparin in 3171 patients with unstable angina pctoris or non-Q-wave myocardial infarction.[51] The primary outcome of the trial was a combined endpoint of death, myocardial infarction, or recurrent angina at 14 days of follow-up. The composite endpoint was also examined at 48 hours, 14 days, and 30 days. The incidence of major and minor hemorrhage was also examined. Of note was the observation that within 12–24 hours of randomization, only 46% of the patients in the unfractionated heparin group had an activated partial thromboplastin time of 55–85 seconds. The combined triple endpoint was significantly lower in patients randomized to enoxaparin at both 14 and 30 days. Furthermore, 30 days after randomization, the need for coronary revascularization was significantly less frequent among patients assigned to the enoxaparin group than in those in the unfractionated heparin group. There was no significant difference between the two treatment groups with regard to serious hemorrhagic complications; however, there was an increased incidence in the exonaparin group in minor hemorrhagic events.

Although together the outcomes of the trials using LMWHs in acute coronary syndromes differ, their use seems to be associated with a more favorable outcome.[51–5] This apparent benefit is achieved without an increase in major hemorrhagic complications. More data are needed to determine long-term efficacy and safety of these drugs. It will be interesting to see future applications of the LMWHs in the treatment of acute coronary syndromes, as in the ongoing Hypertension Audit of Risk Factor Therapy (HART-II) trial, which will compare unfractionated heparin with enoxaparin as adjunctive antithrombin therapy for patients receiving a front-loaded TPA regimen for ST segment elevation myocardial infarction.

The current revised ACC/AHA guidelines have expanded the recommendations for the treatment of acute coronary syndromes to include the LMWHs.[56] Specifically, LMWHs may be used instead of standard unfractionated heparin in patients with non-ST segment elevation myocardial infarction. Furthermore, the recommendations call for LMWHs as an alternative to subcutaneous unfractionated heparin in all patients not treated with thrombolytic therapy who do not have a contraindication to heparin. In high-risk patients (left ventricular thrombus, large anterior myocardial infarction, atrial fibrillation, or previous embolus), intravenous heparin is preferred.

THROMBOLYTIC AGENTS

The role of thrombotic occlusion in acute myocardial infarction has been well documented angiographically.[57] This observation led to a great interest in the 1980s in the use of potent direct-acting and indirect-acting thrombolytic agents in the therapy of acute myocardial infarction. The thrombolytic (fibrinolytic) agents all work enzymatically to convert the single-chain plasminogen molecule to the double-chain plasmin, exposing the active enzymatic center of the molecule, which then works as a potent stimulator of fibrinolysis. They also differ from each other in dose, circulating half-life, cost, risk profile, and relative effiacy. These differences are summarized in Table 20.4.

Table 20.4 *Comparison of US FDA-approved thrombolytic agents*

	Streptokinase	Alteplase (TPA)[a]	Reteplase (r-TPA)[a]
Dose	1.5 MU in 30–60 minutes	100 mg in 90 minutes[b]	10 U × 2 over 30 minutes
Bolus	No	No	Yes
Antigenic	Yes	No	No
Allergic reactions	Yes	No	No
90 minute patency rates (%)	Approximately 50	Approximately 75	Approximately 75
TIMI 3 flow (%)	32	54	60
Mortality rate (%) – US trials	7.3	7.2	7.5
Cost per dose (US$) in 2000	538	2750	2750

[a]TPA = tissue plasminogen activator; r-TPA = recombinant tissue plasminogen activator.
[b]Accelerated TPA given as follows: 15-mg bolus, then 0.75 mg/kg over 30 minutes (maximum 50 mg), then 0.50 mg/kg over 60 minutes (maximum 35 mg).
Adapted from Ryan et al. 1999 update: Management of Acute Myocardial Infarction: ACC/AHA published guidelines JACC Vol. 34, No. 3, 1999: 890–911.

The mortality benefit afforded by the use of fibrinolytic agents in acute myocardial infarction has been well documented in clinical trials. The Fibrinolytic Trialists Collaborative Group (FTT), compared 5-week mortality results in the nine largest randomized trials pitting fibrinolytic therapy with no therapy in patients with suspected acute myocardial infarction. They found a mortality benefit for a wide range of patients, in particular patients receiving 12 hours or less after the onset of symptoms, and, whereas the absolute benefit of therapy appeared to be greatest for those patients with anterior ST segment elevation, there was also a significant mortality benefit extended to all patients with ST segment elevation on the echocardiogram (ECG).[58]

In patients presenting with symptoms of more than 12 hours duration, the data on the efficacy of thrombolytic therapy are less clear. In most studies looking at the efficacy of thrombolytic therapy, individuals presenting with symptoms of duration more than 12 hours were excluded. Generally, there is a proportionally smaller benefit for reperfusion therapy in these patients, and therapy should be given only to selected patients with ongoing ischemic pain and persistent ST segment elevation.[59] The reduction in mortality with thrombolytics is generally most pronounced in the subgroup of patients with new bundle branch block on the ECG, and/or ST segment elevation. There is no proven benefit in patients with ST segment depression on the ECG, and these patients actually tend to do worse with therapy (Fig. 20.5). With regard to age, there are no data supporting routinely withholding thrombolytic therapy based on age criteria alone. Although younger patients achieve a greater relative risk reduction in mortality compared to patients older than 75, the absolute reduction in mortality in this group still favors fibrinolytic therapy.[58] Furthermore, the FTT review demonstrated a mortality benefit with thrombolytics in certain other 'high-risk' patients such as those with hypotension or tachycardia.[58] Thus, hemodynamic instability should not be considered a contraindication to thrombolytic therapy in cases when angiography is not readily available.

Certainly, the most feared complication of thrombolytic therapy is the small but not insignificant risk of intracranial hemorrhage. Clinical variables that predict an

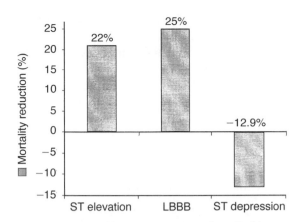

Figure 20.5 *Effect of thrombolytic therapy on mortality according to admission electrocardiogram. LBBB = Left Bundle Branch Block*

increased risk of intracranial hemorrhage include advanced age (greater than 65 years), low body weight (less than 70 kg), hypertension on presentation (systolic blood pressure > 180 mmHg, diastolic blood pressure >110 mmHg), and with the use of alteplase.[60,61] Stroke rates of 1% or less have been seen in most clinical trials evaluating thrombolytic therapy. Clinicians must weigh the net risk/benefit ratio before administering these potent but potentially dangerous drugs.

There have been several studies that have compared the efficacy of different thrombolytic regimens. The largest of these trials (GISSI-2, ISIS-3, and the GUSTO trials) compared streptokinase with a TPA-based regimen (see Table 20.4) with stroke, reinfarction, and death from all causes as the major clinical endpoints. Taken together, these trials revealed an increased rate of stroke in the TPA-based regimen, which was significantly increased in the older group (> 75 years) and the hypertensive patients. The difference in mortality between the groups was not statistically significant; however, a trend toward better early outcome in the TPA group was seen. If one looks at mortality not related to stroke in these trials, the TPA-based regimens were associated with significantly lower mortality rates.

Current clinical practice relies heavily on data obtained from the GUSTO trial.[45] This trial demonstrated that accelerated TPA (alteplase) plus intravenous heparin had a significant, although modest, survival benefit compared to streptokinase with either intravenous or subcutaneous heparin dosing (absolute risk reduction of 1%, relative risk reduction of 14%, $p = 0.0001$). There were also fewer documented complications, including allergic reaction, clinical left ventricular dysfunction, and arrhythmia, in the TPA group. In general, there was no subgroups in which TPA performed significantly worse than the streptokinase regimen, but in those patients less than 75 years of age, or with an anterior myocardial infarction, a greater survival benefit was seen with TPA. Again, the risk of intracranial hemorrhage in the TPA group was slightly higher than with streptokinase (0.2% absolute difference). However, net benefit was still achieved with TPA compared with streptokinase, with nine fewer deaths or disabling strokes per 1000 patients treated.

Thus, based on results of both the GUSTO and Thrombolysis in Myocardial Infarction (TIMI) 4 trials,[62] the most effective therapy for achieving early coronary perfusion in the setting of acute myocardial infarction seems to be accelerated alteplase (TPA) with intravenous heparin. One must keep in mind this regimen is associated with a higher cost per patient and a slight increase in the risk of intracranial hemorrhage. The current ACC/AHA guidelines on the management of acute myocardial infarction recommended this regimen in patients presenting early after symptom onset with a large area of injury (e.g., acute anterior myocardial infarction) and a low risk of intracranial hemorrhage.[59] Other groups, such as those at greater risk for intracranial hemorrhage or patients with smaller absolute survival benefit, may be candidates for streptokinase therapy. A physician with experience in administering these drugs should make these decisions. Lastly, the ACC/AHA guidelines recommend avoiding the reuse of streptokinase for at least 2 years (preferably indefinitely), due to a high prevalence of potentially neutralizing antibody titers.

CHRONIC ANTICOAGULATION AFTER ACUTE CORONARY SYNDROMES

The risks of recurrent unstable angina, myocardial infarction, and death after patients present with unstable angina are high, probably reflecting continued or recurrent plaque instability and thrombus formation. Event rates are only partially improved by aspirin therapy. Oral anticoagulation in addition to aspirin has been investigated for this problem in an attempt to target not only the platelets' role, but also that of thrombin activation. Long-term combination warfarin and aspirin following acute coronary syndromes has been demonstrated to reduce subsequent events in several randomized trials.[63–5] A reduction in risk of death (24%), reinfarction (34%), and strokes was found over an average follow-up of 37 months among survivors of acute myocardial infarction compared with aspirin alone.

The occurrence of serious bleeding was slightly more common when warfarin was combined with aspirin (0.6% per year).[63] However, lower levels of anticoagulation added no protection over aspirin alone.[66] Fixed-dose warfarin (3 mg/day) resulted in median INR levels that ranged during 6-months' follow-up from 1.19 to 1.51. Comparing 1-year follow-up data, there was no improvement in the rate of myocardial infarction, stroke, or cardiovascular death.

In clinical practice, it is not uncommon for patients with acute coronary syndromes to have other indications for anticoagulation. In many of these cases, the decision regarding combination therapy, is whether to add aspirin to ongoing oral anticoagulation. There are limited data that address this. Several head-to-head comparisons between oral anticoagulation and aspirin failed to demonstrate a motality difference.[67,68] As the above risk and efficacy comparison shows an advantage of combination therapy, 80 or 160 mg of aspirin daily should be considered for patients with acute coronary syndromes already receiving warfarin who are not felt to be at high risk for bleeding complications.

LEFT VENTRICULAR THROMBOSIS AND THROMBOEMBOLISM AFTER MYOCARDIAL INFARCTION

Anticoagulation in patients who have sustained myocardial infarction may prevent thrombus formation not only in the coronary arteries, but also in the left ventricular chamber, thereby preventing systemic embolization. Stroke rates have been reported of between 1% and 3% of all myocardial infarctions, and of between 2% and 6% for anterior wall infarction.[69] Characteristics that identified a higher risk of thromboembolism include anterior location of myocardial infarction, poorer left ventricular function, and older age of patients. In a cohort study of post-myocardial infarction patients, at 4 years of follow-up, the incidence of stroke among those with left ventricular ejection fractions greater than 35% was 4.1%, whereas patients with left ventricular ejection fractions less than 29% had an incidence of 8.9%.[70] The embolic potential of thrombi associated with myocardial infarction appears to be much greater early postinfarction. In another retrospective study, when a thrombus was evident on echocardiography early after myocardial infarction (< 3 weeks), 29% of patients had embolic events, compared to 19% that were detected later.[71] Although thrombi can be seen later after myocardial infarction, especially in akinetic or dyskinetic walls, most embolization occurs in the first few weeks postmyocardial infarction.[69]

Echocardiography provides a fairly accurate means of detecting infarct-associated mural thrombi. In an analysis comparing the direct observation of thrombi after aneurysmectomy or autopsy with prior echocardiography, the test was 92% sensitive and 88% specific. However, the majority of thrombi do not lead to clinically apparent embolic events. The incidence of thrombi from aneurysm resection studies has been from 48% to 66%.[72,73]

Heparin administered immediately following myocardial infarction decreases the incidence of thrombus formation and of stroke in the early postinfarction period.[74,75] A cohort analysis of the Survival and Ventricular Enlargement Trial showed protection from stroke by long-term warfarin therapy in all subgroups of severity of left ventricular dysfunction. If the left ventricular ejection fraction was <28%, the relative risk (RR) was 0.17; if 29–35%, the RR was 0.14; and if > 35% the RR was 0.23.[70]

Studies of thrombi complicating chronic left ventricular aneurysms found very low late event rates that were not affected by anticoagulation therapy.[76] On that basis, warfarin is not clearly beneficial as prophylaxis of thromboembolism in chronic aneurysms. Further investigation is needed to define the optimal length of anticoagulation after myocardial infarction in high-risk patients.

Ventricular thrombosis in left ventricular dysfunction

There are several factors inherent to heart failure that predispose patients with left ventricular dysfunction to thrombus formation in the left ventricular cavity. They include heightened platelet activity and elevated levels of circulating procoagulant factors, enhanced by low blood flow, especially near the apex.[77,78] Echocardiography provides a means of visualization of larger thrombi in the heart. Technical advances that improve resolution are likely to continue to increase its sensitivity, and hence the frequency of diagnosis of left ventricular thrombi. Echocardiography has also advanced our understanding of the prevalence and natural history of this complication of heart failure. One study showed that 44 of 129 (34%) patients with severe left ventricular dysfunction had thrombi that were recognized by echocardiography.[79]

This prevalence was the same whether or not coronary disease was present. A prospective study using serial echocardiography on 25 patients with nonischemic cardiomyopathy, not receiving warfarin, demonstrated a left ventricular thrombus in 11 (44%) on their initial study.[80] Over 9–30-months follow-up, two thrombi disappeared and two additional patients developed thrombi. The study showed that approximately one-third of patients with thrombi identified on echocardiography had embolic events during their follow-up, most of which were strokes.

From echocardiography studies, it has also been found that several characteristics of thrombi are associated with a higher likelihood of embolism. Patients who had left ventricular thrombi on echocardiography following myocardial infarction were most likely to suffer embolic events if the thrombus was freely mobile or protruding.[73] Another study found that those features, as well as central lucency of thrombi, were associated with higher rates of embolization.[71] The central lucency appears to result from a liquid center, demonstrated on one postmortem examination.

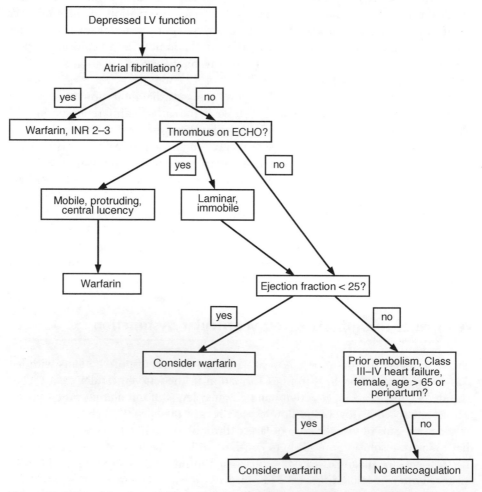

Figure 20.6 *Algorithm for consideration of anticoagulation in left ventricular (LV) dysfunction. (ECHO = echocardiography; INR = International Normalized Ratio.)*

There are no controlled trials of anticoagulation for the prophylaxis of thromboembolism in heart failure. However, in light of the potential for embolization when high-risk features of a known thrombus are evident, unless contraindicated, long-term warfarin should be strongly considered (Fig. 20.6).

Prophylactic anticoagulation in left ventricular dysfunction

Many arterial embolic events in patients with severe heart failure probably result from thrombi that are not visible on echocardiography. Autopsy studies have shown that most left ventricular thrombi are not visible on echocardiography. Furthermore, the resolution and recurrence of thrombi over time limit the usefulness of echocardiography as a measure of long-term embolic risk. Retrospective data have helped to quantify the risk and to identify factors that stratify patients' risk. The reported incidence of embolic events from large clinical trials, in which anticoagulation was not controlled, ranges from 1.5 to 2.5 per 100 patient-years, and in a smaller retrospective study was 3.5 per 100 patient-years.[70,81,82] Features that identified higher risk included poorer functional capacity, female gender, and advanced age. Among patients with severe left ventricular dysfunction, ejection fraction did not usually further stratify the risk of embolic events. Autopsy studies of patients with dilated cardiomyopathy show a much higher incidence of embolism (37%), suggesting that most embolic events are subclinical.[83] Peripartum cardiomyopathy stands out among etiologies of heart failure as one in which embolic disease is substantially more common.[84] This might result from the altered coagulative state during pregnancy.

Variable results of the efficacy of warfarin prophylaxis in dilated cardiomyopathy have been reported from retrospective analyses. No studies had randomized the use or dose of anticoagulants, hence it is likely that patients with known thrombi, atrial fibrillation, and other risks for embolism were treated more often. Despite this potential bais, most studies have shown a significantly lower incidence of embolism among patients on warfarin. One study found the rate of embolization in idiopathic dilated cardiomyopathy to be 3.5 per 100 patient-years among those not on anticoagulation (19 events in 103 patients). In contrast, none of the 32 patients on warfarin suffered an event.[82] In another post-hoc analysis, an 81% risk reduction in stroke by warfarin was seen in the Survival and Ventricular Enlargement (SAVE) trial. However, similar analyses of the Veterans Heart Failure Trial (VeHFT) and the Studies of Left Ventricular Dysfunction (SOLVD) failed to show a reduction in embolic events.[81,85] Interestingly, a separate cohort analysis from the SOLVD data found an association between warfarin use and reduced mortality that was independent of ejection fraction, atrial fibrillation, functional class, or etiology of cardiomyopathy.[86]

Two recent consensus guidelines on the management of heart failure have offered somewhat different approaches for patients with severe left ventricular dysfunction. One recommends considering warfarin use for patients with left ventricular ejection fractions of 35% or less, with consideration of the individual patient's risks and potential benefits.[87] Alternatively, others only suggest consideration of warfarin for secondary prevention in heart failure patients who have had an embolic event, but do not recommend any degree of left ventricular dysfunction or dilatation as an indication to consider anticoagulation.[88] In the absence of controlled trial data, application of the available evidence to stratify the risk of embolism in patients with moderately to severely depressed left ventricular function seems warranted in guiding anticoagulation.

Low molecular weight heparins are effective for short-term prophylaxis in a number of clinical settings, but have not been tested for the prophylaxis of thromboembolism in those at risk of left ventricular thrombus formation.

Antiplatelet therapy in heart failure or asymptomatic left ventricular dysfunction

In patients with heart failure, antiplatelet therapy can gave both beneficial effects and potentially adverse ones. Antiplatelet therapy is an important part of the treatment for atherosclerotic disease. Also, a number of retrospective studies looking at aspirin in patients with heart failure have shown protection from thromboembolism and sudden cardiac death. Others have provided evidence of a possible deleterious interaction with angiotensin-converting enzyme inhibitors.

Among patients with severe heart failure, aspirin use was associated with a lower incidence of thromboembolism than no antiplatelet therapy or anticoagulation in a post-hoc analysis by VeHFT investigators (0.5 versus 2.7 per 100 patients-years).[89] Similarly, a retrospective look at the SAVE trial showed a 56% reduced risk of stroke associated with aspirin use in patients with reduced left ventricular function after myocardial infarction.[70] The effect was most pronounced in individuals with worse left ventricular function. In another cohort study, the protection by aspirin was greater in women.[90] The risk reduction among men in the SOLVD trial was 23%, whereas in women it was 53%. A 24% reduction in risk of sudden cardiac death was also reported.

However, data from some of the same angiotension-converting enzyme inhibitor trials have raised concerns of adverse interactions between aspirin and angiotensin-converting enzyme inhibitors. The Studies of Left Ventricular Dysfunction (SOLVD) trials are among numerous trials that demonstrated improved survival and symptoms in patients with heart failure by angiotensin-converting enzyme inhibition. A retrospective analysis of that study found that patients on antiplatelet therapy gained no survival benefit from the addition of enalapril.[91] Analyses of the CONSENSUS II and GUSTO I trials showed similar effects. Besides inhibiting angiotension II production, angiotensin-converting enzyme inhibitors decrease the metabolism of bradykinin, resulting in a vasodilator effect. The relative importance of that for the clinical benefits of angiotensin-converting enzyme inhibitors is not known, but aspirin's interference of that arm of action could account for possible attenuation of their efficacy. This is reinforced by hemodynamic measurements showing that the effects of angiotensin-converting enzyme inhibition are blunted by aspirin but not by platelet inhibition by the ADP antagonist, ticlopidine.[92] There are no prospective data looking at aspirin–angiotensin-converting enzyme inhibitor interactions. The available evidence is insufficient to conclude whether aspirin negates the benefits of angiotensin-converting enzyme inhibition or whether their benefits simply occur by a similar mechanism of action, and are not additive. The overwhelming evidence of the importance of angiotensin-converting enzyme inhibition in heart failure and of aspirin's benefits in various cardiovascular diseases warrants their use when indicated individually. This approach has been promoted by consensus guidelines for the management of heart failure.[87]

REFERENCES

1 Zareba W, Moss AJ, Raubertas RF. Risk of subsequent cardiac events in stable convalescing patients after first non-Q-wave and Q-wave myocardial infarction. *Coron Artery Dis* 1994; **5**: 1009–18.

2 Graves E. National Hospital Discharge Survey. Annual survey 1966. Series 13, no. 4. Washington, DC: National Center for Health Statistics, 1998.

3 Lincoff AM, Tcheng JE, Califf RM, et al. Sustained suppression of ischemic complications of coronary intervention by platelet GP IIb/IIIa blockade with abciximab: one year outcome in the EPILOG trial. *Circulation* 1999; **99**: 1951–8.

4 Braunwald E, Mark DB, Jones RH, et al. Unstable angina: diagnosis and management. Clinical practice guideline. No. 10. Rockville, MD: Department of Health and Human Services, 1994 (AHCPR publication no. 94-0602).

5 Braunwald E, Willerson JT, et al. Diagnosing and managing unstable angina. *Circulation* 1994; **90**: 613–22.

6 Little WC, Constantinescu M, Applegate RJ, et al. Can coronary angiography predict the site of a subsequent myocardial infarction in patients with mild to moderate coronary artery disease? *Circulation* 1988; **78**: 1157–66.

7 Anbrose JA, Tannenbaum MA, Alexopoulos D, et al. Angiographic progression of coronary artery disease and the development of myocardial infarction. *J Am Coll Cardiol* 1988; **12**: 56–62.

8 Davies MJ, Thomas AC. Plaque fissuring: the cause of acute myocardial infarction, sudden ischemic death, and crescendo angina. *Br Heart J* 1985; **53**: 363–73.

9 Clarkson TB, Prichard RW, et al. Remodeling of coronary arteries in human and nonhuman primates. *JAMA* 1994; **271**: 289–94.

10 Glagov S, Wiesenberg E, et al. Compensatory enlargement of human atherosclerotic coronary arteries. *N Engl J Med* 1987; **316**: 371–5.

11 Fuster V, Lewis A. Mechanisms leading to myocardial infarction: insights from studies of vascular biology. *Circulation* 1994; **90**: 2126–46.

12 Burke AP, Farb A, et al. Coronary risk factors and plaque morphology in men with coronary disease who died suddenly. *N Engl J Med* 1997; **336**: 1267–81.

13 Shah PK, Falk E, et al. Human monocyte derived macrophages induce collagen breakdown in fibrous caps of atherosclerotic plaques: potential role of matrix degrading metallproteinases and implications for plaque rupture. *Circulation* 1995; **92**: 11565–9.

14 Libby P. Molecular bases of the acute coronary syndromes. *Circulation* 1995; **91**: 2844–50.

15 ISIS-2 Collaborative Group. Second international study of infarct survival. *Lancet* 1988; **13**: 348–60.

16 GISIS Investigators. Effectiveness of intravenous thrombolytic treatment in acute myocardial infarction. *Lancet* 1986; **I**: 397–402.

17 Fitzgerald DJ, Catella F, Roy L, Fitzgerald GA. Marked platelet activation in vivo after intravenous streptokinase in patients with acute myocardial infarction. *Circulation* 1988; **77**: 142–50.

18 Kerins DM, Roy L, Fitzgerald DJ. Platelet and vascular function during coronary thrombolysis with tissue type plasminogen activator. *Circulation* 1989; **80**: 1718–25.

19 Reilly IAG, Fitzgerald GA. Inhibition of thromboxane formation in vivo and ex vivo: implications for therapy with platelet inhibitory drugs. *Blood* 1987; **69**: 180–6.

20 Antiplatelet Trialists Collaboration. *BMJ* 1994; **308**: 811.

21 The RISC group. Risk of myocardial infarction and death during treatment with low dose aspirin and intravenous heparin in men with unstable coronary artery disease. *Lancet* 1990; **336**: 827–30.

22 Lewis HD, Davis JW, et al. Protective effects of aspirin against acute myocardial infarction and death in men with unstable angina: results of Veterans Administration Cooperative Study. *N Engl Med J* 1985; **313**: 1369–75.

23 Cairns JA, Gent M, Singer J, et al. Aspirin, sulfinpyrazone, or both, in unstable angina: result of a Canadian multicenter trial. *N Engl Med J* 1985; **313**: 1369–75.

24 Theroux P, et al. Aspirin, heparin, or both to treat acute unstable angina. *N Engl Med J* 1988; **319**: 1105–11.

25 Peto R, Gray R, Collins R, et al. Randomized trial of prophylactic daily aspirin in British male doctors. *BMJ* 1988; **926**: 313–16.

26 The steering committee of the Physicians Health Study Research Group. *N Engl Med J* 1989; **321**: 129–35,

27 Cairns JA, et al. Fifth ACCP Concensus Conference on Antithrombotic Therapy. *Chest* 1998; **114**: 611–35.

28 Lincoff AM, Califf RM, Anderson KM, Weisman HF, Aguirre FV, Kleiman NS, et al. Evidence for prevention of death and myocardial infarction with platelet membrane glycoprotein IIb/IIIa receptor bloackade by abciximab (c7E3 Fab) among patients with unstable angina undergoing percutaneous coronary revascularization. *J Am Coll Cardiol* 1997; **30**: 149–56.

29 The EPIC Investigators. Use of a monoclonal antibody directed against the platelet IIb/IIIa receptor in high risk coronary angioplasty. *N Engl Med J* 1994; **330**: 956–61.

30 Hamm CW, Heeschen C, et al. For the c7E3 Fab Antiplatelet Therapy in Unstable Refractory Angina (CAPTURE) Study Investigators. *N Engl Med J* 1999; **340**: 1623–9.

31 Deckers J, Califf RM, et al. Use of abciximab (Reopro) is not associated with an increase in the risk of stroke: overview of three randomized trials. *J Am Coll Cardiol* 1997; **29**(Suppl. A): abstract 974–89.

32 Comparison of sibrafiban with aspirin for prevention of cardiovasacular events after acute coronary synromes: a randomized trial. *Lancet* 2000; **355**: 337–45.

33 Topol EJ, Ferguson JJ, et al. Long term protection from myocardial ischemic events in a randomized trial of brief integrin Beta3 blockade with percutaneous coronary revascularization. EPIC investigators group. *JAMA* 1997; **278**: 479–84.

34 Leon MB, Baim DS, et al. A clinical trial comparing three antithrombotic-drug regimens after coronary-artery stenting. *N Engl J Med* 1998; **339**: 1665–71.

35 Thebault JJ, Blatrix CE, Blanchard JF, Panak EA. The interactions of ticlopidine and aspirin in normal subjects. *J Int Med Res* 1997; **5**: 405–11.

36 Uchiyama S, Sone R, Nagayama T, Shibagaki Y, Kobayashi I, Maruyama S, et al. Combination therapy with low-dose aspirin and ticlopidine in cerebral ischemia. *Stroke* 1989; **20**: 1643–7.

37 Darius H, Veit K, Rupprecht HJ. Synergistic inhibition of platelet aggregation by ticlopidine plus aspirin following intracoronary stent placement (Abstract). *Circulation* 1996; **94**(Suppl. I): 1–257.

38 Balsano F, Rizzon P, et al. Antiplatelet treatment with ticlopidine in unstable angina. A controlled multicenter clinical trial. *Circulation* 1990; **82**: 17–26.

39 McTavish D, Faulds D, Goa KL. Ticlopidine. An update review of its pharmacology and therapeutic use in platelet-dependent disorders. *Drugs* 1990; **40**: 238–59.

40 Bennett CL, Weinberg PD, et al. Thrombotic thrombocytopenia purpura associated with ticlopidine. A review of 60 cases. *Ann Intern Med* 1998; **128**: 541–4.

41 CAPRIE steering committee. A randomized, blinded study of clopidigrel versus aspirin in patients at risk of ischemic events. *Lancet* 1996; **348**: 1329–39.

42 Weitz JI. Low molcular weight heparins. *N Engl J Med* 1997; **337**: 688–9.

43 Gruppo Italiano per lo Studio della Sopravivenza nell'Infarto Miocardico. GISSI-2: a factorial randomised trial of alteplase versus streptokinase and heparin vesus no heparin among 12 490 patients with acute myocardial infarction. *Lancet* 1990; **336**: 65–71.

44 ISIS-3: a randomised comparison of streptokinase versus tissue plasminogen activator versus anistreplase and of aspirin plus heparin versus aspirin alone among 41 299 cases of suspected acute myocardial infarction. *Lancet* 1992; **339**: 753–70.

45 The GUSTO Investigators. An international randomized trial comparing four thrombolytic strategies for acute myocardial infarction. *N Engl J Med* 1993; **329**: 673–82.

46 The Global Use of Strategies to Open Occluded Coronary Arteries (GUSTO) IIa Investigators. Randomized trial of intravenous heparin versus recombinant hirudin for acute coronary syndromes. *Circulation* 1994; **90**: 1631–7.

47 Oler A, Whooley M, Oler J, Grady D, Adding heparin to aspirin reduces the incidence of myocardial infarction and death in patients with unstable angina: a meta-analysis. *JAMA* 1996; **276**: 811–15.

48 Antman EM. Hirudin in acute myocardial infarction: Thrombolysis and Thrombin Inhibition in Myocardial Infarction (TIMI) 9B trial. *Circulation* 1996; **94**: 911–21.

49 Theroux P, Waters D, Lam J, Juneau M, McCans J. Reactivation of unstable angina after the discontinuation of heparin. *N Engl J Med* 1992; **327**: 141–5.

50 Warkentin TE, Levine MN, et al. Heparin induced thrombocytopenia in patients treated with low molecular weight heparin or unfractionated heparin. *N Engl J Med* 1995; **332**: 1330–5.

51 Cohen M, Demers C, et al. A comparison of low molecular weight heparin with unfractionated heparin for unstable coronary artery disease. *N Engl J Med* 1997; **337**: 447–52.

52 Klien W, Buchwald A, et al. Fragmin in unstable angina or in non-Q-wave myocardial infarction (the FRIC study). *Am J Cardiol* 1997; **80**: 30E–34E.

53 Fragmin during Instability in Coronary Artery Disease (FRISC) Study Group. *Lancet* 1996; **347**: 561–8.

54 Fragmin and fast revascularization during instability in coronary artery disease (FRISC II) investigators. Low molecular-mass heparin in unstable coronary artery disease: FRISC II prospective randomised multicenter study. *Lancet* 1999; **354**: 701–7.

55 Antman EM, et al. Enoxaparin prevents death and cardiac ischemic events in unstable angina/non-Q-wave myocardial infarction: result of the (TIMI) 11B trial. *Circulation* 1999; **100**: 1593–1601.

56 Ryan TJ, Antman EM, et al. 1999 Update: ACC/AHA guidelines for the management of patients with acute myocardial infarction. Report of the American College of Cardiology/American Heart Association task force on practice guidelines (committee on management of acute myocardial infarction). *J Am Coll Cardiol* 1993; **34**: 890–911.

57 DeWood MA, Spores J, et al. Prevalence of total coronary occlusion during the early hours of transmural myocardial infarction. *N Engl J Med* 1980; **303**: 897–902.

58 Fibrinolytic Therapy Trialists' (FTT) Collaborative Group. Indications for fibrinolytic therapy in suspected acute myocardial infarction: collaborative overview of early mortality and major morbidity results form all randomised trials of more than 1000 patients. *Lancet* 1994; **343**: 311–22.

59 Ryan TJ, Anderson JL, et al. ACC/AHA guidelines for the management of acute myocardial infarction. A report of the American College of Cardiology/American Heart Association task force on practice guidelines (committee on management of acute myocardial infarction). *J Am Coll Cardiol* 1996; **28**: 1328–428.

60 Simoons ML, Maggioni AP, et al. Individual risk assessment for intracranial hemorrhage during thrombolytic therapy. *Lancet* 1993; **342**: 1523–8.

61 De Jaegere PP, Arnold AA, Balk AH, Simoons ML. Intracranial hemorrhage in association with thrombolytic therapy: incidence and clinical predictive factors. *J Am Coll Cardiol* 1992; **19**: 289–94.

62 Cannon CP, McCabe CH, et al. Comparison of front loaded tissue-type plasminogen activator, anistreplase, and combination thrombolytic therapy for acute myocardial infarction: results of the Thrombolysis in Myocardial Infarction (TIMI) 4 trial. *J Am Coll Cardiol* 1994; **24**: 1602–10.

63 Smith P, Arnesen H, et al. The effect of warfarin and reinfarction after myocardial infarction. *N Engl Med J* 1990; **323**: 147–52.

64 Cohen M, Adams PC, et al. Combination antithrombotic therapy in unstable rest angina and non-Q-wave infarction in non-prior aspirin users. *Circulation* 1994; **89**: 81–8.

65 Anand SS, Yusuf S, Pogue J et al. Long-term oral anticoagulant therapy in patients with unstable angina or suspected non-Q-wave myocardial infarction. *Circulation* 1998; **98**: 1064–70.

66 Coumadin aspirin re-infarction study investigators. Randomised double-blind trial of fixed low-dose warfarin with aspirin after myocardial infarction. *Lancet* 1997; **350**: 389–96.

67 The EPSIM research group. A controlled comparison of aspirin and oral anticoagulants in prevention of death after myocardial infarction. *N Engl J Med* 1982; **307**: 701–8.

68 Julian DG, Chamberlain DA, et al. A comparison of aspirin and anticoagulation following thrombolysis for myocardial infarction: a multicenter unblinded randomised clinical trial. *BMJ* 1996; **313**: 1429–31.

69 Weinrich DJ, Burke JF, et al. Left ventricular mural thrombi complicating acute myocardial infarction: long-term follow-up with serial echocardiography. *Ann Intern Med* 1984; **86**: 35–9.

70 Loh E, Sutton MS, et al. Ventricular dysfunction predicts stroke following myocardial infarction. *N Engl J Med* 1997; **336**: 251–7.

71 Haugland JM, Asinger RW, et al. Embolic potntial of left ventricular thrombi detected by two-dimensional echocardiography. *Circulation* 1984; **70**: 588–98.

72 Reeder GS, Lengyel M, et al. Mural thrombus in left ventricular aneurysm: incidence, role of angiography, and relation between anticoagulation and embolization. *Mayo Clin Proc* 1981; **56**: 77–81.

73 Visser CA, Han G, et al. Embolic potential of left ventricular thrombus after myocardial infarction: a two-dimensional echocardiographic study of 119 patients. *J Am Coll Cardiol* 1985; **5**: 1276–80.

74 Veterans Administration Cooperative Study. Anticoagulation in acute myocardial infarction: results of a cooperative clinical trial. *JAMA* 1973; **225**: 724–9.

75 Turpie AGG, Robinson JG, et al. Comparison of high-dose with low-dose subcutaneous heparin to prevent left ventricular mural thrombus in patients with acute transmural anterior myocardial infarction. *N Engl J Med* 1989; **320**: 352–7.

76 Lapeyre AC, Steele PM, et al. Sytemic embolization in chronic left ventricular aneurysm: incidence and the role of antocoagulation. *J Am Coll Cardiol* 1985; **6**: 534–8.

77 Jafri SM, Ozawa T, et al. Platelet function, thrombin and fibrinolytic activation in patients with heart failure. *Eur Heart J* 1993; **14**: 205–12.

78 Yamamoto K, Ikeda U, et al. The coagulation system is activated in idiopathic cardiomyopathy. *J Am Coll Cardiol* 1995; **25**: 1634–40.

79 Gottdiener JS, Gay JA, et al. Frequency and embolic potential of left ventricular thrombus in dilated cardiomyopathy: assessment by two dimensional echocardiography. *Am J Cardiol* 1993; **52**: 1281–5.

80 Falk RH, Foster E, et al. Ventricular thrombi and thromboembolism in dilated cardiomyopathy: a prospective follow-up study. *Am Heart J* 1992; **123**: 136–42.

81 Dunkman WB, Johnson GR, et al. Incidence of thromboembolic events in congestive heart failure. *Circulation* 1993; **87**(Suppl. VI): 94–101.

82 Fuster V, Gersh BJ, et al. The natural history of idiopathic dilated cardiomyopathy. *Am J Cardiol* 1981; **47**: 525–31.

83 Roberts WC, Siegal RJ, et al. Idiopathic dilated cardiomyopathy: analysis of 152 patients. *Am J Cardiol* 1987; **60**: 1340–55.

84 Julian DG, Szekely P. Peripartum cardiomyopathy. *Prog Cardiovasc Dis* 1985; **27**: 233–40.

85 Dries DL, Rosenberg Y, et al. Ejection fraction and risk of thromboembolic events in patients with systolic dysfunction and sinus rhythm: evidence for gender differences in the studies of left ventricular dysfunction trials. *J Am Coll Cardiol* 1997; **29**: 1074–80.

86 Al-Khadra AS, Salem DN, et al. Warfarin anticoagulation and survival: a cohort analysis from the studies of left ventricular dysfunction. *J Am Coll Cardiol* 1998; **31**: 749–53.

87 Heart Failure Society of America guidelines for management of patients with heart failure caused by left ventricular systolic dysfunction – pharmacologic approaches. *J Cardiac Failure* 1999; **5**: 357–82.

88 Consensus recommendations for the management of chronic heart failure. *Am J Cardiol* 1999; **83**

89 Dunkman WB, Johnson GR, et al. Incidence of thromboembolic events in congestive heart failure. *Circulation* 1993; **87**(Suppl. VI): 94–101.

90 Dries DL, Rosenberg Y, et al. Ejection fraction and risk of thromboembolic events in patients with systolic dysfunction and sinus rhythm: evidence for gender differences in the studies of left ventricular dysfunction trials. *J Am Coll Cardiol* 1997; **29**: 1074–80.

91 Al-Khadra AS, Salem DN, et al. Antiplatelet agents and survival: a cohort analysis from the Studies of Left Ventricular Dysfunction (SOLVD) trial. *J Am Coll Cardiol* 1998; **31**: 419–25.

92 Spaulding C, Charbonnier B, et al. Acute hemodynamic interaction of aspirin and ticlopidine with enalapril: results of a double-blind, randomized comparative trial. *Circulation* 1998; **98**: 757–65.

21

Establishing and operating an anticoagulation program

SUSAN LYNCH

INTRODUCTION

Oral anticoagulants were introduced in the USA over 50 years ago. Now, over 1 million patients in the USA are prescribed warfarin annually. As indications for warfarin continue to increase, so will the need for appropriate monitoring of patients to achieve safe and effective patient outcomes. In countries such as the Netherlands and Great Britain, coordinated anticoagulation programs have a long-standing tradition. Anticoagulation services are gaining more popularity in the USA, but there are still many physicians reluctant to use such services. Three main barriers to greater chronic anticoagulation use have been identified: (1) gaps in knowledge of or belief in its effectiveness; (2) concerns about its safety; and (3) concerns about the difficulty of managing patients on anticoagulation.[1]

Through a series of Consensus Conferences, the American College of Chest Physicians (ACCP) has attempted to reduce the first two barriers.[1] However, the more difficult task of alleviating the physicians' fears remains. Based on the accumulating evidence, anticoagulation services are demonstrating improved clinical outcomes with a reduction in the incidence of hemorrhagic and thromboembolic events, thereby leading to a more cost-effective therapy.[1-11] In addition, these data support the reduction in utilization of hospital services when patients' care is managed by an anticoagulation service, a cost saving of from $800 to $1400 per patient-year to the healthcare system.[1-11] Similar data are reported by Chiquette et al.,[11] which indicate a reduced rate of complications, hospitalizations, and emergency room visits, and a yearly cost saving of $162 000 per 100 patients followed in a pharmacist-managed anticoagulation clinic, compared to routine medical care.

NETWORKING

When implementing an anticoagulation service, one should first explore the many issues involved with running such a service successfully. This can be achieved through local networking. Observing the daily operations of an established program is very beneficial. It will allow you to see first hand how an effective service operates, to identify potential barriers, and how to plan for them. Most importantly, it will allow for the establishment of realistic expectations to identify what might work for your organization. In addition, there are several national educational programs offered yearly, including the American Society of Health Systems Pharmacists, which sponsors traineeship programs. The Anticoagulation Forum is another national multidisciplinary organization comprising physicians, pharmacists, and nurses involved in anticoagulation programs.

DEVELOPMENT

Establishing an anticoagulation service in your practice can result in increased safety and efficacy of anticoagulation through comprehensive monitoring, patient education, and follow-up, provided the necessary personnel and resources are committed to the venture. This service is attractive because anticoagulation management can be done without interfering with the overall management of patients provided by their primary care providers. In order to establish an anticoagulation service, one must first determine the practice site. Table 21.1 summarizes the locations of the services for which management can be rendered. One must also determine who will manage the service. Will a single-disciplinary or a multidisciplinary team manage this service? Advantages to having single-disciplinary management of the program are individual continuity of care and possible patient preference to identify one contact person. However, with a multidisciplinary approach, there is more continuous coverage of the

Table 21.1 *Location of service*

Hospital inpatient service
Physician's office
Clinic
Long-term care facility
Pharmacy

Table 21.2 *Management of service*

Physician
Registered nurse
Nurse practitioner
Pharmacist
Physician's assistant

practice, ample staffing, and more reimbursable services. Table 21.2 identifies the different disciplines able to manage an anticoagulation service.

The primary role of the physician can be one of a consultant/supervisor; however, the availability and accessibility of the physician may be crucial in some practice sites. The drug therapy management for patients can be delegated to support staff who have been trained in managing anticoagulation therapy. Currently, there is only one Certificate Program available to healthcare providers in the area of anticoagulation therapy management. Sponsored by The Anticoagulation Forum and developed by the National Certification Board for Anticoagulation Providers (NCBAP), this program consists of a 40-hour continuing education program that is organized into five content modules. Participants who pass the certification examination earn the Certified Anticoagulation Care Provider (CACP) credential.

When establishing an anticoagulation service, it is helpful to know what features are important to build into the system. Table 21.3 outlines the key components of an adequate anticoagulation service management system.

Table 21.3 *Key components of service*

Determine appropriateness of anticoagulation therapy
Thorough clinical assessment and frequent INR testing
Systematic monitoring of patients for tracking PT/INR results
Continuous patient education regarding warfarin, diet, safety measures, and concomitant drug therapy
Prompt patient feedback regarding test results and patient complications
Collection of quality assurance data
Communication between all healthcare providers involved in patient care

INR, International Normalized Ratio; PT, prothrombin time.

IMPLEMENTATION

One of the key aspects to establishing a well-functioning anticoagulation service is developing standard operating procedures that will ensure consistency in managing patients and organizing patient flow. Policies and procedures for the program should address the mechanisms for referrals, provide an overview of daily operations, and outline the management of noncompliant patients. A description of the program goals and objectives should be the first item in a written policy and procedure. Although programs will probably share the common goal of reducing anticoagulant

Table 21.4 *Issues and questions to consider*

Identify patient population
Patient admission: criteria for admission into service? Indications, intensity and duration of treatment?
Patient assessment: information to be obtained? Management of minor and major complications?
Initiation of treatment: how will dosing regimens be determined and recorded?
Monitoring of INR: guidelines for obtaining and frequency of PT/INR; identify laboratory requirements
Dosage adjustments: who will make adjustments? How will adjustments be made? How will they be documented and communicated to patient and other healthcare providers?
Patient education: who will do the teaching? What will be taught? How often will patients be educated on anticoagulation issues?
Noncompliant patients: how will they be managed? Legal issues?
Discharging noncompliant patients from service: who will discharge patients?
Performance outcomes: who will collect data? How will data be collected? How will it be monitored? How often will it be monitored?

INR, International Normalized Ratio; PT, prothrombin time.

therapy complications while improving efficacy, the individual policies and procedures will vary depending on the setting (inpatient versus outpatient), type of practice, and patient population. Table 21.4 addresses some issues to consider when developing policies and procedures.

Logistical issues such as appointment times, days of operation, length of office visits, telephone consultations, and billing procedures must also be addressed. Clearly defined job descriptions and the development of systematic approaches will increase confidence, prevent conflicts, anticipate staffing needs, and promote teamwork and cooperation.

The roles and responsibilities of all staff positions, clinical and nonclinical, should be delineated; authorization for refilling prescriptions and making warfarin-dosing adjustments should be granted to qualified personnel. Regardless of the autonomy granted to staff members, Anticoagulation service providers only have the authority to operate within their scope of practice. Secretarial support is essential in practices with a large patient volume and can also relieve the anticoagulation service provider of clerical tasks, including mailing reminder letters, scheduling return visits and laboratory blood draws, obtaining laboratory results, and coordinating home healthcare visits. Table 21.5 is a sample of policies and procedures developed for an anticoagulation service at Thomas Jefferson University Hospital.

BUDGET

When developing a budget, all anticipated costs for operating the anticoagulation service should be identified. Salary support, operating costs, equipment and supplies, plus any unique costs for prothrombin time/International Normalized Ratio (PT/INR) monitoring require consideration. Revenue generated through inpatient

Table 21.5 *Jefferson anticoagulation therapy service policies and procedures*

The anticoagulation program is a service directed by a physician and staffed by registered nurses and pharmacists with specific knowledge of anticoagulation therapy. Oral anticoagulant care is managed under the supervision of physicians in the Department of Internal Medicine.

I. Purpose
   A. To manage oral anticoagulant therapy (warfarin) by evaluating the prothrombin time (PT) and/or the International Normalized Ratio (INR) and instructing patients or family of appropriate dosage of warfarin.
   B. To assess patients for possible complications related to anticoagulant therapy.
   C. To provide comprehensive and ongoing education to patients and/or family members about anticoagulant therapy with specific attention to signs and symptoms to report.

II. Policy
   A. Evaluation of patients
     1. Initial evaluation of patients will occur after a physician consult is called to the anticoagulation program from the Department of Internal Medicine.
     2. Consults are preferably made prior to the inpatient's discharge so as to allow adequate time for chart review and patient education.
     3. Patient chart will be reviewed, and the following information will be obtained for clinic chart:
       a. past medical/surgical history
       b. hospital course
       c. medications
       d. allergies
       e. anticoagulation therapy received and date of initiation
       f. primary physician
       g. patient telephone number, address, and emergency contact.
     4. Patient will be seen by a member of the anticoagulation program (RN, Pharm D, RPh) who will review the following:
       a. clinic policy and procedure
       b. comprehensive patient education according to guidelines established for patient education.
     5. Patients will sign anticoagulation program contract, which will outline their responsibilities as participants in the program.
   B. Target PT/INR range
     1. Target PT/INR ranges will be determined by the physician according to individual patient indication and need. Changes in these therapeutic ranges will be made as indicated by the primary or clinic physician.
   C. Expected duration of therapy
     1. Expected length of anticoagulant therapy will be determined by primary or clinic physician and will be made on an individual basis, depending on indication. When therapy has reached the expected discontinuation date, the primary physician will evaluate the need for continuation of warfarin and the decision will be documented in the patient's chart.
   D. Frequency of PT/INR testing*
     1. When anticoagulation therapy has been initiated or when a patient has been recently discharged after hospitalization, the PT/INR will be checked one or two times weekly until stable.
     2. When the PT/INR and dose of warfarin remain stable for two testing days, the PT/INR will be checked weekly.

3. When the PT/INR and dose of warfarin remain stable for two weeks, the PT/INR will be checked every two weeks.
4. When the PT/INR and dose of warfarin remain stable for four weeks, the PT/INR will be checked in one month.
5. All patients must have their PT/INR checked at least monthly.
6. After a change in dose is made, all patients are required to have their PT/INR checked at least weekly until stable.
   Note: These are only general monitoring guidelines applied to patients. Frequency of PT/INR will depend on individual patient condition and overall treatment plan.

III. Eligibility criteria
  A. Patients must be able to attend clinic appointments.
  B. If patients are not able to meet this requirement, the final decision to accept the patient will be made by the program director. The patient will be classified as a 'phone patient.'
  C. Patients must agree to come in for appropriate comprehensive follow-up visits with a physician in the Department of Internal Medicine.
  D. The patient or family members should have the capacity to understand the patient's condition and implications of anticoagulant therapy.
  E. Patients must be willing to be active participants in their health maintenance.
  F. Patients must be able to travel to and from clinic appointments.
  G. Patients must be accessible by telephone.
  H. Patients must have a documented need for anticoagulant therapy.

IV. Clinic visits
  A. Clinic visits are by appointment only. If patients are unable to keep an appointment, they are to notify the office and reschedule.
  B. Patients will have PT/INR checked by fingerstick with a portable INR machine.
  C. Patients will then be seen by the nurse or pharmacist and the following will be assessed:
    1. signs/symptoms of bleeding episodes (gingival bleeding, epistaxis, ecchymoses, hematuria, melena, blood per rectum, etc.)
    2. signs/symptoms of a thrombotic event (shortness of breath, pain/swelling of extremity, numbness, tingling, headache, etc.)
    3. significant changes in diet
    4. any changes in concomitant drug therapy (including over-the-counter medications and intermittent antibiotic therapy)
    5. compliance with anticoagulant therapy
    6. signs/symptoms of intolerance of drug (nausea/vomiting/diarrhea, rash, skin necrosis, etc.).
  D. Based on these assessments and the PT/INR, dosage changes in anticoagulant therapy will be made if necessary and patients will be counseled on these changes.
  E. Dosage changes are to be supervised by clinic physician as evidence by co-signature beside the documented change.
  F. Patient education will be reinforced.
  G. Patients will be instructed on when to return for clinic appointments.
  H. Patients will be referred to the physician on site for any of the following:
    1. signs/symptoms of thrombosis
    2. signs/symptoms of serious bleeding episodes
    3. significant adverse drug reactions
    4. significantly subtherapeutic or elevated PT

5. any other acute problem related or unrelated to anticoagulant therapy.
I. Prescription for anticoagulant therapy may be renewed by telephone by the nurse or pharmacist, with documentation in the patient's chart, which is to be signed by the primary physician.

V. Phone patients
A. Patients who are unable to attend clinic because of immobility, geographic inaccessibility, or patient condition may have their PT/INR drawn by a laboratory other than the clinic and are classified as phone patients.
B. Phone patients are only accepted into the program at the discretion and approval of the program director.
C. Patients must have access to transportation in the case of suspected anticoagulation complications that might require medical attention.
D. Anticoagulation clinical personnel will make arrangements for blood draws for the homebound patient. Patients who are not homebound may have their blood drawn at a local hospital or laboratory in their area.
E. A clinic chart will be kept on these patients as well as a PT laboratory check file. The file will include the patient's name, telephone number, name of laboratory, laboratory telephone number, and date that next PT is to be drawn. This card will be filed under the date of the month that the blood is to be drawn plus one day. This allows the laboratory one working day to process the blood. The PT laboratory check file will be reviewed daily.
F. Anticoagulation members will obtain results from the laboratory used by the patient.
G. The patient will then receive instructions by telephone from the nurse or pharmacist during clinic hours.
H. Patients will be interviewed for complications (see Clinic visits section).
I. Patients will be required to call the office for instructions if they do not receive a telephone call within 48 hours after a blood test.
J. Patients are still required to be followed by their primary physician or a physician within the Department of Internal Medicine. If a patient is to take a three- to six-month course of therapy, the patient is to see his or her physician in the middle of therapy and at completion of therapy. If the patient is on long-term therapy, he or she is to see the primary physician every six months.

VI. Documentation
A. Anticoagulant therapy will be documented on the monitoring flowsheet.
B. Assessments of patients during clinic visits will also be documented in the progress notes.
C. Prescription renewals and scheduled laboratory draws will be documented.
D. Letters will be forwarded to the primary physician if requested, stating the PT, ratio, INR, and dosage change.

These policies and procedures were developed and mutually agreed upon by the following:

Program Director	Date

Registered Nurse	Date

Pharmacist	Date

consults by attending physicians may help offset the operating costs for those practices affiliated with hospitals. In addition, practices with hospital affiliations may solicit the support of hospital administrators for funding. Reviewing inpatient adverse drug reaction data and documenting the numbers of adverse outcomes attributed to anticoagulation therapy can often support the justification of the need for this specialized service. Additionally, examining the readmission rates for patients recently started on anticoagulants who have a subsequent hemorrhagic complication, and conducting an anticoagulant-focused drug usage evaluation are useful measures for gaining necessary administrative approval. Risk management and quality assurance personnel are other sources for obtaining institution-specific data.

An anticoagulation service can yield important financial benefits; however, these benefits may not be immediately apparent. Attention must be given to the improved patient care and to the medical costs avoided through the use of the anticoagulation service. Preparing a financial analysis will identify the start-up costs, fixed and variable costs, revenue from optimal reimbursement, cost avoidance, cost efficiencies, and break-even analysis. Investigating these areas will evaluate whether the implementation of an anticoagulation service can be financially justified. Table 21.6[12] shows the results of the financial analysis performed at Overlake Hospital Medical Center, Bellevue, Washington, to justify an anticoagulation service at their institution. From this analysis, at least 300

Table 21.6 *Financial assessment of anticoagulation clinic*

Variable	Low volume[a] ($)	High volume[b] ($)
Revenue		
Patient charge per visit[c]	33	33
Estimated monthly gross clinic revenue	6600	9900
Bad debt to revenue[3]	−92	−139
Billing services cost[e]	−305	−458
Estimated clinic revenue, monthly	4025	6036
Estimated net clinic revenue, annually	48 300	74 232
Expenses		
Annual wages and benefits[f]	61 100	61 100
Annual supply costs[g]	12 000	18 000
Expense reduction[h]	12 548	18 822
Net loss or profit[i]	−12 252	12 154

[a]Two hundred visits monthly or 10 visits daily Monday through Friday.
[b]Three hundred visits monthly or 15 visits daily Monday through Friday.
[c]Clinic visit plus laboratory charge.
[d]Based on hospital-wide rate of 1.4%.
[e]Seven percent of receivables.
[f]One full-time equivalent pharmacist at $29.25/hour, including benefits.
[g]Estimated at $5 per visit.
[h]Estimated annual savings to health system resulting from prevention of one admission for gastrointestinal bleeding per 100 patient visits (total savings per admission is $6274, a fully allocated cost excluding physician costs and charges).
[i]Depreciation of laboratory and computer equipment not included.
Originally published in *Establishing an outpatient anticoagulation clinic in a community hospital* © 1996. American Society of Health-System Pharmacists, Inc. All rights reserved. Reprinted with permission (R 9964).

monthly patient visits are needed to generate a profit. However, with the prevention of one treatment-related hospitalization, the health system can save $6274 annually per 100 patients. This again demonstrates that an anticoagulation service is a cost-effective service.

REIMBURSEMENT

Major insurance payers have been reluctant to reimburse for anticoagulation services; however, reimbursement for anticoagulation services is gaining more acceptance. Nonphysicians may bill for ambulatory office visits using CPT code 99211, a face-to-face patient interaction requiring minimal or no physician presence. The costs for venipuncture and PT/INRs can be charged separately. All telephone management of patients is not reimbursable by any payer. With respect to managed healthcare organizations, an anticoagulation service may secure specific contracts based on a discounted fee-for-service formula or on a capitated basis that will allow reimbursement for non-face-to-face encounters. Inadequate reimbursement for cognitive services that are provided by anticoagulation services is an issue currently being addressed on a national level through the American Pharmaceutical Association (APhA). Additional information on coding and billing guides is available from the APhA (1-800-632-0123) and DuPont Pharma (1-800-4PHARMA).

LABORATORY

The specific laboratory procedure required for the practice setting, including whether INRs will be assessed by venipuncture or by a portable fingerstick device, must be clearly outlined in the policies and procedures. Several hand-held instruments, such as CoaguChek/Coumatrak monitors (Roche Diagnostics 1-800-852-8766) or Protime monitors (ITC 1-800-631-5945), determine the PT/INR within a few minutes.[13,14] These devices are similar to bedside glucose monitors and offer the advantage of immediate results, allowing dosing adjustments while the patient is in the office. The need for a follow-up phone call is thus eliminated. These machines are attractive from the aspect of patient convenience (particularly for those patients with limited venous access) and staff efficiency. Medicare, managed health care, and private insurance provide reimbursement for these tests. When the portable PT monitor is used in the outpatient setting, federal and state clinical regulations must be followed. A separate policy and procedure describing the preferred patient-testing method and containing laboratory certifications and quality-control documentation can be incorporated into the main policy and procedure.

PATIENT EDUCATION

The critical foundation of an anticoagulation service is a comprehensive patient educational program. Patient education must be individualized to accommodate a wide range of intellectual and reading capabilities. Ideally, patients should receive counseling when anticoagulant therapy is initiated. Informing the patient of the risks and benefits of therapy will enhance patient compliance. For practices that are hospital affiliated, education must begin before hospital discharge, with major principles of anticoagulation therapy re-emphasized at the first outpatient follow-up appointment. Alternatively, initial teaching may begin in the outpatient setting or by telephone consultation. Family members or caregivers are encouraged to participate in the educational process to further enhance patient compliance. Education is an ongoing process, and even those patients maintained on long-term anticoagulant therapy should occasionally receive a 'refresher course.' Patients should also be periodically tested with regard to their anticoagulation knowledge through a series of patient tests to ascertain their present knowledge base.

Components of a comprehensive teaching program should include, but not be limited to, expected duration of treatment, signs and symptoms of subtherapeutic/supratherapeutic anticoagulation, signs and symptoms of thrombosis, risks of noncompliance, drug–drug and drug–food interactions, and the frequency of laboratory testing. Educational material may be custom made or commercially purchased. Several types of patient education items are available through DuPont Pharma and Barr Laboratories. These include booklets, weekly pillboxes, and bilingual materials/audio and videotapes. Patients receiving long-term anticoagulation are encouraged to purchase medic alert bracelets, available at retail pharmacies in the community.

PATIENT OFFICE VISITS

The typical patient visit encompasses determining the PT/INR, assessing patient compliance, evaluating complications, and assessing changes in concomitant medications. In addition, inquiries should be made regarding the use of over-the-counter medications or herbal products, dietary habits, alcohol consumption, and concurrent illness. After interviewing the patient, adjustments in the warfarin dosage regimen are made and the return visit is scheduled. An outpatient practice can provide thorough evaluations of minor complications, including assessing for occult blood in the urine or stool. When necessary, appropriate referrals or triage to other medical services can be provided to patients. The need for medical intervention for the evaluation of both acute complications of anticoagulant therapy and other emerging acute disease exacerbations should be anticipated.

For warfarin dosage changes, an office-based protocol can be developed, or one of several published dosing nomograms may be followed.[15] General principles based on warfarin pharmacokinetics and pharmacodynamics recommend increasing or decreasing the warfarin dose by no more than 10–20% of the total weekly dose at each visit.[16] To avoid patient confusion and enhance patient compliance, it is suggested that one warfarin strength is dispensed, incorporating dosing changes from that tablet strength. For example, dosing changes that may be incorporated from 5-mg tablets include 2.5 mg, 7.5 mg, 10 mg, etc.

The frequency of follow-up visits for PT/INR testing and for physician evaluation should be specified. Although guidelines will depend on individual patient compliance and the overall treatment plan, general recommendations can be made. For example, a patient may be required to see their primary care provider at the initiation of therapy, then at least every 3 months during the course of warfarin treatment, and finally at the cessation of therapy. When therapy is first started, the PT/INR should be drawn at least twice during the first week, and then weekly until two consecutive INRs are therapeutic. Thereafter, the interval between tests can be increased.

Practices with a large patient volume spread over a wide geographic region may necessitate managing patients over the telephone. Additionally, patients who are immobilized secondary to orthopedic procedures or spinal cord injuries may also be candidates for telephone follow-ups. The same principles discussed previously apply to managing patients over the telephone.[17] Forming alliances with the local home healthcare agency or independent laboratories is beneficial for providing home laboratory draws.

DOCUMENTATION

Documenting all clinical information is important for an anticoagulation service to run efficiently. Flow sheets are recommended to record laboratory results, warfarin dosing changes, prescription refills, and follow-up visits. Table 21.7 provides a flow sheet sample form.

Table 21.7 *Flow sheet*

Patient Name				MR#		DOB		
Phone Home				LAB				
Phone Work				LAB				
Phone Relative				VNA				
Diagnosis				PHARMACY				
MD				TAB SIZE				
INR RANGE				DURATION		DATE DC		
DATE	CURRENT DOSE	PT	INR	NEW DOSE	NEXT APPT.	INITIAL	COMMENTS	

A progress note employing the standard 'SOAP' format (subjective, objective, assessment, plan) is entered into the patient's chart and cosigned by the attending physician for all patient anticoagulation visits. Additionally, the attending physician on the flow sheet cosigns all telephone consultations. Details of the next scheduled patient visit are readily available by checking the flow sheet, which reduces the likelihood that a patient will be lost to follow-up. Providing laboratory data and warfarin dosage adjustments to the patient's primary care provider or specialists, such as cardiologists or neurologists, is easily done with a standard written letter, which is completed and faxed following each patient visit. There is a wide range of patient-tracking mechanisms that can be used, depending on the patient population size and the available start-up expenses. Tracking mechanisms can be as simple as index cards, with patient information filed according to the date of the next visit, to sophisticated computer

Table 21.8 *Management of 'no-shows'*

I.   The patient is responsible for rescheduling all missed appointments.

II. The first time a patient misses a scheduled appointment:
   A. The patient will be notified by telephone.
   B. Another appointment will be scheduled.
   C. A note will be written in the progress notes of the patient's chart stating that the appointment was missed.

III. The second consecutive time a patient misses a scheduled appointment:
   A. The patient will be notified by telephone.
   B. Another appointment will be scheduled.
   C. A letter will be sent to the patient.
   D. A copy of above letter will be placed in the correspondence section of the patient's chart.
   E. A note will be written in the progress notes of the patient's chart stating that the appointment was missed.

IV. The third consecutive time a patient misses a scheduled appointment:
   A. The patient will be notified by telephone.
   B. Another appointment will be scheduled. The urgency and importance of this will be stressed.
   C. The program director will be notified.
   D. A letter cosigned by the program director will be sent to the patient's primary physician.
   E. A copy of above letter will be placed in the correspondence section of the patient's chart.
   F. A letter will be sent to the patient.
   G. A copy of above letter will be placed in the correspondence section of the patient's chart.
   H. A note will be written in the progress notes of the patient's chart stating that the appointment was missed, and that the program director and the primary physician were notified.

V.   The fourth consecutive time a patient misses a scheduled appointment:
   A. The patient will be notified by telephone. The patient will be told that a letter will be sent by certified mail. If the patient fails to respond after letter sent, then patient will be terminated from the anticoagulation program.
   B. A letter signed by the program director outlining alternative forms of care will be sent via certified mail.
   C. A copy of above letter will be placed in the correspondence section of the patient's chart.
   D. A note will be written in the progress notes of the patient's chart stating that the appointment was missed, and that a letter was sent via certified mail.

VI. If the patient has not contacted the office within 10 working days:
   A. The program director will be notified.
   B. A letter will be sent to the patient's primary physician stating that the patient has been terminated from the anticoagulation program.
   C. A termination note will be written in the progress notes of the patient's chart.

software programs. Computerized methods can include an individualized database (Filemaker Pro) or commercial software such as Dawn AC or DuPont Pharma's CoumaCare program.

Noncompliant patients are a reality of every anticoagulation service. It is imperative that guidelines be developed for managing this patient population. Table 21.8 provides a sample policy for noncompliant patients. The steps involved can range from documenting the reason for noncompliance to terminating a patient's involvement in the anticoagulation service. Every attempt should be made to determine the underlying reason for the noncompliant behavior. This behavior may be due to such things as inadequate patient education, denial of the medical condition requiring anticoagulation, and the lack of support systems, including transportation required for appointments. Documenting each incidence of noncompliance is important for liability issues.

Patients must demonstrate to the anticoagulation service staff that they are active participants in their own care by agreeing to modify their lifestyle, notify staff of adverse effects, and report for regularly scheduled follow-up appointments. Contracts can be devised to document the willingness of patients to comply with the anticoagulation service instructions and their ability to share in the responsibility for their care. Alternative methods of anticoagulation or treatments may be needed for those patients who are unwilling or unable to comply with the required follow-up visits and warfarin dosing instructions. When the risks of anticoagulant therapy outweigh the benefits, the final decision regarding patient treatment rests with the attending physician. The decision to terminate a patient's involvement in the anticoagulation service can only be made by the primary care provider, and the patient must be notified via certified mail or personal contact.

MARKETING THE SERVICE

Marketing your anticoagulation service is an important factor for its success. There are a variety of marketing approaches that can be employed to increase clinical referrals as well as build professional awareness and help to promote patient interest. Marketing the program should be a continuous process. Table 21.9[18] identifies some marketing tools that are useful.

Table 21.9 *Marketing tools*

Grand round presentations
Hospital inservices
Announcement letters
Physicians
Patients
Presentations to hospital board members and physician group practices
Press release/newsletter announcement
Posters
Open house reception
Electronic mail announcements

Evaluating your anticoagulation service can be achieved through the following resources:

- Patient outcomes
- Decrease in hospitalizations and adverse events
- Clinic utilization
- Cost avoidance
- Medical staff acceptance/satisfaction
- Measuring patient satisfaction through focus groups and questionnaires.

Demonstrating the benefits of your service will increase support for its continued operation. In addition, this will allow for a better understanding of the service's impact on the patients, achieve valuable marketing information, and obtain quality measures that are useful in gaining reimbursement for your service.

EXPANDING THE SERVICE

One unique area that offers the potential for expanding services beyond the traditional anticoagulation service practice is the outpatient prophylaxis and treatment of deep vein thrombosis/pulmonary embolism with low molecular weight heparin (LMWH). The Food and Drug Administration has approved the use of various LMWHs in unstable angina, the treatment of deep vein thrombosis, and deep vein thrombosis prophylaxis for orthopedic and abdominal surgeries. With healthcare reform and the need to decrease the number of days in hospital, LMWHs may be used to treat patients at home, without any hospital admission being necessary.

The framework for a home treatment program must be established, and adherence to the protocol is necessary to prevent adverse complications. A referral system, inclusion and exclusion criteria, and a thorough clinical pathway for home monitoring must be developed.

Another area to investigate for additional revenues for your practice may be a potential teaching site for healthcare professionals in the area of anticoagulation therapy management. Offering an anticoagulation certificate program and sponsoring seminars and/or conferences can be a financial asset to any program. Consideration as a research site may be an added bonus. Pharmaceutical grants can be obtained in a wide variety of areas, and participation in follow-up studies is another possibility for potential financial resources.

CONCLUSION

Anticoagulation services managed by nurses, pharmacists, or physician assistants are recognized as an effective mechanism for monitoring patients receiving anticoagulant therapy. As the indications for anticoagulant therapy continue to expand, the numbers of patients receiving this therapy will also increase. Specialized anticoagulation services offer a means for coordinating and providing intensive patient education and follow-up, thus ultimately improving patient outcomes and reducing the risks of complications.

REFERENCES

1   Ansell J, Buttaro M, Thomas O, Knowlton C, and the Anticoagulation Task Force. Consensus guidelines for coordinated outpatient oral anticoagulation therapy management. *Ann Pharmacother* 1997; **31**: 604–15.
2   Lee YP, Schommer JC. Effect of a pharmacist-managed anticoagulation clinic on warfarin-related hospital admissions. *Am J Health-Syst Pharm* 1996; **53**: 1580–3.
3   Cortelazzo S, Finazzi G, Viero P, et al. Thrombotic and hemorrhagic complications in patients with mechanical heart valve prosthesis attending an anticoagulation clinic. *Thromb Haemost* 1993; **69**: 316–20.
4   Kornblitt P, Senderoff J, Davis-Erickson M, Zenk J. Anticoagulation therapy: patient management and evaluation of an outpatient clinic. *Nurse Pract* 1990; **15**: 21–32.
5   Bussey HI, Rospond RM, Quandt CM, Clark GM. The safety and effectiveness of long-term warfarin therapy in an anticoagulation clinic. *Pharmacotherapy* 1989; **9**: 214–19.
6   Conte RR, Kehoe WA, Nielson N, Lodhia H. Nine-year experience with a pharmacist-managed anticoagulation clinic. *Am J Hosp Pharm* 1986; **43**: 2460–4.
7   Garabedian-Ruffalo SM, Gray DR, Sax MJ, Ruffalo RL. Retrospective evaluation of a pharmacist-managed warfarin anticoagulation clinic. *Am J Hosp Pharm* 1985; **42**: 304–8.
8   Ansell JE. The value of an anticoagulation service. In: Ansell JE, Oertal LB, Whittkowsky A, eds *Managing oral anticoagulant therapy: clinical and operational guidelines*. Gaithersburg, MD: Aspen Publishing Co., 1997; 2:1–2:5.
9   Ansell JE, Hughes R. Evolving models of warfarin management: anticoagulation clinics, patient self-monitoring, and patient self-management. *Am Heart J* 1996; **132**: 1095–100.
10 Ansell JE. Anticoagulation management as a risk factor for adverse events: grounds for improvement. *J Thromb Thrombolysis* 1998; **5**: S13–S18.
11 Chiquette E, Amato MG, Bussey HI. Comparison of an anticoagulation clinic with routine medical care. *Circulation* 1995; **92**(Suppl. I): 1686.
12 Norton JL, Gibson DL. Establishing an outpatient anticoagulation clinic in a community hospital. *Am J Health-Syst Pharm* 1996; **53**: 1151–8.
13 CougaChek Plus System. Roche Diagnostic, 9115 Hague Road, PO Box 50457, Indianapolis, IN 46250-0457.
14 ProTime Microcoagulation System. International Technidyne Corporation, 8 Olsen Ave, Edison, NJ 98820.
15 Saltiel E, Shane R. Evaluating costs of a pharmacist-run thromboprophylaxis program. *Formulary* 1996; **31**: 276–90.
16 Ansell JE. Oral anticoagulation therapy: 50 years later. *Arch Intern Med* 1993; **153**: 586–96.
17 Wasson J, Gaudette C, Whaley F, Asuvigne A, Baribeau P, Welch HG. Telephone care as a substitute for routine clinic follow-up. *JAMA* 1992; **267**: 1788–93.
18 *Anticoagulation service implementation guide*. DuPont Pharma, Wilmington, DE, 1997: 16.

Index